Psychological Aspects of Sport-Related Concussions

Recognition of concussion as a serious injury, informed by neurological and physiological research, is now commonplace in sport. However, research on the psychology of concussive injury—its psychological implications and outcomes, and psychological interventions for prevention and recovery—has largely been overlooked. This is the first book to explicitly and authoritatively focus on psychological aspects of sport-related concussions from a multidisciplinary and global perspective.

The book attempts to offer a global understanding of the injury by presenting an historical overview; exploring the psychological implications of sport-related concussion and the influence of gender and sociocultural context on concussive injury and recovery; setting out practical guidance on working with special populations suffering from concussive injuries; and discussing the theoretical and methodological considerations for research on concussion and future directions for this research.

Written by a group of leading international experts and offering a hitherto underdeveloped perspective on this area of sports injury research, this book is crucial reading for any upper-level student, researcher, sport scientist, coach, or allied health professional working on sport-related concussion. It is also valuable reading for students and researchers interested in the psychosocial processes that impact injury and recovery or general professional practice in sport psychology.

Gordon A. Bloom is a professor of sport psychology at McGill University, Canada, who has worked with the world's leading coaches and athletes as both a researcher and sport psychology practitioner for over 20 years. He is currently the director of the McGill Sport Psychology Research Laboratory, which is focused on applied and theoretical research within the areas of sport, physical activity, and health promotion. The primary goal of his program of research is to create positive sport environments so that athletes can reach their ideal states of human performance and well-being. He has co-authored nearly 100 coaching and sport science publications and is regularly invited as a featured speaker at national and international events.

Jeffrey G. Caron is an assistant professor in the School of Kinesiology and Physical Activity Sciences at Université de Montréal, Canada. Prior to his appointment, Jeff obtained a Ph.D. in Kinesiology and Physical Education from McGill University in 2016, and he was subsequently a postdoctoral fellow at McGill University (2016–2017) and Yale University (2017–2018). Jeff's research program focuses on better understanding psychosocial aspects of sport-related concussions. In particular, he investigates the dissemination of concussion information to the members of the sport community and strategies to assist athletes during their recovery and return to sport, school, and daily life.

Routledge Research in Sport and Exercise Science

The *Routledge Research in Sport and Exercise Science* series is a showcase for cutting-edge research from across the sport and exercise sciences, including physiology, psychology, biomechanics, motor control, physical activity and health, and every core sub-discipline. Featuring the work of established and emerging scientists and practitioners from around the world, and covering the theoretical, investigative and applied dimensions of sport and exercise, this series is an important channel for new and ground-breaking research in the human movement sciences.

Available in this series:

Complex Sport Analytics
Felix Lebed

The Science of Figure Skating
Edited by Jason Vescovi and Jaci VanHeest

The Science of Judo
Edited by Mike Callan

Modelling and Simulation in Sport and Exercise
Edited by Arnold Baca and Jürgen Perl

The Exercising Female
Science and Application
Edited by Jacky J. Forsyth and Claire-Marie Roberts

Genetics and the Psychology of Motor Performance
Sigal Ben-Zaken, Veronique Richard and Gershon Tenenbaum

Psychological Aspects of Sport-Related Concussions
Edited by Gordon A. Bloom and Jeffrey G. Caron

For more information about this series, please visit: https://www.routledge.com/sport/series/RRSES

Psychological Aspects of Sport-Related Concussions

Edited by Gordon A. Bloom and Jeffrey G. Caron

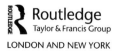

Routledge
Taylor & Francis Group

LONDON AND NEW YORK

First published 2019
by Routledge
2 Park Square, Milton Park, Abingdon, Oxon OX14 4RN

and by Routledge
605 Third Avenue, New York, NY 10017

First issued in paperback 2020

Routledge is an imprint of the Taylor & Francis Group, an informa business

British Library Cataloguing-in-Publication Data
A catalogue record for this book is available from the British Library

Library of Congress Cataloging-in-Publication Data
Names: Bloom, Gordon A., editor. | Caron, Jeffrey G., editor.
Title: Psychological aspects of sport-related concussions/edited by
Gordon A. Bloom and Jeffrey G. Caron.
Description: Milton Park, Abingdon, Oxon; New York, NY: Routledge,
2019. | Includes bibliographical references and index.
Identifiers: LCCN 2018050140| ISBN 9780815391869 (hardback) |
ISBN 9781351200516 (ebook)
Subjects: LCSH: Brain—Concussion. | Head—Wounds and injuries. |
Sports injuries—Psychological aspects.
Classification: LCC RC394.C7 P79 2019 | DDC 617.5/1044—dc23
LC record available at https://lccn.loc.gov/2018050140

ISBN 13: 978-0-367-73118-2 (pbk)
ISBN 13: 978-0-8153-9186-9 (hbk)

Typeset in Galliard
by Deanta Global Publishing Services, Chennai, India

Dedication

Gordon Bloom: To my three wonderful children—Jacob, Alexis, and Noah—who continue to amaze and inspire me each day.

Jeffrey Caron: To all those who have shared their concussion experiences with me. You are the reason why I am passionate about this work and why I am invested in helping find ways to make sport safer.

Contents

Figures

Tables

Contributors

Osman Hassan Ahmed is a physiotherapist and lecturer in physiotherapy and sports therapy at Bournemouth University, the United Kingdom. He has an extensive research background focusing on concussion in sport and has also researched into eHealth and online interventions. His post-doctoral research spans across a range of outputs, including peer-reviewed papers, book chapters, and invited presentations at international sports and medical conferences. He is a senior associate editor at the *British Journal of Sports Medicine* and is a member of the International Blind Sports Association medical committee. He has worked extensively as a clinician in disability football and accompanied the England Cerebral Palsy Football squad to the 2008 Paralympic Games in Beijing and the 2016 Paralympic Games in Rio de Janeiro as team physiotherapist. He has also worked with many other disability football squads (including amputee/deaf/blind/partially sighted/learning disabled), and currently works with the Football Association in England with their elite disability football program. He helped establish the FA Centre for Disability Football Research and was a co-lead on the world's first "Disability Football" module run by FIFA for their Diploma in Football Medicine.

Morgan Anderson is a second-year Ph.D. student at Michigan State University, the United States. Her research interests include the neuropsychological, psychosocial, and physical effects of sport-related concussion. She completed her master's degree in kinesiology in exercise science at the University of Arkansas in 2017. Her thesis compared before-school and after-school neurocognitive performance and symptoms to determine the optimal time to administer computerized neurocognitive testing. Anderson is currently a research assistant in the Department of Kinesiology at Michigan State University.

Jamie B. Barker is a senior lecturer in sport psychology at Loughborough University, the United Kingdom. He has an international research profile with research interests centered on applied (sport and performance) psychology research. Barker has over 60 scholarly publications (including 45 peer-reviewed papers, 12 book chapters, and 4 books). He is associate editor for the *Journal of Applied Sport Psychology*, whilst also serving on the editorial boards of *The Sport Psychologist* and the *International Review of Sport and Exercise*

Psychology. As a consultant, he has 20 years of experience working in business and professional sport. For example, he has consulted with Sony Europe, Sony Mobile, Impact International, the Football Association, the England and Wales Cricket Board, Nottinghamshire County Cricket Club, and Great Britain Rowing. Recently, Barker has worked in disability football and was the sport psychologist to the Great Britain Cerebral Palsy Football team at the Rio 2016 Paralympics.

Tracy Blake is a registered physiotherapist in Canada, where she maintains an active clinical practice in acute inpatient care, private practice, and high-performance sport. She is an instructor in the Department of Physical Therapy at the University of Toronto, Canada, where she facilitates experiential learning and clinical skills development for students in the entry-level Master of Science (Physical Therapy) program and the Ontario Internationally Educated Physical Therapy Bridging (OIEPB) program. Blake's scholarly work focuses primarily on sport medicine and sport physiotherapy, including an emphasis on concussion in youth ice hockey. She is an associate editor at the *British Journal of Sports Medicine*. As a consultant, Blake has developed evidence-informed content and recommendations for the Canadian Injury Prevention Curriculum and the Active and Safe Central website, and she has provided onsite clinical training and evaluation for healthcare professionals and staff participating in spinal cord research throughout North America.

Abigail C. Bretzin is a fourth-year Ph.D. student interested in sport-related concussion at Michigan State University, the United States. Currently, her focus is neurocognitive deficits and sex differences following a sport-related concussion, as well as investigating long-term effects of both sport-related concussion and head impacts below the threshold of a concussion. Her master's thesis evaluated the relationship of head impact kinematics and strength of various muscle groups in the cervical spine in soccer athletes. Bretzin is currently a research assistant in the Sport Concussion Research Laboratory and teaching assistant in the Department of Kinesiology, Michigan State University. Bretzin was recently awarded the National Athletic Trainers Association Research and Education Foundation Memorial Scholarship in recognition of her work at Michigan State University.

Tracey Covassin is a full professor and licensed athletic trainer in the Department of Kinesiology at Michigan State University, the United States. She is also the director of the Sport Concussion Research Laboratory, where her research focuses on sex differences in concussion outcomes, epidemiology, and risk factors associated with sports-related concussion. Dr. Covassin currently directs a multi-site high school and college sport-concussion outreach program in the Mid Michigan area. Dr. Covassin has over 100 professional publications and 150 professional presentations and has received over $2 million in external funding as a principal investigator. In 2013 she was appointed to the Institute of Medicine (IOM) and National Research Council Sport-Related Concussion in Youth Committee. The committee reviewed current literature on concussions, their causes, and the relationship of hits to the head during sport, effectiveness of protective devices and equipment, screening and diagnosis, prevention, management, and treatment. In 2014, Dr. Covassin was invited to the White House for President Obama's Healthy Kids and Safety Sports Concussion Summit.

J. Scott Delaney practices emergency medicine and sport medicine at McGill University , Montreal, Canada. He completed residencies in both family medicine and emergency medicine at McGill University, Montreal, before completing a fellowship in sport medicine. He is an associate professor at McGill University, Montreal, and is a team physician for the Montreal Alouettes, Montreal Impact, Cirque du Soleil, and McGill Football and Soccer teams. He was the team physician for Montreal's professional lacrosse team (Montreal Express) and continues to look after a number of Olympic athletes. Dr. Delaney is a member of the editorial board for the *Clinical Journal of Sport Medicine*, and his research interests include concussions and neck injuries in both the athletic and emergency department populations. In 2010 he was awarded the Dr. Tom Pashby Sports Safety Award, which recognizes outstanding contributions towards the prevention of catastrophic injuries in sport and recreational activities.

Natalie Durand-Bush works as a sport psychology professor, scientist, and practitioner in the School of Human Kinetics at the University of Ottawa, Canada. As a mental performance consultant for the past 23 years, she has helped amateur and professional athletes and coaches of all ages, sports, and levels achieve their performance and well-being goals. A relentless advocate for the field of sport psychology, Dr. Durand-Bush has co-founded and chaired the Canadian Sport Psychology Association and has served as the Vice President of the International Society of Sport Psychology. She currently is a member of the Executive Board of the Association for Applied Sport Psychology in the United States. Dr. Durand-Bush's areas of specialization include psychological skills training and assessment, coaching psychology, and mental health. She has recently co-founded the Canadian Centre for Mental Health in Sport (CCMHS), a not-for-profit organization supporting the mental health and performance of competitive and high-performance athletes and coaches. The CCMHS is the first Centre in Canada to offer collaborative sport-focused mental health care services designed to help athletes and coaches strengthen their mental health and well-being, recover from mental illness and physical injuries, and achieve their performance goals.

Dave Ellemberg is a neuroscientist and professor at the University of Montreal, Canada and Sainte-Justine Children's Hospital. He is also a clinical neuropsychologist and the director of the Concussion Institute, Montreal, Quebec. Dr. Ellemberg holds a bachelor's degree in psychology from McGill University, Montreal, a master's degree (sciences) from McMaster University, Hamilton, as well as a doctorate in clinical neuropsychology from Université de Montréal, and he has completed two post-doctorate fellowships. Dr. Ellemberg leads several research projects investigating the effects of sport-related traumatic brain injuries, as well as the resilience of the human brain during development. He has presented his work in more than 100 international conferences in the United States, Europe, and Asia, and has over 60 publications in peer-reviewed scientific journals. He is the recipient of numerous prizes, including the Certificate of Excellence from the Canadian Psychological Association, the Brain Star Award from the Canadian Institutes of Health Research, and the E. A. Baker award from the Medical Research Council of Canada.

Camille Guertin is a Ph.D. student in experimental psychology at the University of Ottawa, Canada. Her research focuses on the motivational processes that are involved in the initiation and maintenance of health behaviors (such as healthy eating and physical activity), the etiology of body image and dysfunctional eating, and the promotion of health behaviors through message framing and tailoring. Her research also focuses on validating measures to assess healthy and unhealthy eating behaviors and understanding the various factors that are involved in the prediction of healthy and unhealthy eating in women. In her future work, she is interested in advancing knowledge on the positive and negative strategies that individuals use to regulate their eating behaviors and their effects on health, and on promoting the maintenance of healthy eating in individuals at risk for chronic illnesses.

Chris Hammer is the head triathlon coach and an adjunct professor in the Department of Sport Sciences at Davis and Elkins College in Elkins, West Virginia, the United States. His research emphasis is on posttraumatic growth for individuals with acquired disabilities and the potential role that physical activity and sport may have in shaping these experiences. Dr. Hammer, a congenital amputee, is a two-time Paralympian, having competed in London in 2012 and Rio de Janeiro in 2016. In his free time, Dr. Hammer enjoys traveling, camping, and playing board games with his family.

Adam Harrison is currently a doctoral student in the Department of Exercise Science at the University of South Carolina, the United States. He received his bachelor's degree in psychology from Illinois Wesleyan University, Bloomington, before moving to the University of South Carolina, where he earned his master's in exercise science in 2015. His primary research objectives focus on identifying neuropsychological and functional outcomes following neurological injuries. He is currently working on projects aimed at identifying both neurophysiological (i.e., EEG and HRV) and behavioral markers that can be used to detect and monitor deficits following concussive injuries. He is also interested in investigating the utility of exercise and other neurorehabilitative therapies as supplements to enhance recovery from neurological injury. In addition to concussive injuries, Harrison has been involved with several research projects aimed at identifying cognitive, visual, and motor deficits, following other neurological conditions (e.g., stroke, Parkinson's disease, and PTSD) and how they relate to task performance within an interactive virtual environment.

John Heil is a clinical and sport psychologist at Psychological Health Roanoke, Virginia, the United States. He is the author of *The Psychology of Sport Injury* and numerous other works on pain and injury. He works with Olympic, professional, and youth athletes and has consulted at three Olympic Games. Dr. Heil is a lecturer at the Virginia Tech Carilion School of Medicine and at the Roanoke Police Academy, Virginia. He is a member of the Sport Science Board of the International Swim Coaches Association and served as Director of Sports Medicine for the Virginia State Games for over 20 years and as Chair of Sports Medicine and Science with USA Fencing for over 15 years. He is past president of the American Psychological Association Division of Sport, Exercise and Performance Psychology.

Jacob J. M. Kay is a doctoral student with particular interests in physical activity, cognition, and brain health at the University of South Carolina, the United States. He holds a master's degree in psychology (emphasis of behavioral neuroscience) from University of Wisconsin-Milwaukee, where he used optical imaging techniques to examine exercise-induced changes in the rodent cerebrovascular system. He is currently working toward his Ph.D. in exercise science (with an emphasis of rehabilitation science) at the University of South Carolina, where he conducts research on the psychophysiological benefits of exercise and on advancing the assessment, management, and rehabilitation of concussion. He is currently working on projects aimed at identifying factors that predict recovery outcomes (e.g., age, sex, *a priori* health conditions) following concussive brain injury. Additionally, he is interested in evaluating the effectiveness of various rehabilitation strategies, including: behavioral (e.g., exercise, biofeedback) and neuropharmacological interventions (e.g., cannabidiol). For his dissertation, Kay aims to use advanced brain imaging techniques (i.e., fMRI and DTI) to evaluate structural and functional brain recovery, pre-post intervention.

Anthony P. Kontos is research director for the UPMC Sports Medicine Concussion Program and Associate Professor in the Departments of Orthopedic Surgery and Sports Medicine and Rehabilitation at the University of Pittsburgh, Pennsylvania, the United States. He has specialized in concussion research for 13 years and has 211 professional publications and 290 professional presentations. His research is funded by the National Institutes of Health and Department of Defense and focuses on risk factors; neurocognitive/neuromotor effects; psychological issues; treatment; and concussion in military, pediatric, and sport populations. Dr. Kontos is a fellow and past president of the Society for Sport, Exercise & Performance Psychology (APA-Div47), and a fellow of the National Academy of Kinesiology, Association for Applied Sport Psychology, and Eastern Psychological Association. He is also the lead co-author (with Dr. Collins) of *Concussion: A Clinical Profiles Based Approach to Assessment and Treatment.*

Emily Kroshus is a research assistant professor in the Department of Pediatrics and Seattle Children's Research Institutes Center for Child Health, Behavior, and Development at the University of Washington, the United States. Prior to coming to the University of Washington, she was a post-doctoral research fellow at the National Collegiate Athletic Association's Sport Science Institute, where she worked on research and program development related to concussion and mental health in college sport. Her research interests include social and contextual determinants of health-related behaviors, including risk-taking and help-seeking, as well as intervention design and evaluation.

Lynda Mainwaring is an associate professor in the Faculty of Kinesiology and Physical Education at the University of Toronto, Canada, and she is a registered psychologist with training in both human kinetics and psychology. Her research interests include psychological aspects of physical injury and recovery, the emotional impact of mild traumatic brain injury in sport, perfectionism, performance enhancement, and qualitative methodology. She initiated the Concussion Program at the University of Toronto in 1999 and conducts research on the emotional impact of sport-related concussion. She has been instrumental in raising awareness about the psychological impact of injury to international audiences and has published and presented over 200 works related to performance, sport, and dance psychology. She is a member of the College of Psychologists of Ontario, the Ontario Psychological Association, the American Psychological Association, and the Research Committee for the International Association for Dance Medicine and Science. Her teaching and practice emphasizes optimal wellness and performance enhancement.

Dominic Malcolm is reader in the sociology of sport in the School of Sport, Exercise and Health Sciences at Loughborough University, the United Kingdom. He has published widely in the sociology of sport, including the *Sage Dictionary of Sports Studies* (2008), *Sport and Sociology* (2012), and *Sport and Society: A Student Introduction* (2016, co-edited with Barrie Houlihan). His core research interests draw on and apply the theoretical ideas of Norbert Elias's figurational sociology to two substantive areas: the social development of cricket; and sport, health, and medicine. His research on sport, medicine, and health explores a variety of sport- and health-related policies, the embodied experiences of injury, practices harmful to athletes' health, and the problems of practicing medicine within sport. He has published *The Social Organization of Sports Medicine* (2012, co-edited with Parissa Safai), has recently completed a book titled *Sport, Medicine and Health: The Medicalization of Sport?*, and is currently working on a book called *The Concussion Crisis in Sport*. He is the editor-in-chief of the *International Review for the Sociology of Sport*.

Emilie Michalovic is a Ph.D. candidate in the Department of Kinesiology and Physical Education at McGill University, Montreal, Canada. She is working under the supervision of Dr. Shane Sweet in the Theories and Interventions in Exercise and Health Psychology Laboratory. She is studying exercise and health psychology, where her focus is on physical activity participation in special populations, especially those living with chronic obstructive pulmonary disease. With this research, she is exploring the role of peers and interpersonal behaviors in this population and how individuals' participation varies as their disease progresses. As well, her research is focused on identifying the needs of individuals living with disease or disability to better conduct future research and inform clinical practice. Outside of this research, Michalovic also examines exercise promotion for inactive adults through the use of persuasive messages, the needs of individuals living with a disability in the community, and the application of theory to better understand health behaviors.

Robert Davis Moore is currently an assistant professor in the Department of Exercise Science and Institute for Mind and Brain at the University of South Carolina, the United States. Dr. Moore completed his undergraduate degree in psychology and his master's degree in exercise psychology at the University of Georgia. He then completed his Ph.D. in kinesiology at the University of Illinois, followed by a post-doctoral fellowship at the University of Montreal, Canada. Dr. Moore's primary line of research focuses on concussive injuries. He uses a variety of psychophysiological, behavioral, and clinical measures to investigate the short- and long-term outcomes of concussion. Through his research, he aims to: 1) create more comprehensive and sensitive assessment protocols; 2) identify factors that moderate injury outcomes; and 3) develop active rehabilitation protocols for post-concussion syndrome. Dr. Moore's secondary line of research focuses on the influence of health factors such as physical activity, fitness, and obesity on neuropsychological health and development.

Michael Orenstein is a family medicine doctor who is currently completing a fellowship in sport and exercise medicine at the University of British Columbia (UBC) in Vancouver, Canada. He completed his undergraduate degree at McGill University in Montreal, with a major in anatomy and cell biology while minoring in kinesiology. He then completed his medical school training and family medicine residency at McGill University, Montreal. Currently, as a sport medicine fellow at UBC, Vancouver, he is directly involved in the care of the school's varsity athletes as well as providing event medical coverage for a variety of national and international level sporting events. His research interests include concussions and physical activity promotion. He is a former rower at McGill University, Montreal. He enjoys spending his free time playing basketball, volleyball, and staying active outdoors.

Kaleigh Ferdinand Pennock is a Ph.D. candidate in the Faculty of Kinesiology and Physical Education at the University of Toronto, Canada. She completed a double master's degree from the European Masters in Sports and Exercise Psychology (EMSEP) program, earning a Master of Sports Science in Sport

Psychology from Lund University, Sweden, and a Master of Science with a specialization in Diagnostics and Intervention from Leipzig University, Germany. Her doctoral work focuses on concussion under-reporting by adolescent athletes and considers individual, interpersonal, and sociocultural factors that may contribute to an athlete's reluctance to report concussion symptoms. Her research and teaching interests include sport and performance psychology, psychology of athletic injury, perfectionism in sport and dance, and qualitative and mixed methods research. She is an editor for the *Undergraduate Journal of Exercise Sciences* and a member of the North American Society for Sociology in Sport, the Association for Applied Sport Psychology, and the Canadian Society for Psychomotor Learning and Sport Psychology.

Kyle M. Petit is a third-year Ph.D. student who currently serves as a research and teaching assistant in the Department of Kinesiology at Michigan State University, the United States. His research interests primarily focus around rest and activity after a sports-related concussion. Petit is particularly interested in assessing how manipulations to physical and cognitive rest affect concussion recovery. He is also interested in the use of cognitive and physical activity when managing athletes with a sports-related concussion. His recent work evaluated athletic trainers' perceptions of rest and activity when managing athletes with a sports-related concussion.

Leslie Podlog is a faculty member at the University of Utah, the United States. Dr. Podlog's research focuses on health psychology issues, primarily the psychological aspects of injury rehabilitation and athlete burnout. He has published over 85 peer reviewed journal articles and book chapters. His interests in the psychology of injury recovery stem from his personal injury experiences as a former amateur wrestler at Simon Fraser University in Burnaby, Canada. Following completion of his doctoral studies (2006) at the University of Western Australia, Australia, Dr. Podlog held faculty positions at Charles Sturt University, Bathurst, Australia, the German Sport University, Cologne, Germany, and Texas Tech University, Texas, the United States. He has been a faculty member at the University of Utah since 2011, where he teaches classes in sport psychology and the psychology of sport injury. Outside of work, Dr. Podlog enjoys hiking, skiing, and spending time with his family.

Stefanie Podlog is an assistant professor at the University of St. Augustine for Health Sciences, Florida, the United States, where she teaches various courses (e.g., Evidence-Based Concussion Management) in the interprofessional and post-professional programs. She has over 20 years of experience as a nurse, educator, researcher, and consultant in the health and injury fields. Her Ph.D. dissertation at the German Sport University, Cologne, Germany, focused on blood-based biomarkers of sports-related concussion. Following her doctoral program, she completed a postdoctoral fellowship with the National Center for Veterans Studies at the University of Utah, to broaden her research interests to the military setting. In her recreational time, Dr. Podlog enjoys yoga, outdoor activities, and spending time with her family.

Laura Purcell practices pediatric sport medicine at the Grand River Sports Medicine Centre in Kitchener, Ontario, Canada. She obtained her medical degree from McMaster University, Hamilton, and completed a residency in pediatrics at Dalhousie University, Halifax. She then completed a sport medicine fellowship at Fowler Kennedy Sport Medicine Clinic at Western University, Ontario. She is an Associate Clinical Professor in the Department of Pediatrics at McMaster University, Hamilton. Dr. Purcell has authored many articles, chapters, and position statements on concussion in sport in pediatric patients, including the Canadian Paediatric Society concussion position statement first published in 2006, with revisions published in 2012 and 2014. She was an invited speaker and panelist at the third and fourth International Consensus Conferences on Concussion in Sport and was an invited attendee at the fifth International Consensus Conference on Concussion in Sport in October 2016. She was involved in the development and revision of the ChildSCAT assessment tool and has presented on pediatric sport-related concussion locally, nationally, and internationally.

Scott Rathwell is an assistant professor in the Department of Kinesiology and Physical Education at the University of Lethbridge, Alberta, Canada. His research interests revolve around three main streams: (a) the personal and psychosocial development of university athletes, (b) the psychosocial factors related to master's athletics and lifelong sport participation, and (c) concussion prevention and rehabilitation. From a methodological perspective, Dr. Rathwell has expertise on both quantitative measurement and design. More specifically, he has created and validated a number of psychometric measurement tools related to coaching and athlete development. Moreover, he has created and evaluated interventions aimed at promoting concussion awareness and positive youth development through sport, and he has utilized randomized controlled trial designs for his research. Finally, Dr. Rathwell teaches research methods in kinesiology and physical education at the University of Lethbridge, Alberta.

Meredith Rocchi is a postdoctoral scholar in the Department of Kinesiology and Physical Education at McGill University, Montreal, Canada. She completed her Ph.D. in psychology at the University of Ottawa, and her research focuses on examining the role of interpersonal relationships and how they promote positive or negative outcomes in sport, health, and education settings. She is also an expert in psychometrics, and her research has contributed to the advancement of measurement and assessment of sport and exercise psychology constructs. Through her research, she has contributed to the validation of a number of published measures and incorporated novel advanced statistical analysis approaches into her work. Dr. Rocchi also teaches research methods and advanced statistics courses and runs a popular statistics tutorial channel on YouTube. Outside of her research, Dr. Rocchi is an active member of the Canadian figure skating community, where she works as a Skate Canada professional coach.

Jennifer L. Savage is currently a fourth-year Ph.D. student in kinesiology with a concentration in athletic training at Michigan State University, the United States. Her interest includes examining simulated driving performance among concussed high school and collegiate athletes and the self-efficacy of certified athletic trainers in the use of concussion assessment and management. She completed her master's degree in sports medicine in 2015 at Georgia State University, and her bachelor's degree in athletic training in 2013 at Western Carolina University. Savage received the 2018 Doctoral Research Assistant Grant from the National Athletic Trainers' Association Research and Education Foundation to support her ongoing work investigating simulated driving performance in high school and collegiate athletes following a sport-related concussion. She serves as a teaching and research assistant in the Department of Kinesiology at Michigan State University.

Cassandra M. Seguin is currently a doctoral candidate in the School of Human Kinetics at the University of Ottawa, Canada, studying under the supervision of Dr. Diane Culver. Her research interests include sport psychology, concussions, coaching, and high-performance/elite sport. She has also been actively working as a mental performance consultant since the completion of her Master of Human Kinetics degree, under the supervision of Dr. Natalie Durand-Bush. As a student member of both the Association for Applied Sport Psychology and the Canadian Sport Psychology Association, Seguin strives to positively represent and advocate for the field through her work with athletes, musicians, academics, and other professionals. Prior to her graduate education, Seguin studied at Princeton University, where she pursued education in the fields of molecular biology, neuroscience, and psychology. As a former National Team and NCAA Division I goaltender in hockey, Seguin maintains a passion for the high-performance domain. This passion has also fueled her pursuit of coaching opportunities; following in her father's footsteps, Seguin has coached at both the Canadian national and provincial levels.

Veronik Sicard is a doctoral student in exercise sciences in the Department of Kinesiology at the Université de Montréal, Canada. Under the supervision of Dr. Dave Ellemberg, her current research aims to improve the acute and long-term assessment of sport-related concussions. Specifically, she is developing a standardized protocol to help determine when an athlete can make a safe return to play, in addition to other concussion projects that focus on sex differences, sub-concussive impacts, pediatric concussions, slow-to-recover athletes, and ADHD. Sicard has presented her work at over a dozen conferences across America and has won several student prizes. She obtained her bachelor's degree in microbiology and immunology at the Université de Montréal and studied molecular biology at the Louis Pasteur Institute of the Université de Strasbourg, France. Upon recommendation by the advisor, Sicard was approved for a fast track to the Ph.D. program.

Matthew Slater is a senior lecturer in sport and exercise psychology and an internationally recognized researcher at Staffordshire University, Stoke-on-Trent, the United Kingdom. Dr. Slater's main expertise focuses on leadership and team functioning and the application of psychological skills for performance and health. Dr. Slater's work focuses primarily on the social identity approach to leadership and team functioning, and these endeavors inform his undergraduate and postgraduate teaching, Ph.D. supervision, enterprise activities, and consultancy links. Dr. Slater is a chartered psychologist (CPsychol) with the British Psychological Society (BPS). Dr. Slater has published over 20 peer-reviewed papers, five book chapters, regularly speaks at international and national conferences, and delivers workshops in the application of the social identity approach. His research has also received international public reach through the media (e.g., The Conversation, TalkSport, Cape Town radio, and coverage in *The Times* and *The Independent* newspapers, and on the BBC).

Rebecca Steins is a second-year master's student at McGill University, Montreal, Canada working under the supervision of Dr. Gordon Bloom. She completed her undergraduate degree at Drury University in Springfield, Missouri, with a double major in exercise science and psychology and a minor in behavioral neuroscience. Her master's thesis focuses on exploring the coping efforts used by female collegiate athletes who suffer long-term concussion symptoms. Other research interests include the neuropsychology of concussions and the promotion of concussion education. Steins grew up in St. Louis, Missouri, where she played basketball throughout her life, including at the university level. Her interests include cooking, the St. Louis Blues, music, and being an advocate for the environment.

Shane Sweet is an assistant professor in the Department of Kinesiology and Physical Education at McGill University, Montreal, Canada and the co-director of the Theories and Interventions in Exercise and Health Psychology Laboratory. Dr. Sweet is an exercise and health psychologist and a disability and community-based researcher who utilizes theories across his research program. The overarching goal of his program of research is to enhance the lives of adults, whether healthy or living with chronic conditions/disease (e.g., adults with cardiovascular disease, spinal cord injury). He aims to (a) understand physical activity participation and well-being by testing and integrating theory and developing conceptual models; (b) promote physical activity participation and enhance well-being via theory-based interventions; and (c) engage the community in research to co-construct and disseminate knowledge as well as evaluate knowledge translation initiatives. He is also a sports enthusiast, enjoys reading fiction, and is an emerging comic book fan.

Katherine A. Tamminen is an assistant professor in the Faculty of Kinesiology and Physical Education at the University of Toronto, Canada. Her research in sport psychology focuses on two main areas: stress, coping, and emotion in sport; and young athletes' experiences in sport. Her current research examines how adolescent athletes learn to cope with stressors in sport and how parents and coaches influence athletes' coping. She also conducts research on inter-personal emotion regulation and social processes of coping in team sports. Her work also focuses on the use of qualitative research approaches in sport psychology. Her research has been funded through the Social Sciences and Humanities Research Council of Canada (SSHRC), the Province of Ontario Ministry of Research and Innovation (Early Researcher Award), the Canadian Foundation for Innovation (John R. Evans Leaders Fund) and the Ontario Research Foundation, and by the University of Toronto (Connaught New Researcher Award). She is currently an associate editor for the *International Review of Sport and Exercise Psychology* and serves on the editorial board for the journal *Psychology of Sport and Exercise*.

1 Introduction

Gordon A. Bloom and Jeffrey G. Caron

> If you hit your head hard enough, things can get really confusing. Things can come unraveled and you have no control ... People don't understand going from, in their eyes, a hockey celebrity to the point where you can't walk out of your house. You can't shave. You have no desire to do anything. You're depressed.
>
> (Excerpt from an interview with a retired professional athlete; see Caron et al., 2013, p. 173)

Broadly speaking, researchers in psychology study the relationship between the brain and behavior. Since the 1980s, there has been a great deal of psychological research on sport-related performance, well-being, and injuries. In particular, athletic injuries have become an area of specialization within psychology, evidenced by an ever-increasing number of peer-reviewed articles (e.g., Forsdyke et al., 2016) and textbooks (e.g., Arvinen-Barrow & Walker, 2013), which have provided key information about the antecedents, determinants, and outcomes associated with psychological aspects of athletic injuries. Concussions are a specific type of athletic injury that have become recognized as a serious injury in a variety of sports (Johnson, Partridge, & Gilbert, 2015). Recent documentaries and films such as *Concussion*, which depicted Dr. Bennett Omalu's discovery of chronic traumatic encephalopathy among deceased former professional football athletes, along with increased media coverage of high-profile athletes with severe concussions (e.g., Canadian professional ice hockey player Sidney Crosby), have also increased the public's awareness of this injury (Hainline & Ellenbogen, 2017; McGannon, Cunningham, & Schinke, 2013). Despite the increased attention, researchers and clinicians are still learning about the short- and long-term health implications of sport-related concussions.

A concussion is defined as a traumatic brain injury (TBI) that results from biomechanical forces transmitted via a direct or indirect blow to the face, head, or elsewhere on the body (McCrory et al., 2017). On the spectrum of TBI, concussions are considered "mild" because they are closed head injuries that are typically not life-threatening. However, the term "mild" is a rather paradoxical way to describe an injury that has been linked to serious adverse health consequences (Manley et al., 2017; Moore, Kay, & Ellemberg, 2018). The majority of sport-related concussions occur as a result of participating in contact or collision sports like American football, rugby, and ice hockey. Concussed athletes experience one or more of the following after injury: physical signs, behavioral changes, balance and cognitive impairment, and sleep disturbance, as well as somatic, cognitive, and emotional symptoms (McCrory et al., 2017). Most concussed adult athletes recover within 10–14 days, whereas symptomatology for children and adolescent athletes typically resolves within 30 days (McCrory et al., 2017). A smaller percentage of athletes are slow to recover and can experience concussion symptoms for longer periods of time that can last from months to years (Martini & Broglio, 2018), an issue that continues to be at the forefront of research on concussions.

Scientists have been interested in concussions dating back as far as 1700 bce, when a case involving a patient who had symptoms of coma, stupor, and confusion was described in the Edwin Smith medical document (see Chapter 2 for a more detailed historical overview). The term "concussion" first appeared in the medical literature when Nichols and Smith (1906) wrote about "concussions of the brain" in an editorial commentary for the *Boston Medical and Surgical Journal* (p. 3). The authors reported on their experiences providing care for Harvard University football players during the 1905 season (Nichols & Smith, 1906). Although there was research on sport-related concussions in the 20th century, much of the exponential growth in research that we are currently experiencing can likely be attributed to the Concussion in Sport Group (CISG), who first met in the early 2000s. The CISG is an assembly of leading clinical and research experts from various backgrounds including (but not limited to) sports medicine, neurology, neuropsychology, and sports science. The CISG has held five meetings to date: Vienna in 2001, Prague in 2004, Zurich in 2008 and 2012, and Berlin in 2016 (cf. McCrory et al., 2017). These meetings have largely shaped "best practice" for the evaluation and management of concussion worldwide.

The vast majority of research has centred on the pathophyisiological diagnosis, evaluation, and management of sport-related concussions. However, researchers have also become interested in the psychological aspects of sport-related concussions. In fact, there is now a large body of evidence demonstrating that concussed athletes may concurrently suffer from psychological sequelae such as depression, isolation, irritability, and anxiety, which can exacerbate the overall effect of a concussion (e.g., Henry, Tremblay, & De Beaumont, 2017; Ptito, Chen, & Johnston, 2008). Contemporary thinking and research on the psychological aspects of concussion owes much to the pioneering work of neuropsychologist Dr. Jeffrey Barth and colleagues, who studied individuals involved in motor vehicle accidents in the 1980s (e.g., Barth et al., 1983; Rimel et al., 1981). The authors found that 34% of these individuals who sustained a mild head injury had not returned to work three months after injury. Moreover, these individuals with mild head injuries were found to be experiencing emotional stress and deficits associated with their attention, concentration, memory, and judgment. Almost a decade later, Barth et al. (1989) were among the first to issue warnings about the long-term effects of sport-related head injuries after studying more than 2,000 college and professional football athletes.

There is now an ever-growing body of evidence suggesting that individuals who sustain sport-related concussions can experience psychological symptoms that can last for days, weeks, or in some severe cases, persist from months to years (e.g., Caron et al., 2013). Unlike most musculoskeletal injuries, however, a concussion is an "invisible injury," meaning there are typically no visible signs of trauma (Bloom et al., 2004). Consequently, it is difficult for casual observers to identify the athlete as being injured. Additionally, athletes with musculoskeletal injuries are often provided with a timeline for recovery and regimented rehabilitation protocol, whereas athletes diagnosed with a concussion have no definitive timeline for recovery, and they often leave the doctor with a minimally structured return to activity schedule. Currently, there is work underway to enhance clinicians' ability to predict timelines for recovery through the use of neuroimaging, fluid biomarkers, and genetic testing (see McCrea et al., 2017 for a review).

Although research on psychological aspects of sport-related concussions has continued to grow since Barth and colleagues' work in the 1980s, many questions remain unanswered. In a recent special issue on sport-related concussions in the journal *Sport, Exercise, and Performance Psychology*, editor Anthony Kontos (2017) noted: "the role of psychological factors in predicting outcomes following a concussion is not well understood. We also know little about the psychological sequelae that often accompany concussion" (p. 215). Given that sport-related concussions have reached an epidemic level and are widely regarded as a serious public health issue, the time is right to highlight the current understanding of psychological implications of the injury and recovery process.

About the editors

I [GB] have been working as a sport psychology researcher and consultant for over 20 years. As a consultant, I work with athletes and teams at a variety of competitive levels. A significant amount of this work has involved consulting with injured athletes, including helping them cope with isolation, pain, anxiety, and disruption of daily life as a result of their injuries. When I first started working in the Department of Kinesiology and Physical Education at McGill University in 2000, I was asked to give a talk to a group of medical doctors at a local hospital about the psychology of athletic injuries. One of the attendees that day was Dr. Karen Johnston, a neurosurgeon who specialized in sport-related concussions. After the talk, Dr. Johnston and I agreed that the role of psychology had largely been absent from the literature on the management of sport-related concussions. Additionally, we felt that psychological skills training, which I had been using in my professional practice with injured athletes, had great potential in solving some of the practical issues facing clinicians (i.e., diminishing persistent concussion symptoms). Soon after that initial meeting, we started working on a series of projects. Interestingly, the same year that Dr. Johnston, myself, and our co-authors published our first papers on the psychological aspects of sport-related concussions (Bloom et al., 2004; Johnston et al., 2004), so too did colleagues in Canada (Mainwaring et al., 2004) and the United States (Kontos, Collins, &

Russo, 2004).[1] Since then, my work has continued to encourage researchers to account for psychological factors related to athletic, academic, and social factors associated with concussive injury and recovery.

After my undergraduate degree, I [JC] was interested in pursuing graduate work in the area of sport-related concussions because I had experienced a number of head injuries during my career as a high-performance ice hockey player. As I began learning about the expanse of research on the topic, I realized there was a relative dearth of empirical literature on psychosocial aspects of sport-related concussions—especially using qualitative methodologies. My first publication explored the effects of multiple concussions on retired professional ice hockey players using interpretative phenomenological analysis, a type of qualitative methodology that allowed me to explore the mens' injury experiences alongside my own (Caron et al., 2013). The results of this research highlighted the depths of symptomatology experienced by these men (e.g., depression, suicidal ideation), as well as the profound impact that the injury and recovery process had on participants' personal and professional lives. Reflecting on these findings, it became clear that there was (and remains) a need for concussion education programming and outreach. As a result, my doctoral work developed, implemented, and assessed a concussion education intervention for adolescent athletes (Caron et al., 2018). In my current role as a faculty member at Université de Montréal, my research program on sport-related concussions continues to examine the dissemination of education information and also how psychosocial strategies could help us to better understand and improve recovery and return to activity experiences.

About this book

We were fortunate to have such a renowned group of authors agree to contribute to this book. We believe that the various chapters facilitate a more comprehensive understanding of the psychological aspects of concussions and recovery processes. A wide range of topics are covered in this book, which are briefly summarized below.

The book begins with a contribution from Podlog and colleagues in Chapter 2. The information in their chapter effectively provides a contextual backdrop for the rest of this book by discussing historical aspects of concussions. Chapter 3 was co-authored by Ellemberg and colleagues, who provide an overview of the role of neuropsychology in concussive injury and management, which includes a discussion of the neurophysiological cascade in concussion and contemporary neuroimaging techniques. Following this, in Chapter 4, Kontos examines common psychological issues that occur following a sport-related concussion, such as anxiety, depression, and malingering. The chapter also discusses a novel approach that clinicians can use to inform targeted management and treatment strategies for concussed athletes.

In Chapter 5, Caron summarizes contemporary concussion education efforts. He also discusses the ways in which this knowledge has been disseminated to members of the sport community, including some suggestions for future research and practice. Chapter 6 from Michalovic and colleagues is a natural extension of Chapter 5, as it examines how theory can (and should) be used to better understand and improve concussion-related behaviors. The authors also detail how theory has been used in other health-related domains and how it could inform concussion research. In Chapter 7, Seguin and Durand-Bush describe a novel approach to assisting concussed athletes during their recovery. Specifically, the authors outline a psychological skills training intervention they developed for athletes suffering from sport-related concussions.

Ahmed and colleagues contributed Chapter 8, which discusses concussions among athletes with disabilities. The authors highlight several concepts (i.e., symptom disclosure, adherence to treatment, and implications for concussion management) that have rarely been discussed in the sport-concussion literature. In Chapter 9, Covassin and colleagues review sex differences as they relate to risk, recovery, and treatment of sport-related concussions. They also expand on research that has found female athletes are at a higher risk of sustaining a concussion than males in sex-comparable sports.

The next three chapters (10–12) all examine concussion research for different age cohorts. In Chapter 10, Purcell provides an overview of concussions among child and adolescent athletes. This includes unique considerations for returning child and adolescent athletes to school and sport. In Chapter 11, Kroshus reviews the ever-growing body of research on collegiate athletes. Framed using the social ecological model, the chapter discusses this body of literature in relation to three time periods: (1) pre-injury, (2) at the time of injury, and (3) and post-injury. In Chapter 12, Delaney and colleagues address concussion research and practice in the professional sport setting. They also outline some of the clinical issues related to working in professional sports.

In Chapter 13, Malcolm describes the ways in which sociocultural analyses enhance the understanding of sport-related concussions. In particular, Malcolm applies a sociological lens to concussion-related research, such as athletes' experiences, medical practice, medical knowledge, public health, and cultural representations. Chapters 14 and 15 review concussion research that has used both quantitative and qualitative research designs. In Chapter 14, Rocchi and colleagues review quantitative research designs that have been used in the literature to date. Significantly, the authors discuss the advantages, disadvantages, and implications of each approach. Chapter 15, written by Pennock and colleagues, reviews the small yet growing body of literature that has used qualitative research designs to study sport-related concussions. The authors also discuss some of the current trends and future directions for qualitative research on sport-related concussions.

Based on our experiences working together and learning from many of the authors who contributed to this book, we felt that the time was right to pull together the knowledge of psychological aspects of sport-related concussions. We envision that some of the content in this book will have application to other publications on athletic injury. However, this is the only book to our knowledge with an explicit focus on psychological aspects of sport-related concussions from a multidisciplinary perspective. As a result, we hope that the content of this book is of interest to students at the undergraduate and graduate levels, post-secondary academics and researchers, sports scientists, and allied health professionals. We also believe this book could be of interest to coaches, athletic directors, and sport program administrators in high school, club, college, and elite amateur and professional settings. In sum, we have both enjoyed the process of editing this book, and we thank Routledge for supporting our desire to contribute to a comprehensive thematic landscape of the psychology of sport-related concussions.

Note

1 Of interest, both Dr. Lynda Mainwaring and Dr. Anthony Kontos have co-authored chapters in this book.

References

Arvinen-Barrow, M., & Walker, N. (Eds.). (2013). *The psychology of sport injury and rehabilitation*. New York, NY: Routledge.

Barth, J. T., Alves, W. M., Ryan, T. V., Macciocchi, S. N., Rimel, R. W., Jane, J. A., & Nelson, W. E. (1989). Mild head injury in sports: Neuropsychological sequelae and recovery of function. In H. S. Levin, H. M. Eisenberg, and A. L. Benton (Eds.), *Mild head injury* (pp. 257–275). New York, NY: Oxford University Press.

Barth, J. T., Macciocchi, S. N., Giordani, B., Rimel, R., Jane, J. A., & Boll, T. J. (1983). Neuropsychological sequelae of minor head injury. *Neurosurgery, 13*, 529–533. doi:10.1227/00006123-198311000-00008.

Bloom, G. A., Horton, A. S., McCrory, P., & Johnston, K. M. (2004). Sport psychology and concussion: New impacts to explore. *British Journal of Sports Medicine, 38*, 519–521. doi:10.1136/bjsm.2004.014811.

Caron, J. G., Bloom, G. A., Johnston, K. M., & Sabiston, C. M. (2013). Effects of multiple concussions on retired National Hockey League players. *Journal of Sport and Exercise Psychology, 35*, 168–179. doi:10.1123/jsep.35.2.168.

Caron, J. G., Rathwell, S., Delaney, J. S., Johnston, K. M., Ptito, A., & Bloom, G. A. (2018). Development, implementation and assessment of a concussion education programme for high school student-athletes. *Journal of Sports Sciences, 36*, 48–55. doi:10.1080/02640414.2017.1280180.

Forsdyke, D., Smith, A., Jones, M., & Gledhill, A. (2016). Psychosocial factors associated with outcomes of sports injury rehabilitation in competitive athletes: A mixed studies systematic review. *British Journal of Sports Medicine, 50*, 537–544. doi:10.1136/bjsports-2015-094850.

Hainline, B., & Ellenbogen, R. G. (2017). A perfect storm. *Journal of Athletic Training, 52*, 157–159. doi:10.4085/1062-6050-51.10.04.

Henry, L. C., Tremblay, S., & De Beaumont, L. (2017). Long-term effects of sports concussions: Bridging the neurocognitive repercussions of the injury with the newest neuroimaging data. *The Neuroscientist, 23*, 567–578. doi:10.1177/1073858416651034.

Johnson, L., Partridge, B., & Gilbert, F. (2015). Framing the debate: Concussion and mild traumatic brain injury. *Neuroethics, 8*, 1–4. doi:10.1007/s12152-015-9233-8.

Johnston, K. M., Bloom, G. A., Ramsay, J., Kissick, J., Montgomery, D., Foley, D., Chen, J. K., & Ptito, A. (2004). Current concepts in concussion rehabilitation. *Current Sports Medicine Reports, 3,* 316–323.

Kontos, A. P. (2017). Concussion in sport: Psychological perspectives. *Sport, Exercise, and Performance Psychology, 6,* 215–219. doi:10.1037/spy0000108.

Kontos, A. P., Collins, M., & Russo, S. A. (2004). An introduction to sports concussion for the sport psychology consultant. *Journal of Applied Sport Psychology, 16,* 220–235. doi:10.1080/10413200490485568.

Mainwaring, L. M., Bisschop, S. M., Green, R. E. A., Antoniazzi, M., Comper, P., Kristman, V., Provvidenza, C., & Richards, D. W. (2004). Emotional reaction of varsity athletes to sport-related concussion. *Journal of Sport and Exercise Psychology, 26,* 119–135.

Manley, G., Gardner, A. J., Schneider, K. J., Guskiewicz, K. M., Bailes, J., Cantu, R. C., ... & Dvořák, J. (2017). A systematic review of potential long-term effects of sport-related concussion. *British Journal of Sports Medicine, 51,* 969–977. doi:10.1136/bjsports-2017-097791.

Martini, D. N., & Broglio, S. P. (2018). Long-term effects of sport concussion on cognitive and motor performance: A review. *International Journal of Psychophysiology, 132,* 25–30. doi:10.1016/j.ijpsycho.2017.09.019.

McCrea, M., Meier, T., Huber, D., Ptito, A., Bigler, E., Debert, C. T., ... & McAllister, T. (2017). Role of advanced neuroimaging, fluid biomarkers and genetic testing in the assessment of sport-related concussion: A systematic review. *British Journal of Sports Medicine, 51,* 919–929. doi:10.1136/bjsports-2016-097447.

McCrory, P., Meeuwisse, W., Dvorak, J., Aubry, M., Bailes, J., Broglio, S., ... & Davis, G. A. (2017). Consensus statement on concussion in sport—the 5th international conference on concussion in sport held in Berlin, October 2016. *British Journal of Sports Medicine, 51,* 838–847. doi:10.1136/bjsports-2017-097699.

McGannon, K. R., Cunningham, S. M., & Schinke, R. J. (2013). Understanding concussion in socio-cultural context: A media analysis of a National Hockey League star's concussion. *Psychology of Sport and Exercise, 14,* 891–899. doi:10.1016/j.psychsport.2013.08.003.

Moore, R. D., Kay, J. J., & Ellemberg, D. (2018). The long-term outcomes of sport-related concussion in pediatric populations. *International Journal of Psychophysiology, 132,* 14–24. doi:10.1016/j.ijpsycho.2018.04.003.

Nichols, E. D., & Smith, H. B. (1906). The physical aspect of american football. *Boston Medical and Surgical Journal, 154,* 1–8. doi:10.1056/NEJM190601041540101.

Rimel, R. W., Giordani, B., Barth, J. T., Boll, T. J., & Jane, J. A. (1981). Disability caused by minor head injury. *Neurosurgery, 9,* 221–228. doi:10.1227/00006123-198109000-00001.

2 Historical perspectives of athletic injuries and concussions

Leslie Podlog, John Heil, Stefanie Podlog, and Chris Hammer

Introduction

Sport concussion research and media coverage of the injury have proliferated in recent years. Recognition of concussion-like symptoms among sport participants, however, dates back many centuries. This chapter seeks to provide a historical perspective on concussions in order to contextualize research developments on the psychosocial aspects of concussion highlighted in subsequent chapters. Scholars and health practitioners from a variety of disciplines have contributed to concussion knowledge, education, and management. This chapter includes literature spanning sports medicine, neuropsychology, sociology, and sport psychology. The chapter is divided into four main sections. In section one, we provide a long-term historical perspective on the first accounts of concussive symptoms in sport and performance domains. In section two, we describe more recent events (over the past 40 years) which have moved concussion issues into the forefront of popular consciousness and transformed sport concussion into a social issue—one requiring appropriate management and intervention on the part of sport organizations and government agencies. In section three, we examine the extent to which contemporary research has impacted social change and public policy efforts. These pragmatic issues bear consideration as scholars consider their role—and that of their research—in promoting concussion awareness, education, and enhanced management. Finally, section four provides summary conclusions and future research directions.

Recognition of concussion as a sport injury

The modern term "concussion" is derived from two Latin terms, the first, *concutere*, meaning "to shake violently" (Pearce, 2008), and the second, *concussus*, interpreted as the "action of striking together" (Brooks & Hunt, 2006). Although concussion is often thought of as a contemporary sport issue, evidence of concussion symptoms including coma, stupor, and confusion were recognized as early as 1700 bce in the Edwin Smith Papyrus, an ancient medical document describing 48 cases of injuries, fractures, wounds, dislocations, and tumors (Kamp et al., 2012). Many centuries later, in 400 bce, the Latin term for concussion, *commotio cerebri,* appeared for the first time in the *Hippocratic Corpus*—a collection of medical works from ancient Greece—to refer to a "commotion of the brain" (Masferrer et al., 2000; Tuke, 1910). Hippocrates observed this "commotion of the brain" in ancient Greek wrestlers and fist fighters, noting that "in cerebral concussion, whatever the cause, the patient becomes speechless, … falls down immediately, loses their speech, and cannot see and hear" (as cited in McCrory & Berkovic, 2001, p. 284). Hippocrates also stated that "no head injury is too trivial to ignore," the irony of which echoes across the centuries and into the modern era (Wason & Reich, 1979).

By the 10th century ad, the Arabic physician Rhazes described concussion as a problem of brain function in the absence of gross structural injury (McCrory & Berkovic, 2001). The distinction between concussion as a temporary state of altered brain function versus an injury related to ongoing structural impairment was a critical turning point in understanding the nature of concussive injury. Later, in the 13th century ad, Lanfrancus, a European physician, confirmed Rhazes' finding that an abnormal physiological state could be caused by the shaking of the brain, employing Hippocrates' term of brain *commotion,* a description that is still used in contemporary medical texts. Despite Lanfrancus' verification of Rhazes' discovery, other Renaissance physicians failed to appreciate the distinctions between a concussion and gross structural brain damage, given an absence of objective findings in vivo (McCrory & Berkovic, 2001).

One century later, da Carpi (1460–1530) and Paré (1510–1590), two renowned European surgeons, treated members of high Royal Courts with concussion-like symptoms following jousting events in which two mounted armored knights charged each other with blunted lances (da Carpi, 1518; Dowling & Goodrich, 2016; Park, 1896). da Carpi reported signs such as vomiting, loss of speech, vertigo, falling down, and "stupor of the mind" (da Carpi, 1518; Dowling & Goodrich, 2016; Park, 1896). Both da Carpi and Paré noted the distinction between temporary symptoms experienced by individuals sustaining a concussion during sports participation versus those experiencing a structural injury of the brain. They also observed that problems with speech and memory were common following a sport-related concussion, in addition to the more apparent symptoms of dizziness, imbalance, and a loss of consciousness (da Carpi, 1518; Meehan, 2017; Park, 1896).

The development of the microscope in the early 17th century was a milestone in concussion research, enabling scientists to categorize concussion as a unique transient clinical syndrome separate from moderate and severe head injuries (McCrory & Berkovic, 2001). The microscope allowed physicians to explore underlying physical and structural mechanisms of concussion by examining brain samples of deceased patients with a history of concussion (McCrory & Berkovic, 2001). Through examination of deceased patients' brain tissue, physicians could objectively confirm the pathological differences between a concussion and a moderate or severe brain injury on a cellular level (e.g., absence of gross anatomic lesions or bleedings; as described in Signoretti et al., 2011). The pathophysiological, microscopic changes in the brain were characterized by softening or inflammation of the brain tissue, which was linked to athletes' behavioral change (Harrison, 2014). The absence of gross structural damage explained why a resolution of concussion symptoms such as photophobia, tinnitus, and headache, was typically reported within two weeks (Abernethy, 1825; McCrory & Berkovic, 2001).

In 1863, John Hilton was the first to recommend rest and withdrawal from sports following concussion (Hilton, 1891). Despite recognition that concussion represented an injury at the cellular level, during much of the 19th and 20th century, post-concussive symptoms were often ascribed to a patient's deficient personality. Such beliefs persisted given the absence of objective diagnostic tools (Courville, 1953). By 1927, scientists observed lingering concussive symptoms in various athletes. Osnato and Giliberti (1927) described 100 cases of concussed patients, suggesting that if symptoms did not completely resolve, a degeneration of the brain might occur. Shortly after, Martland (1928) used the term "punch drunk" (dementia pugilistica) to describe long-term sequelae of repeated concussions in boxers. Specifically, he noted boxers who appeared to experience early Parkinson-like symptoms, characterized by postural instability such as dysfunctional shuffling, speech problems, or inappropriate or explosive behavior, occasionally forcing a boxer into retirement or even commitment to a mental institution (Martland, 1928; Rabadi & Jordan, 2001). In 1933, the NCAA heeded Hilton's previous suggestions recommending rest until concussion symptoms had resolved.

Parker (1934) coined the clinical term *traumatic encephalopathy* to characterize a persistent or progressive state of neurological or neurobehavioral degeneration following repetitive blows to the head in reference to boxers, who had been colloquially described as punch-drunk (Victoroff, 2013). In an effort to further specify the nature of boxers' unresolved symptoms, Romanis and Mitchiner (1934) used the term *traumatic encephalitis* to describe inflammatory cerebral reactions caused by repetitive trauma to the brain tissue. Given the variety of terms used to describe what Martland (1928) first called the *punch drunk* syndrome, Critchley (1937) and Johnson (1969) advocated use of the term *chronic traumatic encephalopathy* (CTE) due to lingering symptoms with a striking tendency for gradual worsening. However, subsequent scholars suggested the label CTE might be misleading, as it implied a particular clinical course. Accordingly, Victoroff and Baron (2012) recently suggested employing Parker's original term, *traumatic encephalopathy*, as it encompassed pathologies including, but not limited to, inflammatory processes.

Beaussart and Beaussart-Boulengé (1970) conducted clinical examinations and electroencephalography of 123 amateur boxers before and immediately following matches. Although no pathological changes were observed, even when boxers experienced loss of consciousness, arterial blood pressure showed significant variations. Kelly (1981) was among the first in the modern era to acknowledge that prolonged concussion symptoms could be due to a failure to acknowledge and treat the problem. Kelly asserted that in the absence of injury recognition and medical treatment, patients who suffered from persisting post-concussive symptoms were at risk for a secondary iatrogenic injury due to the increased vulnerability to reinjury.

The current system of field-side evaluation of head injury was first recommended in an American Psychological Association (APA) boxing-related position statement in 1985. In 1991, the Colorado Medical Society published a concussion grading system that was incorporated by the NCAA and high school football.

The history of concussion diagnosis and treatment is a remarkably long and circuitous one, notable for persistent and diligent attention to the most prized and distinctly human of organs, the brain. Yet there is also a puzzlingly persistent resistance to fully embrace the underlying science and to taking action in response. In a telling story from the history of neuroscience, physician Marc Dax observed that a cavalry officer with a right-sided head injury suffered language deficits, which sparked continuing study on his part. He eventually presented his accumulated work on lateralization and localization of brain function in 1836, well in advance of the work of Broca in 1863, who is recognized as the pioneer. Clearly controversy is not new to the science of the brain.

The psychology of sport injury and the emergence of sport concussion as a contemporary social issue

Sports medicine and science evolved as dedicated disciplines in North America, beginning in the 1950s with the formation of the National Athletic Trainers Association (NATA) and the American College of Sports Medicine (ACSM). The seminal sport psychology organization, the International Society of Sport Psychology (ISSP), was formed in 1965. However, the field was not solidified until two decades later with the formation of the Association for the Advancement of Applied Sport Psychology (AAASP, now AASP) in 1985 and Division 47 of the American Psychological Association (APA) in 1986, now the Society for Sport, Exercise & Performance Psychology. Although injury was central to the mission of NATA and ACSM from the onset, the tipping point for injury as a focus within sport psychology came with the publication of the *Psychology of Sport Injury* (Heil, 1993) and the *Psychological Bases of Sport Injuries* (Pargman, 1993).

The publication of Heil (1993) and Pargman's (1993) books reflected a growing recognition among sport and health practitioners that beyond the physical toll of injury, a range of emotional, behavioral, and social implications were also apparent (Brewer et al., 1995; Crossman, 1997; Gordon, Milios, & Grove, 1991). By the late 1980s and mid-to-late 1990s, sport psychology researchers began to develop and test conceptual models aimed at better understanding the potential role of psychological factors in injury onset (Andersen & Williams, 1988); rehabilitation (Heil, 1993; Wiese-Bjornstal et al., 1998); and return to play (Taylor & Taylor, 1997). Much of the research testing these models focused on acute musculoskeletal injuries among recreational and competitive athletes (e.g., 18 and above; Brewer, Linder, & Phelps, 1995; Taylor & May, 1996). In 1998, Britton Brewer edited a special edition of the *Journal of Applied Sport Psychology* examining various theoretical, empirical, and applied issues.

As highlighted below, it was not until the new millennium that sport psychology researchers began to focus on sport-related concussion in earnest. A key turning point occurred in the 1980s with the seminal work of Barth and colleagues (Barth et al., 1983; 1989; Boll & Barth, 1983; Rimel et al., 1981), who identified the utility of neuropsychological assessment of concussion in sport. Their work paved the way for the adoption of neuropsychological assessment protocols in the National Football League (NFL) in 1993 (beginning with the Pittsburgh Steelers), and in the National Hockey League (NHL) in 1996 (Johnson, Kegel, & Collins, 2011). Other notable developments in sport concussion management followed, including Major League Baseball's adoption of neuropsychological assessment protocols in 2004 (Johnson et al., 2011), and NATA's 2004 position statement outlining salient concussion information and medical care recommendations (updated in 2014).

In 2001, the first International Concussion in Sport Group (CISG) conference took place in Vienna, Austria, with programs ongoing (Prague, 2004; Zurich, 2008 & 2012; and Berlin, 2016). The CISG conferences generated a series of consensus statements yielding recommendations on concussion recognition, evaluation, and management. These statements have been influential in guiding clinical practice, identifying directions for future research, emphasizing the importance of individualized concussion management, and promoting the value of knowledge translation strategies (Berlin, 2016).

Preliminary sport psychology research identified emotional responses to sport-related concussion among varsity athletes (Mainwaring et al., 2010) and highlighted the efficacy of a social support group in mitigating post-concussion mood disturbance (Horton, Bloom, & Johnston, 2002). Similarly, several conceptual papers underscored the importance of social support in mitigating concussion-related stressors and uncertainties, and the potential role of sport psychology providers in facilitating post-concussion adjustment, recovery, and return to play (Bloom et al., 2004; Johnston et al., 2004; Kontos, Collins, & Russo, 2004).

Other important work on the incidence and prevention of concussion in sport includes: the development of injury surveillance systems (e.g., the National Center for Catastrophic Sport Injury Research [NCCSIR], formed in 1982); public education campaigns designed to prevent head and spinal cord injuries (e.g., the ThinkFirst National Injury Prevention Foundation, started in 1986); and the work of industrial and consumer products standards groups, such as ASTM (originally, the Association for the Study of Testing and Materials). Also, the media plays an influential role. For example, ESPN discontinued its "Jacked Up!" program in 2006, which included a regular segment highlighting the hardest and most spectacular hits in the weekend's football.

From a retrospective view, it does not appear that any of these broad-based efforts had a significant influence on the Zeitgeist of the times. Even as change came to high-profile sport, awareness of the problem of concussion failed to penetrate the mass consciousness of sport. For example, in an epidemiological study of 566 school-age athletes, although 55% reported at least 1 concussion-related symptom following an injury to the head, and only 13.6% reported a concussion, due in part to the perception that being "dinged" or "getting your bell rung" was not a concussion, but rather, a normal part of the game (Valovich McLeod et al., 2008). It was not until the film *Concussion* in 2015, based on the neuro-pathologist Bennett Omalu's 2005 publication in the journal *Neurosurgery*, that awareness of concussion as a health concern erupted in the public consciousness. Though the accuracy of the storyline may be debated, the movie's positive impact on the recognition and prevention of head injury is noteworthy. That a popular film may have been a turning point in the conversation on sport concussion, despite all the preceding science, points to the limits that science faces in bringing issues to the public and to policymakers.

Just as increased media attention helped raise the profile of concussion in public awareness, such coverage also appears to have intensified research efforts regarding the psychosocial aspects of concussion. Indicative of the growing interest in the area, the journal *Sport, Exercise, and Performance Psychology* devoted a 2017 special edition to the topic. Edited by leading concussion researcher Anthony Kontos, the issue highlighted the influence of psychosocial factors (e.g., mood, anxiety, motivation, personality) on a range of concussion issues, including: decisions related to playing concussion-risk sports (Murphy, Askew, & Summer, 2017); baseline testing (Schatz et al., 2017); concussion-history (Beidler et al., 2017); concussion symptomology (O'Rourke et al., 2017); emotional responses following concussion (André-Morin, Caron, & Bloom, 2017; Turner et al., 2017); and treating psychological issues in concussed athletes (Sandel et al., 2017). Most recently, scholars have examined the value of various educational strategies (including use of social media platforms) in promoting enhanced concussion knowledge, attitudes, and reporting intentions/behaviors (Caron et al., 2018), as well as the importance of knowledge translation strategies in bridging the gap between science and public awareness (Mrazik et al., 2015). The extent to which recent scholarship has played a role in social change efforts is examined in the next section.

Has scientific research played a role in social change efforts? Considerations for researchers moving forward

The gap between knowledge of concussion and the willingness to take action on this knowledge spans the history of the study of brain injury. In antiquity, Hippocrates stated that "no head injury is too trivial to ignore." By 1518, da Carpi had identified the symptoms of impaired speech and memory, as well as dizziness and imbalance, as key indicators of concussive damage. It was not until 1991, however, that such symptoms were uniformly examined as part of field-side assessment protocols (Colorado Medical Society, 1991). In 1863, John Hilton recommended rest and withdrawal from sports following concussion, a practice that did not truly come into place untill recent years (Hilton, 1891). The disconnect between scientific evidence, public perception, and organizational response has persisted into the 21st century and is puzzling given the crescendo of emerging scientific knowledge. Understanding why this is and how to remedy it offers the promise of more timely and effective solutions.

While the exact causes are unclear, the disconnect between concussion knowledge and social action is likely a consequence of a variety of factors including the shortcomings with the way in which scientists share information with the public, deeply engrained cultural schema which may implicitly drive prevailing expectations about sport, and the social politics that emerge at the intersection of sport, health, and business. Sport is subject to a set of contemporary and historic forces ranging from embedded cultural beliefs like the warrior ethos (Nixon, 1992, 1993) to the practical realities of the brand and the bottom line. The warrior ethos has deep roots in sport, as is reflected in the legend of the Greek soldier, Pheidippides, who collapsed and died after bringing news to Athens from the battle of Marathon, and whose run is memorialized in the classic race of endurance (Perseus Digital Library Project, n.d.). In the 19th century, Hilton (1891) notes that despite an emerging body of scientific evidence, the symptoms of those who suffered concussions was commonly attributed to a deficient personality. The minimization of symptoms has continued until recently, influenced by positively toned euphemisms for brain injury ranging from the "punch drunk" label of Martland (1928) to more recent references to "getting your bell rung."

Both the sport and the healthcare systems are formidable enterprises driven by distinct values, perspectives, and objectives, which may potentially be in concert or in conflict. Each is composed of constituent groups (patients and athletes, coaches and medical providers, insurance carriers and sponsors, equipment suppliers and governing bodies) which drive these respective systems. As an entity functioning within the vast sport enterprise, the delivery of healthcare will be subject to the influences—positive and negative—of the sport system and its constituent groups. While both the sport and medical systems are business enterprises driven by a bottom line, in healthcare there is a strong ethical code which poses potential constraints when the welfare of the individual and that of the organization are in conflict.

The failure of the science to have an impact commensurate with the body of evidence may ultimately be a function of poor knowledge translation efforts. Knowledge translation refers to the synthesis, dissemination, exchange, and practical application of knowledge for the purpose of improving the lives of individuals with injury or disabilities (Canadian Institutes of Health Research, 2018). Unfortunately, the practical application piece is often neglected by scholars, many of whom are rewarded and incentivized to publish work in scholarly outlets but often lack the interest or incentives to communicate their findings to the lay public, health practitioners, or policymakers. Moreover, the extent to which public policymakers are informed of, or influenced by, scientific findings when policy decisions are made remains unknown. Greater efforts to foster interactions (presentations, forums, meetings) between researchers, health practitioners, and public policymakers are needed. If concussion scholars wish to have a societal impact in promoting greater concussion awareness, education, and prevention efforts, then communication of findings beyond academic outlets—to include social media platforms—seems prudent.

An additional reason for the limited impact of concussion scholarship on social awareness relates to scholars' failure to consider contextual barriers and challenges involved in implementing their work. For example, Klügl, Shrier, and

McBain (2010) reviewed over 10,000 sport injury prevention studies and found that while 75% of the research focused on incidence, less than 4% examined the impact of implementation. Research by Harmer (2015) also demonstrated the obstacles encountered in applying science to change in organizational policy. The goal of the project was framed as balancing the moral obligation to protect fencers from injury with the fiduciary duty to protect the integrity of the sport for the benefit of the membership at large. The full cycle of scientific investigation and implementation was interrupted as the work group settled on a solution prematurely, which Harmer (2015) suggested was a consequence of the majority of the group not coming from a research background. Researchers are cautioned that solutions based on best evidence may not prevail because scholars may fail to appreciate the political, financial, and social forces that hold sway in policy decisions (Harmer, 2015). Such cautions are not intended to suggest that future research efforts are unnecessary or unimportant, but rather, as Kerr and colleagues (2014) have highlighted, to make researchers aware of the need to consider the wider social context within which their research occurs and impacts the likelihood of such findings influencing policy decisions.

Conclusions and future research directions

This chapter has provided a long-term and recent historical perspective on the emergence of concussion as a sport-related injury. A confluence of factors, but in particular social and popular media, have helped move concussion into the forefront of public consciousness. As argued above, if scientists are to influence the culture of concussion policy and promote wider social change, then we hope some of the cautionary tales described above figure into action research efforts moving forward. With that in mind, further work examining various stakeholders' receptiveness to implementing concussion policies based on available evidence would be beneficial. Similarly, the relevance of social-contextual and ideological influences impacting concussion occurrence and management is warranted, as is further examination of the reward structures which encourages athletes to deny, downplay, or continue playing despite concussive injury. Moreover, the efficacy of knowledge translation strategies in impacting concussion knolwedge, attitudes, and reporting behaviors in various sport contexts is needed. Other avenues for future research include examination of the psychosocial implications of concussion for athletes, the impact of particular cognitions (efficacy beliefs, motivations to recover, attributions for recovery) on the quality and timeliness of concussion recovery, and the efficacy of sport psychology interventions (e.g., goal, setting, imagery, social support) in mitigating concussion symptomology and enhancing psychological responses.

References

Andersen, M. B., & Williams, J. M. (1988). A model of stress and athletic injury: Prediction and prevention. *Journal of Sport & Exercise Psychology, 10*, 294–306.

Abernethy, J. (1825). *The surgical and physiological works of John Abernethy.* Hartford: Reprinted by Oliver D. Cooke & Company.

André-Morin, D., Caron, J. G., & Bloom, G. A. (2017). Exploring the unique challenges faced by female university athletes experiencing prolonged concussion symptoms. *Sport, Exercise, and Performance Psychology,* 6, 289–303.

Barth, J. T., Alves, W. M., Ryan, T. V., Macciocchi, S. N., Rimel, R. W., Jane, J. A., & Nelson, W. E. (1989). Mild head injury in sports: Neuropsychological sequelae and recovery of function. In H. S. Levin, H. M. Eisenberg, & A. L. Benton (Eds.), *Mild head injury* (pp. 257–275). New York, NY, U.S.: Oxford University Press.

Barth, J. T., Macciocchi, S. N., Giordani, B., Rimel, R., Jane, J. A., & Boll, T. J. (1983). Neuropsychological sequelae of minor head injury. *Neurosurgery,* 13, 529–533.

Beaussart, M., & Beaussart-Boulengé, L. (1970). "Experimental" study of cerebral concussion in 123 amateur boxers, by clinical examination and EEG before and immediately after fights. *Electroencephalography and Clinical Neurophysiology,* 29, 529–530.

Beidler, E., Donnellan, M. B., Covassin, T., Phelps, A. L., & Kontos, A. P. (2017). The association between personality traits and sport-related concussion history in collegiate student-athletes. *Sport, Exercise, and Performance Psychology,* 6, 252–261.

Bloom, G. A., Horton, A. S., McCrory, P., & Johnston, K. M. (2004). Sport psychology and concussion: New impacts to explore. *British Journal of Sports Medicine,* 38, 519–521.

Boll, T. J., & Barth, J. (1983). Mild head injury. *Psychiatric Developments,* 1, 263–275.

Brewer, B. W., Linder, D. E., & Phelps, C. M. (1995). Situational correlates of emotional adjustment to athletic injury. *Clinical Journal of Sport Medicine,* 5, 241–245.

Brewer, B. W., Van Raalte, J. L., Petitpas, A. J., Sklar, J. H., & Ditmar, T. D. (1995). A brief measure of adherence during sport injury rehabilitation sessions. *Journal of Applied Sport Psychology,* 7, S44.

Broca, P. (1863). Localisations des fonctions cérébrales. Siège de la faculté du langage articulé. *Bulletin de la Société d'Anthropologie,* 4, 200–208.

Brooks, D., & Hunt, B. M. (2006). Current concepts in concussion diagnosis and management in sports: A clinical review. *British Columbia Medical Journal,* 48, 453.

Canadian Institutes of Health Research. Retrieved June 6, 2018, from www.cihr-irsc. gc.ca/e/29529.html.

Caron, J. G., Rathwell, S., Delaney, J. S., Johnston, K. M., Ptito, A., & Bloom, G. A. (2018). Development, implementation, and assessment of a concussion education programme for high school student-athletes. *Journal of Sport Sciences,* 36, 48–55.

Crossman, J. (1997). Psychological rehabilitation from sports injuries. *Sports Medicine,* 23, 333–339.

Courville, C. B. (1953). *Commotio cerebri; cerebral concussion and the postconcussion syndrome in their medical and legal aspects.* Los Angeles, CA: San Lucas Press.

Colorado Medical Society. (1991). *Report of the Sports Medicine Committee: Guidelines for the Management of Concussion in Sports (revised).* Denver, CO: Colorado Medical Society.

Critchley, E. (1937). Nervous disorders in boxers. *Medical Annual,* 318–320.

da Carpi, J. B. (1518). Tractatus de fractura calve sive cranei (d. B. H. Ed.). Bologna.

Dax, M. (1836). Lésions de la moitié gauche de l'encéphale coïncident avec l'oubli des signes de la pensée (lu à Montpellier en 1836). *Bulletin hebdomadaire de médecine et de chirurgie*, 2me série, 1865, 2, 259–62.

Dowling, K. A., & Goodrich, J. T. (2016). Two cases of 16th century head injuries managed in royal European families. *Neurosurgical Focus, 41*, E2.

Gordon, S., Milios, D., & Grove, J. R. (1991). Psychological aspects of the recovery process from sport injury: The perspective of sport physiotherapists. *Australian Journal of Science and Medicine in Sport, 23*, 53–60.

Harrison, E. A. (2014). The first concussion crisis: Head injury and evidence in early American football. *American Journal of Public Health, 104*, 822–833.

Harmer, P. A. (2015). Preventing penetrating hand injuries in sabre fencing: An application and critique of the van Mechelen model by the Fédération Internationale d'Escrime. *British Journal of Sports Medicine, 49*, 1138–1143.

Heil, J. (1993). *Psychology of sport injury*. Champaign, IL: Human Kinetics.

Hilton, J. (1891). *Rest and pain. A course of lectures*, 2nd ed. Cincinnati, OH: P. W. Garfield.

Horton, A., Bloom, G. A., & Johnston, K. (2002). The impact of support groups on the psychological state of athletes experiencing concussions. *Medicine & Science in Sports and Exercise, 34*, S99.

Johnson, J. (1969). Organic psychosyndromes due to boxing. *The British Journal of Psychiatry, 115*, 45–53.

Johnson, E. W., Kegel, N. E., & Collins, M. W. (2011). Neuropsychological assessment of sport-related concussion. *Clinics in Sports Medicine, 30*, 73–88.

Johnston, K. M., Bloom, G. A., Ramsay, J., Kissick, J., Montgomery, D., Foley, D., Chen, J., & Ptito, A. (2004). Current concepts in concussion rehabilitation. *Current Sports Medicine Reports, 3*, 316–323.

Kamp, M., Tahsim-Oglou, Y., Steiger, H.-J., & Hänggi, D. (2012). Traumatic brain injuries in the ancient Egypt: Insights from the Edwin Smith Papyrus. *Journal of Neurological Surgery Part A: Central European Neurosurgery, 73*, 230–237.

Kelly, R. (1981). The post-traumatic syndrome. *Journal of the Royal Society of Medicine, 74*, 242–245.

Kerr, Z. Y., Register-Mihalik, J. K., Marshall, S. W., Evenson, K. R., Mihalik, J. P., & Guskiewicz, K. M. (2014). Disclosure and non-disclosure of concussion and concussion symptoms in athletes: Review and application of the socio-ecological framework. *Brain Injury, 28*, 1009–1021.

Klügl, M., Shrier, I., McBain, K. (2010). The prevention of sport injury: An analysis of 12,000 published manuscripts. *Clinical Journal of Sport Medicine, 20*, 407–412.

Kontos, A. P., Collins, M., & Russo, S. A. (2004). An introduction to sports concussion for the sport psychology consultant. *Journal of Applied Sport Psychology, 16*, 220–235.

Mainwaring, L. M., Bisschop, S., Comper, P., Hutchison, M., & Richards, D. W. (2010). Emotional response to sport concussion compared to ACL injury. *Brain Injury, 24*, 589–597.

Martland, H. S. (1928). Punch drunk. *Journal of the American Medical Association, 91*, 1103–1107.

Masferrer, R., Masferrer, M., Prendergast, V., & Harrington, R. (2000). Grading scale for cerebral concussions. *Barrow Neurological Institute Quarterly, 16*, 4–9.

McCrory, P., & Berkovic, S. (2001). Concussion: The history of clinical and pathophysiological concepts and misconceptions. *Neurology, 57*, 2283–2289.

Meehan, W. (2017). *Concussions.* Santa Barbara, CA: Greenwood.

Mrazik, M., Dennison, C. R., Brook, B. L., Yeates, K. O., Babul, S., & Naidu, D. (2015). A qualitative review of sports concussion education: prime time for evidence-based knowledge translation. *British Journal of Sports Medicine, 49,* 1548–1553.

Murphy, A. M., Askew, K. L., & Summer, K. E. (2017). Parents' intentions to allow youth football participation: Perceived concussion risk and the theory of planned behavior. *Sport, Exercise, and Performance Psychology, 6,* 230–242.

Nixon, H. L. (1992). A social network analysis of influences on athletes to play with pain and injuries. *Journal of Sport and Social Issues, 16,* 127–135.

Nixon, H. L. (1993). Accepting the risks of pain and injury in sport: Mediated cultural influences on playing hurt. *Sociology of Sport Journal, 10,* 183–196.

Omalu, B. I., DeKosky, S. T., Minster, R. L., Kamboh, M. I., Hamilton, R. L., & Wecht, C. H. (2005). Chronic traumatic encephalopathy in a National Football League player. *Neurosurgery, 57,* 128–134.

O'Rourke, D. J., Smith, R. E., Punt, S., Coppel, D. B., & Breiger, D. (2017). Psychosocial correlates of young athletes' self-reported concussion symptoms during the course of recovery. *Sport, Exercise, and Performance Psychology, 6,* 262–276.

Osnato, M., & Giliberti, V. (1927). Postconcussion neurosis-traumatic encephalitis: A conception of postconcussion phenomena. *Archives of Neurology & Psychiatry, 18,* 181–214.

Pargman, D. (1993). *Psychological bases of sports injuries.* Morgantown, WV: Fitness Information Technology.

Park, R. (1896). *Surgical diseases and injuries of the head.* In R. Park (Ed.). A treatise on surgery by American authors: For students and practitioners of surgery and medicine (Vol. 2) (pp. 17–85). Philadelphia, PA: Lea Brothers & Co.

Parker, H. L. (1934). Traumatic encephalopathy ('Punch Drunk') of professional pugilists. *Journal of Neural Psychopathology, 15,* 20–28.

Pearce, J. M. S. (2008). Observations on concussion. *European Neurology, 59,* 113.

Perseus Digital Library Project. (2004, August 13). Retrieved from www.perseus.tufts.edu/Olympics/index.html.

Rabadi, M. H., & Jordan, B. D. (2001). The cumulative effect of repetitive concussion in sports. *Clinical Journal of Sport Medicine, 11,* 194–198.

Rimel, R. W., Giordani, B., Barth, J. T., Boll, T. J., & Jane, J. A. (1981). Disability caused by minor head injury. *Neurosurgery, 9,* 221–228.

Romanis, W., & Mitchiner, P. (1934). *The science and practice of surgery,* Vol 2, 5th edn, Philadelphia, PA: Lea and Febiger.

Sandel, N., Reynolds, E., Cohen, P. E., Gillie, B. L., & Kontos, A. P. (2017). Anxiety and mood clinical profile following sport-related concussion: From risk factors to treatment. *Sport, Exercise, and Performance Psychology, 6,* 304–323.

Schatz, P., Elbin, R. J., Anderson, M. N., Savage, J., & Covassin, T. (2017). Exploring sandbagging behaviors, effort, and perceived utility of the ImPACT Baseline Assessment in college athletes. *Sport, Exercise, and Performance Psychology, 6,* 243–251.

Signoretti, S., Lazzarino, G., Tavazzi, B., & Vagnozzi, R. (2011). The pathophysiology of concussion. *Physical Medicine & Rehabilitation, 3,* S359–S368.

Taylor, A. H., & May, S. (1996). Threat and coping appraisal as determinants of compliance with sports injury rehabilitation: An application of Protection Motivation Theory. *Journal of Sport Sciences, 14,* 471–482.

Taylor, J., & Taylor, S. (1997). Psychological approaches to sports injury rehabilitation. Lippincott Williams & Wilkins.

Tuke, J. (1910). Hippocrates. *Encyclopaedia Britannica, 13*, 517–519.

Turner, S., Langdon, J., Shaver, G., Graham, V., Naugle, K., & Buckley, T. (2017). Comparison of psychological response between concussion and musculoskeletal injury in collegiate athletes. *Sport, Exercise, and Performance Psychology, 6*, 277–288.

Valovich McLeod, T. C., Bay R. C., Heil J., & McVeigh, S. D. (2008). Identification of sport and recreational activity concussion history through the pre-participation screening and a symptom survey in young athletes. *Clinical Journal of Sport Medicine, 18*, 235–240.

Victoroff, J. (2013). Traumatic encephalopathy: Review and provisional research diagnostic criteria. *NeuroRehabilitation, 32*, 211–224.

Victoroff, J., & Baron, D. (2012). Diagnosis and treatment of sports-related traumatic brain injury. *Psychiatric Annals, 42*, 365–370.

Wason, P. C., & Reich, S. S. (1979). A verbal illusion. *The Quarterly Journal of Experimental Psychology, 31*, 591–597.

Wiese-Bjornstal, D. M., Smith, A. M., Shaffer, S. M., & Morrey, M. A. (1998). An integrated model of response to sport injury: Psychological and sociological dynamics. *Journal of Applied Sport Psychology, 10*, 46–69.

3 The role of neuropsychology in understanding, assessing, and managing sport-related concussions

Dave Ellemberg, Veronik Sicard,
Adam Harrison, Jacob J. M. Kay,
and Robert Davis Moore

Introduction

Neuropsychology is the scientific study of human brain functioning. Clinical neuropsychologists study how behavior and cognition are influenced by the brain's functioning and are concerned with the diagnosis and treatment of the behavioral and cognitive deficits caused by neurological disorders. Neuropsychologists have spearheaded the scientific and clinical research aimed at identifying the consequences of concussion, proper injury management, and the return to learn and play regimen (Ott, Bailey, & Broshek, 2018). They developed clinical assessment tools to identify cognitive deficits caused by concussion and to track injury recovery. With distinct training in brain-behavior relationships, psychological assessment, and psychometrics, neuropsychologists are uniquely qualified to evaluate an athlete's cognitive, emotional, and psychological status following a concussion. In fact, in most Canadian provinces and territories, as well as in many states of the United States, the assessment of cognitive and psychological disorders caused by a neurological disorder is an act that is reserved to the clinical neuropsychologists.

In recent years, the role of the clinical neuropsychologist in the assessment, treatment, and management of sport concussion has become more clearly defined as this domain of clinical practice has exploded. This has led to the emergence of a new discipline, known as sport neuropsychology, with a clinician having an interdisciplinary training in clinical psychology, sport psychology, and neuropsychology (Merz, Perry, & Ross, 2018). The critical role of the sports neuropsychologist has also contributed to the creation of the Sports Neuropsychology Society (SNS), a professional organization established in 2012. Its mission is "to advance the field of sports neuropsychology, to generate and disseminate knowledge regarding brain-behavior relationships as it applies to sports, and to promote the welfare of athletes at all levels" (Sports Neuropsychology Society, 2017).

Following a sport concussion, a neuropsychologist can intervene at several time points and can play a decisive role in promoting an optimal treatment and management plan. Clinical experience commands the importance of early detection, diagnosis, and treatment for a better outcome. The objective of this chapter is to describe the consequences of sport-related concussion on brain and cognitive functioning. Firstly, we will present the neurophysiological cascade caused by a concussion. Second, neuro-imaging techniques and their role in injury diagnosis, prognosis, and rehabilitation will be discussed. Finally, we will present the role of the neuropsychological assessment in the management of concussed athletes. We will provide a comprehensive understanding of the neuropsychological deficits that may be present in the acute phase of the injury as well as of those that persist beyond this phase and likely contribute to the post-concussion syndrome (PCS).

Neurophysiological cascade of concussion

A concussion provokes the rapid transfer of kinetic energy caused by a direct impact to the head or an impact to the body that transmits an impulsive force to the head. This transfer of energy causes the brain to move rapidly inside the skull, leading to twisting, compression, and stretching of brain tissue. This may ultimately lead to the shearing of axonal fibers known as diffuse axonal injury (DAI; Giza & Hovda, 2014).

Research from animal studies suggests that DAI may be a biological substrate of clinical signs and symptoms associated with concussion (Greer, McGinn, & Povlishock, 2011). In addition to the axonal damage, pressure inside the skull increases following the concussive impact. Together, the mechanical damage and the increased intracranial pressure disrupt the electric and metabolic equilibrium of neurons, leading to mass depolarization of neurons (Giza & Hovda, 2014). Other processes, including excessive release of neurotransmitters, calcium accumulation, oxidative stress, decreased cerebral blood flow, and brain tissue inflammation likely also contribute to the alteration of brain function following a concussion (Giza & Hovda, 2014). These alterations seem to resolve within a month in rats.

The consequences of a concussion on the human brain are likely different than those found in the animal model due to fundamental difference in the biomechanics of the impact and in brain morphology. In animals, this metabolic cascade seems to be rather transient, whereas metabolic depression and decreased cerebral blood flow appears to persist longer in humans (Meier et al., 2015). There is also evidence in humans of widespread lesions of white matter tracts or DAI, observed particularly in the brain stem, the corpus callosum, and the frontal lobes (Ajao et al., 2012). Human autopsy studies suggest this axonal pathology as a key feature of concussive injuries and a physiological substrate of clinical symptoms (Meythaler et al., 2001; Sharp & Ham, 2011). As previously mentioned, most athletes present with deficits in memory, attention, and executive functions in the days following a concussion. Cognitive functions rely on a distributed network of neurons; thus, uttermost functioning depends on white matter integrity and neuronal activity, which are disrupted by concussive injuries (Hammeke et al., 2013). DAI may interfere with both efficiency and speed of nerve impulse transmission between brain areas giving rise to cognitive functions.

The general understanding of the pathophysiology of concussion has improved significantly in the last three decades. Recent evidence tells us that a single concussion can trigger physiological changes in the brain (Kraus et al., 2017;

Moore et al., 2015). Importantly, alterations in several nerve cells and brain functions are observed beyond the previously suggested period of seven to ten days for recovery. Further research is needed to understand the link between the physiological disturbances and clinical consequences of concussion.

Neuroimaging and concussion

Although traditional imaging techniques such as computed tomography (CT) and low-resolution magnetic resonance imaging (MRI) are commonly used to assess and manage neurological conditions, their utility for evaluating concussive injuries is limited (Iverson et al., 2012). This is because the diffuse and microscopic damage caused by concussion is not detectable with traditional imaging, and the pathology of concussion is largely functional and microstructural (Broglio, Moore, & Hillman, 2011). As such, there is an ongoing search for neuroimaging methods that can aid the evaluation and management of concussion. The following sections will provide an overview of neuroimaging methods, followed by how different methods can advance the diagnosis and prognosis of concussive injuries.

Structural neuroimaging

Structural imaging methods use various means, such as X-rays and magnetic fields, to image the macro- and micro-structure of the brain. These methodologies provide researchers and clinicians with high-resolution contrasts of brain tissues (i.e., grey matter, white matter, cerebral vasculature, and spinal fluid), which are then used to identify and track abnormalities within the brain such as abnormal tissue growth, fluid buildup, and intracranial bleeding. As previously mentioned, traditional structural imaging measures such as CT and MRI are of limited utility for evaluating milder neurological conditions (e.g., concussion). In contrast, a recent variant of MRI known as diffuse tensor imaging (DTI) appears to be sensitive to even mild neurological conditions including concussion (Henry et al., 2011; Miles et al., 2008), and even sub-concussive impacts (Shenton et al., 2012). DTI images white matter integrity by evaluating the movement of water molecules within white matter tracts. By measuring deviations in the preferred movement of water molecules (Brownian diffusion), white matter abnormalities such as cellular swelling, axonal sheering, or Wallerian degeneration can be identified. Researchers and clinicians utilize DTI to detect and track abnormalities of specific white matter tracts and determine how these alterations are associated with functional outcomes following concussion (Alhilali et al., 2015; Hellstrom et al., 2017).

Functional imaging

In contrast to structural imaging techniques, which measure neuroanatomy, functional imaging techniques measure neurophysiology, either by measuring the brain's hemodynamic or electrophysiological activity. When neurons become active, they signal for increased blood flow to meet metabolic demands known as the *hemodynamic response*. By measuring the magnetic (functional MRI; fMRI) or optical (functional near-infrared spectroscopy; fNIRS) properties of this hemo-dynamic response, a functional and three-dimensional image of blood oxygen-level dependent (BOLD) brain activity is derived. This information can then be used to inform researchers and clinicians about abnormal blood flow and oxygen utilization in specific brain regions.

When neurons become active, they also create electromagnetic fields, which can be detected at the scalp by a method known as electroencephalography (EEG). EEG methodologies such as quantitative (Q) EEG, evoked potentials (EPs), and event-related brain potentials (ERPs) are used to gain information about different aspects of the brain's electrophysiology (spectral power, con-nectivity, amplitude, latency). EEG measures are particularly useful for studying neurological conditions, as they are the only measures that directly measure neurophysiology in real time. Furthermore, ERPs are the only imaging method that can parse the stimulus–response relationship into its constituent processes, enabling the direct linkage of neurophysiological phenomena to specific aspects of information processing. Accordingly, numerous concussion studies have utilized ERPs to identify and track specific deficits in sensation, perception, cognition, and motor function, even when patients report to be asymptomatic (Broglio et al., 2011).

Neurometabolic imaging

Neurometabolic imaging measures either the neurometabolism or neurochemis-try of the brain. Neurometabolism is typically measured by either single-photon emission computed tomography (SPECT) or positron emission tomography (PET). Both measures utilize nuclear imaging techniques to provide a three-dimensional image of glucose metabolism and determine where in the brain altered metabolism is occurring. Neurochemistry is measured by a variant of MRI known as magnetic resonance spectroscopy (MRS). MRS uses magnets to evalu-ate the nuclear structure of neuro-metabolites, providing a comprehensive read-out of absolute and neuro-metabolite ratios. Researchers and clinicians use MRS to gain a greater understanding of the metabolic alterations of neurological con-ditions. With respect to concussion, MRS has been used to reveal post-concus-sion variations in the expression of various neuro-metabolites such as glutamate, choline, and N-acetyl aspartate, which correlate with cognitive and psychological deficits (Babikian et al., 2006; Gardner, Iverson, & Stanwell, 2014; Vagnozzi et al., 2008; Yeo et al., 2006).

Clinical applications of imaging

The clinical utility of traditional neuroimaging methods (e.g., CT, low-resolu-tion MRI) is limited (Iverson et al., 2000; Morgan et al., 2015). Thus, a critical problem facing medical professionals is a lack of imaging measures that can facilitate concussion diagnoses (Ellemberg et al., 2009). Furthermore, it is inherently difficult to predict who will have a poor outcome following a concussion, as concussions are heterogeneous in nature and the acute signs and symptoms of concussion are poor predictors of functional outcomes (McCrory et al., 2017). Accordingly, researchers are working diligently to identify imaging modalities that may be used to advance clinical practices. The following section will address how neuroimaging may facilitate injury diagnoses and prognoses.

Concussion diagnoses

Recent advances in neuroimaging techniques hold promise for advancing concussion diagnoses. For example, DTI is more sensitive in identifying concussion neuropathology compared to structural MRI, and alterations in white matter integrity are consistently observed in the acute and sub-acute phase of injury (Henry et al., 2011; Shenton et al., 2012). In addition, alterations in EEG spectral power and connectivity can be used to accurately classify individuals with and without a concussion within the first week of injury (Thatcher et al., 2001; Thompson, Sebastianelli, & Slobounov, 2005). Furthermore, specific alterations in BOLD signals are consistently observed in the acute phase of injury (Guenette, Shenton, & Koerte, 2018). Similarly, research using MRS reveals consistent neurochemical changes in concussed individuals during the acute phase of injury (Gardner, Iverson, & Stanwell, 2014; Vagnozzi et al., 2008). Lastly, both PET and SPECT can accurately detect variations in brain metabolism that coincide with the acute neurometabolic cascade of concussion (Halstead & Walter, 2010). Thus, future diagnoses may rely less on subjective symptomology and more on objective neuroimaging measures.

Concussion prognoses

Although traditional imaging measures are of limited prognostic utility for concussive injuries, they may be of use for identifying chronic brain injuries and neurodegeneration. Indeed, several MRI studies indicate that retired contact athletes exhibit cortical atrophy, which is linked to neurodegeneration and cognitive decline (Koerte et al., 2016). Further, DTI studies indicate that alterations in white matter correlate with symptoms, cognition, and mental health (Alhilali et al., 2015; Hellstrom et al., 2017). Thus, structural imaging may be useful for identifying those with chronic brain injuries.

With respect to functional imaging, research indicates that alterations in frontal EEG activity can predict recovery of cognition and motor control and identify those with persisting mental health issues (Moore, Lepine, & Ellemberg, 2017; Slobounov et al., 2012). Further, multiple ERP studies indicate that component amplitudes correlate with symptom severity and time since injury and can discriminate between sub-concussive and concussive impacts (Gosselin et al., 2006; Moore, Lepine, & Ellemberg, 2017). Indeed, as ERPs are the only imaging method that identify specific deficits in information processing, they are particularly useful for identifying and tracking deficits in perception, cognition, and motor function (Broglio et al., 2011).

Evaluating hemodynamic activity also shows promise for prognosticating injury outcomes. Alterations in fMRI BOLD signals can predict symptom burden and cognitive functioning up to six weeks following injury (Barlow et al., 2016). Additionally, research using fNIRS indicates that alterations in hemodynamic connectivity can accurately classify those with and without persisting symptoms (Hocke et al., 2018). Thus, hemodynamic measures may also be useful for predicting injury outcomes and identifying persisting pathology.

Lastly, neurometabolic imaging appears useful for identifying persisting pathology and those with chronic brain injuries. For example, chronic alterations in neuro-metabolites, such as glutamate and N-acetyl aspartate, correlate with persisting cognitive deficits and depression and may be able to predict chronic traumatic encephalopathy (Alosco et al., 2017). In addition, PET reliably detects persisting neurometabolic changes in active and retired athletes (Barrio et al., 2015), and SPECT demonstrates high sensitivity for predicting who will exhibit persisting cognitive deficits and clinical symptoms (Raji et al., 2014; Romero et al., 2015). Thus, neurometabolic imaging may be useful for predicting and identifying chronic conditions associated with concussion.

In sum, recent advances in microstructural, functional, and neurometabolic imaging hold great potential for advancing the diagnoses and prognoses of concussive injuries. Although promising, more progress needs to be made before these technologies are clinically viable. For example, DTI cannot effectively discriminate between contact athletes with and without a history of concussion, as repetitive sub-concussive impacts also alter white matter integrity (Davenport et al., 2014). Furthermore, functional neuroimaging measures currently lack standardized protocols, and normative databases limit their clinical utility. Also, neurometabolic imaging is unable to distinguish between mild and severe brain injuries (Giza & Hovda, 2014), and exposure to radiation is a drawback. As such, more research is needed to make these measures clinically useful. Regardless, neuroimaging methods are essential for gaining a more accurate understanding of concussion pathology and will continue to advance the diagnoses and prognoses of concussive injuries.

Neuropsychological assessment and management of concussion

The following sections will discuss the role of the clinical neuropsychologist within each phase of clinical recovery. It is noteworthy to mention that all athletes at risk of concussion, including child and adolescent athletes who take part in non-professional sports, should be supported by an interdisciplinary team of certified health professionals and athletic trainers. The following discussion will mainly consider this population, as most professional athletes usually benefit from a team of clinicians with clearly defined roles and responsibilities.

Acute phase of the injury: When to return to learn and to play

As we have seen in the section on the neurophysiological cascade immediately following a concussion, this injury disrupts several physiological systems in the brain that are responsible for the signs, symptoms, and cognitive deficits following the injury. Critical to recovery in the acute phase of this injury is the brain's need for an appropriate period of rest followed by the progressive return to cognitive and physical activities (McCrory et al., 2017). The clinical neuropsychologist has an important role to play in this initial phase of recovery. The first is related to counseling. Athletes, young and old, must understand the importance of cognitive rest. Although this might seem intuitive and straightforward, it is quite challenging for an intellectually, physically, and socially active person to slow down their pace for a few days. Support and education from a credible professional may be required for the patient to understand and accept that seemingly harmless activities like sending text messages or practicing a musical instrument can be very demanding for a brain and can interfere with its recovery.

The athlete also needs to know when and how to gradually reintroduce cognitive tasks as to not exacerbate or trigger symptoms that have abated. With the collaboration of the athlete, the neuropsychologist will engineer an individualized road map that will establish an optimal plan to progressively return to cognitive activities and eventually to school or other professional obligations. To do so, the neuropsychologist will need to be in direct contact with the parents and the person responsible for academic support at school. If need be, the neuropsychologist will recommend several temporary accommodations at school that can range from a reduced course load to the complete exemption from certain tests and exams. This expertise is well established by neuropsychologists, as they have long contributed to developing personalized education plans for students with learning disabilities (Fletcher-Janzen & Reynolds, 2010).

Another dimension to the management of concussion during the acute phase of the injury is to determine when the athlete is ready to make a complete return to learn/school and when the athlete can safely practice their sport again. It is within this context that the brief neuropsychological assessment initially forged its way in the management of sport concussion. First introduced to determine when professional athletes could return to play, the brief neuropsychological assessment has rapidly gained in popularity in the last 15 years. Over half a dozen testing batteries have been commercialized, and they have been promoted among high school, collegiate, and professional sport teams. Most of these batteries contain five to seven tests that assess different cognitive functions, including short-term and working memory, learning, attention, and processing speed. Total administration time typically ranges from 30 to 50 minutes.

The authors of most of the commercial post-concussion testing batteries suggest that athletes should be tested before the beginning of the sporting season to obtain a personalized measure of their cognitive capabilities before a concussion occurs. The results of this baseline test are then compared to tests completed in the hours and days following the athlete's concussion (Iverson, Lovell,

& Collins, 2003; Louey et al., 2014). By obtaining a pre-season baseline, these authors and several others report that high school and collegiate athletes have measurable cognitive deficits in the hours and days following their concussion that generally resolve within two to three weeks (Van Kampen et al., 2006). Thus, once an athlete's results on the cognitive tests return to baseline, this serves as an indication that the athlete may be ready to make a safe return to the regular practice of their sport.

This approach is appealing, as it makes the reassuring promise of a personalized patient care that aims to prevent a hasty return to play that could compromise the athlete's recovery and health. However, there are several limitations and downfalls to this approach. A first question that we can ask is whether it is necessary to obtain a baseline measure from every athlete on a team. Does this expensive and logistically complicated procedure improve the sensitivity of the post-injury assessment? A major concern with this approach is the low reliability of cognitive testing batteries. The test-retest reliability of commonly implemented cognitive assessment tools for concussion in a sample of student-athletes is less than optimal, ranging from 0.23 to 0.61, and it therefore does not meet the accepted threshold for clinical utility (Broglio et al., 2018). Further, standard normative data is as efficient as reliable change from baseline to identify post-concussion cognitive decline (Echemendia et al., 2012; Louey et al., 2014). It is also important to highlight that there are no other clinical conditions for which it is recommended to obtain such a baseline test. Most neuropsychologists would agree that normative data and clinical expertise suffice, regardless of the clinical condition.

Another issue with the commonly implemented cognitive assessment tools concerns their validity. In a thorough review of the literature covering over 5,968 studies, 69 of which met the inclusion criteria, Alsalaheen et al. (2016) did not find any conclusive evidence of discriminant and predictive validity or of diagnostic accuracy. This is particularly concerning for clinical neuropsychologists who are first and foremost interested in the psychometric properties of the tests that they use. There is accumulating evidence that the tests that are part of the commercial concussion batteries might not target the cognitive functions that are the most affected by a concussion. For example, it appears that higher level executive functions, believed to be in the frontal lobes, are altered several weeks and even months after a first concussion (Ellemberg et al., 2007; Halterman et al., 2006; Sicard, Moore, & Ellemberg, 2018).

Some of the brief commercial test batteries do contain tests that tap these higher-level executive functions, however they might not have the requisite sensitivity or enough trials to detect deficits. In a recent study, Sicard, Moore, and Ellemberg (2017) could detect persisting deficits in working memory by using a modified version of a commonly implemented sport concussion test by adding a 2-back task to it. By doing so, they increased the cognitive load of the test and made it more challenging to complete this task. Thus, several months after their concussion, collegiate athletes performed normally on the 1-back task that is normally part of the battery but had significant deficits on the more complex 2-back task. Thus, these deficits would have gone unobserved if only the standard test battery had been used. Together, this indicates that the commonly implemented tests have a high risk of producing false negatives. In other words, some athletes could be classified as recovered when in fact they are still experiencing cognitive impairments secondary to concussion.

Other issues that are raised concerning the commonly implemented computerized concussion tests are that providers promote group administration for baseline testing and that individuals without any qualifications in psychometry are entitled to administer them. An important series of studies has shown that compared to athletes tested in a private-practice neuropsychology center, athletes tested in a group and in a non-clinical setting had higher rates of invalid results and scored significantly lower on verbal memory, visual memory, motor processing speed, and reaction time (Moser et al., 2011). Recently, certain authors have been critical of the fact that it has become common practice for individuals to operate outside their scope of practice and administer cognitive assessments (Ott, Bailey, & Broshek, 2018). Not only should the person administering the tests have the relevant competence in psychometry, but they need to be able to select the most appropriate tests and know how to interpret the test results. Several factors can influence the concussed athlete's performance on the clinical neuropsychological assessment, including a history of brain injury, psychiatric disorders, mood disorders, learning disabilities, an attention deficit disorder, other medical conditions, prescription drugs, performance anxiety, other psychosocial factors, and motivation (Echemendia, 2006). This is where a formal training in psychology is essential, as any one of these factors can introduce extraneous error, invalidating the test results. Thus, all of these factors must be fully taken into consideration and carefully weighted in the interpretation of the test results.

Although there are several caveats with the use of the commonly implemented computerized brief concussion tests and the way they are administered, there are some circumstances for which they can be useful. For many athletes, a neuropsychological assessment conducted by a qualified professional might be critical to establish an individualized plan to progressively return to cognitive activities and eventually to school or other professional obligations. However, this does not mean that all athletes should systematically be tested as soon as they have a concussion. In fact, most athletes who experience a first concussion and have a typical recovery profile likely do not need such an assessment. An attentive appraisal of signs and symptoms often suffices to plan their return to learn and to play.

Among the athletes who do require a neuropsychological assessment following a concussion are those who are slow to recover. Young athletes who still experience symptoms after three to four weeks post-injury should be assessed rapidly by a multidisciplinary team of clinicians. Athletes who no longer experience symptoms, but who are burdened by certain cognitive impairments, including problems with their attention, memory, learning, and mental fatigue, should also be tested. In both cases, the neuropsychological assessment should target the complex brain functions that are important to succeed at school and at work. This assessment aims to verify if the athlete has any cognitive deficits and whether these are secondary to the concussion. If so, the clinical neuropsychologist will determine how these impairments interfere with learning or work, recommend interventions, including cognitive remediation, and if necessary suggest a series of school or workplace accommodations.

Athletes with a history of concussion should also obtain a comprehensive neuropsychological assessment. Along with complete neurological and physical exams, this will help the athlete to make the very important but also very difficult decision of continuing to practice their sport or of moving on to a sporting activity with a significantly lower risk of concussion. The neuropsychologist will provide the necessary psychological counseling that will enable the athlete to understand the clinical facts and to weigh the risks of pursuing their sport.

Chronic phase of the injury: Understanding and managing persistent cognitive symptoms

Concussive injuries are typically viewed as transitory in nature, with few long-term repercussions (McCrory et al., 2009). However, accumulating research suggests that athletes who report having fully recovered from a concussion and have made a complete return to their sport can still present certain enduring cognitive changes. Several studies suggest that concussive injuries can lead to alterations in episodic memory, learning, and attention (Killam, Cautin, & Santucci, 2005; Halterman et al., 2006; Peterson et al., 2003). There is also evidence of deficits in executive functions that persist months to years following injury and that touch more particularly inhibition, flexibility, working memory, and planning (Ellemberg et al., 2007; Howell et al., 2013; Moore et al., 2015; Ozen et al., 2013; Sicard, Moore, & Ellemberg, 2017).

These alterations in cognition were identified with classical neuropsychological tests used during the standard clinical assessment, suggesting that these tests have the requisite sensitivity to pick out persisting deficits caused by a concussion. However, it is important to specify that for the most part these deficits appear to be quite subtle and that they likely do not have functional consequences in the athlete's everyday life. Most neuropsychological tests have been developed to isolate specific cognitive functions, whilst in everyday life one has access to an ensemble of cognitive strategies that enable to compensate for subtle and highly specific deficits. This may explain why most athletes report feeling fine and that they are back to how they were before their injury, that is, back to "normal" (Kerr et al., 2016).

It could be argued that because these mild and isolated cognitive changes have no immediate consequence for the athlete, they are not clinically significant. These findings are nonetheless important as they confirm that a sport concussion does indeed affect the brain. In fact, there is accumulating evidence that the brain is changed by a concussion. For example, the risk of suffering a concussion is three to five times greater in individuals with a history of concussion (Guskiewicz et al., 2003). Moreover, each new concussion seems to be marked by a longer period of recovery (Morgan et al., 2015). These findings of subtle cognitive alterations are also consistent with those from human neuroimaging studies presented in the previous section that provide evidence for enduring neuroanatomical and neurophysiological damage following a sport concussion (Manley et al., 2017). Both clinicians and scientists should pay attention to these findings, as these cognitive and brain changes could be precursors to more important deficits that may manifest with accumulating concussions and with aging. Athletes who experience an average of three concussions in their sporting career appear to be ten times more likely than the general population to develop a neurodegenerative disorder akin to Alzheimer's (Guskiewicz et al., 2005; Randolph, Karantzoulis, & Guskiewicz, 2013). Further, one of the most important risk factors for PCS is a history of prior concussion (Zuckerman et al., 2016).

The post-concussion syndrome

Individuals who present with persistent and debilitating symptoms of their concussion have been identified as the "miserable minority" (Ruff, Camenzuli, & Mueller, 1996). Symptoms like headache, dizziness, and fatigue can be quite burdening as they negatively impact social, academic, and vocational functioning and in many cases can lead to isolation (Makdissi et al., 2013). The International Statistical Classification of Diseases and Related Health Problems, 10th Revision, defines PCS as three or more symptoms persisting for greater than four weeks, and a survey of more than 500 physicians found that the majority of them diagnosed PCS in patients who endorsed at least one symptom for a minimum of four weeks (Rose et al., 2015).

The provenance of PCS remains a topic of debate among clinicians and scientists as it is still often considered to be psychogenic (Carroll et al., 2004). However, the sport concussion literature has brought on a new perspective to this condition. In this case, those who suffer from PCS are healthy young adolescents or adults who are highly motivated to return to their sport and their studies. These student-athletes benefit from little to no secondary gain. Further, imaging studies in humans provide support to the neuropathophysiological etiology of PCS (Hart et al., 2013; Koerte et al., 2016).

Although anecdotal in nature, clinical experience indicates that it is not rare for an athlete with PCS to report cognitive deficits, including problems with concentration and learning. However, few studies investigated cognitive deficits in athletes with PCS. A recent prospective study evaluated patients who experienced a mild traumatic brain injury with a neuropsychological test battery and found deficits in verbal memory and learning that persisted over a 12-month period after the injury. Some of these patients also had structural alterations on magnetic resonance images, which were compatible with diffuse axonal injury (Radoi et al., 2018). Future research must be carried out to determine if athletes who manifest PCS also have persisting cognitive deficits and if so, the nature of these deficits will need to be clearly identified. Despite the paucity of data regarding this issue, an important aspect of clinical practice in neuropsychology is to provide a comprehensive cognitive assessment to individuals with PCS, sport-related or otherwise. This contributes to guiding the patient's management and treatment plan, including rest, cognitive remediation, and academic or work accommodations.

Conclusions

The assessment and management plan of any patient who suffered a concussion, sport-related or otherwise, requires the expertise of a multidisciplinary team. The clinical neuropsychologist is an important part of the concussion management puzzle, and that, equally so for patients who are in the acute phase of their injury, those who are slow to recover, and those with PCS. Thus, the role of the clinical neuropsychologist goes well beyond providing a brief cognitive assessment very early on following the injury with the sole purpose of planning a safe but rapid return to play. Above and beyond signs and symptoms, a concussion likely has its most impactful consequence on an individual's cognitive functioning. The clinical neuropsychologist must therefore identify the unique cognitive profile of each patient to contribute to the management plan and help track recovery. Finally, it is important not to neglect the critical role the neuropsychologist plays with regards to counseling and psychoeducation to help the patient deal with psychological and emotional challenges and guide them through what may be some very important but extremely difficult decisions.

References

Ajao, D. O., Pop, V., Kamper, J. E., Adami, A., Rudobeck, E., Huang, L., ... Badaut, J. (2012). Traumatic brain injury in young rats leads to progressive behavioral deficits coincident with altered tissue properties in adulthood. *Journal of Neurotrauma*, 29, 2060–2074. doi:10.1089/neu.2011.1883.

Alhilali, L. M., Delic, J. A., Gumus, S., & Fakhran, S. (2015). Evaluation of white matter injury patterns underlying neuropsychiatric symptoms after mild traumatic brain injury. *Radiology*, 277, 793–800. doi:10.1148/radiol.2015142974.

Alosco, M. L., Jarnagin, J., Rowland, B., Liao, H., Stern, R. A., & Lin, A. (2017). Magnetic resonance spectroscopy as a biomarker for chronic traumatic encephalopathy. *Seminars in Neurology*, 37, 503–509. doi:10.1055/s-0037-1608764.

Alsalaheen, B., Stockdale, K., Pechumer, D., & Broglio, S. P. (2016). Validity of the immediate post concussion assessment and cognitive testing (ImPACT). *Sports Medicine*, 46, 1487–1501. doi:10.1007/s40279-016-0532-y.

Babikian, T., Freier, M. C., Ashwal, S., Riggs, M. L., Burley, T., & Holshouser, B. A. (2006). MR spectroscopy: Predicting long-term neuropsychological outcome following pediatric TBI. *Journal of Magnetic Resonance Imaging*, 24, 801–811. doi:10.1002/jmri.20696.

Barlow, K. M., Marcil, L. D., Dewey, D., Carlson, H. L., MacMaster, F. P., Brooks, B. L., & Lebel, R. M. (2016). Cerebral perfusion changes in post-concussion syndrome: A prospective controlled cohort study. *Journal of Neurotrauma*, 34, 996–1004. doi:10.1089/neu.2016.4634.

Barrio, J. R., Small, G. W., Wong, K. P., Huang, S. C., Liu, J., Merrill, D. A., ... Kepe, V. (2015). In vivo characterization of chronic traumatic encephalopathy using [F-18]FDDNP PET brain imaging. *Proceedings of the National Academy of Sciences of the United States of America, 112,* E2039–2047. doi:10.1073/pnas.1409952112.

Broglio, S. P., Katz, B. P., Zhao, S., McCrea, M., & McAllister, T. (2018). Test-retest reliability and interpretation of common concussion assessment tools: Findings from the NCAA-DoD CARE Consortium. *Sports Medicine, 48,* 1255–1268. doi:10.1007/s40279-017-0813-0.

Broglio, S. P., Moore, R. D., & Hillman, C. (2011). A history of sport-related concussion on event-related brain potential correlates of cognition. *International Journal of Psychophysiology, 82,* 16–23.

Davenport, E. M., Whitlow, C. T., Urban, J. E., Espeland, M. A., Jung, Y., Rosenbaum, D. A., ... Maldjian, J. A. (2014). Abnormal white matter integrity related to head impact exposure in a season of high school varsity football. *Journal of Neurotrauma, 31,* 1617–1624. doi:10.1089/neu.2013.3233.

Echemendia, R. J. (2006). *Sports neuropsychology: Assessment and management of traumatic brain injury.* New York City, NY: Guilford Press.

Echemendia, R. J., Bruce, J. M, Bailey, C. M., Sanders, J. F., Arnett, P., & Vargas, G. (2012). The utility of post-concussion neuropsychological data in identifying cognitive change following sports-related MTBI in the absence of baseline data. *The Clinical Neuropsychologist, 26,* 1077–1091. doi:10.1080/13854046.2012.721006.

Ellemberg, D., Henry, L. C., Macciocchi, S. N., Guskiewicz, K. M., & Broglio, S. P. (2009). Advances in sport concussion assessment: From behavioral to brain imaging measures. *Journal of Neurotrauma, 26,* 2365–2382. doi:10.1089/neu.2009.0906.

Ellemberg, D., Leclerc, S., Couture, S., & Daigle, C. (2007). Prolonged neuropsychological impairments following a first concussion in female university soccer athletes. *Clinical Journal of Sport Medicine, 17,* 369–374. doi:10.1097/JSM.0b013e31814c3e3e.

Fletcher-Janzen, E., & Reynolds, C. R. (2010). *Neuropsychological perspectives on learning disabilities in the era of RTI: Recommendations for diagnosis and intervention.* Hoboken, NJ: Wiley.

Gardner, A., Iverson, G. L., & Stanwell, P. (2014). A systematic review of proton magnetic resonance spectroscopy findings in sport-related concussion. *Journal of Neurotrauma, 31,* 1–18. doi:10.1089/neu.2013.3079.

Giza, C. C., & Hovda, D. A. (2014). The new neurometabolic cascade of concussion. *Neurosurgery, 75* (Suppl 4), S24–33. doi:10.1227/neu.0000000000000505.

Gosselin, N., Theriault, M., Leclerc, S., Montplaisir, J., & Lassonde, M. (2006). Neurophysiological anomalies in symptomatic and asymptomatic concussed athletes. *Neurosurgery, 58,* 1151–1161. doi:10.1227/01.neu.0000215953.44097.fa.

Greer, J. E., McGinn, M. J., & Povlishock, J. T. (2011). Diffuse traumatic axonal injury in the mouse induces atrophy, c-Jun activation, and axonal outgrowth in the axotomized neuronal population. *Journal of Neuroscience, 31,* 5089–5105. doi:10.1523/jneurosci.5103-10.2011.

Guenette, J. P., Shenton, M. E., & Koerte, I. K. (2018). Imaging of concussion in young athletes. *Neuroimaging Clinics of North America, 28,* 43–53. doi:10.1016/j.nic.2017.09.004.

Guskiewicz, K. M., Marshall, S. W., Bailes, J., McCrea, M., Cantu, R. C., Randolph, C., & Jordan, B. D. (2005). Association between recurrent concussion and late-life cognitive impairment in retired professional football players. *Neurosurgery, 57,* 719–726.

Guskiewicz, K. M., McCrea, M., Marshall, S. W., Cantu, R. C., Randolph, C., Barr, W., & Kelly, J. P. (2003). Cumulative effects associated with recurrent concussion in collegiate football players: The NCAA concussion study. *JAMA, 290,* 2549–2555. doi:10.1001/jama.290.19.2549.

Halterman, C. I., Langan, J., Drew, A., Rodriguez, E., Osternig, L. R., Chou, L. S., & van Donkelaar, P. (2006). Tracking the recovery of visuospatial attention deficits in mild traumatic brain injury. *Brain, 129,* 747–753. doi:10.1093/brain/awh705.

Hammeke, T. A., McCrea, M., Coats, S. M., Verber, M. D., Durgerian, S., Flora, K., ... Rao, S. M. (2013). Acute and subacute changes in neural activation during the recovery from sport-related concussion. *Journal of the International Neuropsychological Society, 19,* 863–872. doi:10.1017/s1355617713000702.

Hart, J., Jr., Kraut, M. A., Womack, K. B., Strain, J., Didehbani, N., Bartz, E., ... Cullum, C. M. (2013). Neuroimaging of cognitive dysfunction and depression in aging retired National Football League players: A cross-sectional study. *JAMA Neurology, 70,* 326–335. doi:10.1001/2013.jamaneurol.340.

Hellstrom, T., Westlye, L. T., Kaufmann, T., Trung Doan, N., Soberg, H. L., Sigurdardottir, S., ... Andelic, N. (2017). White matter microstructure is associated with functional, cognitive and emotional symptoms 12 months after mild traumatic brain injury. *Scientific Reports, 7,* 13795. doi:10.1038/s41598-017-13628-1.

Henry, L. C., Tremblay, J., Tremblay, S., Lee, A., Brun, C., Lepore, N., ... Lassonde, M. (2011). Acute and chronic changes in diffusivity measures after sports concussion. *Journal of Neurotrauma, 28*(10), 2049–2059. doi:10.1089/neu.2011.1836.

Hocke, L. M., Duszynski, C. C., Debert, C. T., Dleikan, D., & Dunn, J. F. (2018). Reduced functional connectivity in adults with persistent post-concussion symptoms: A functional near-infrared spectroscopy study. *Journal of Neurotrauma, 35,* 1224–1232. doi:10.1089/neu.2017.5365.

Howell, D., Osternig, L., Van Donkelaar, P., Mayr, U., & Chou, L. S. (2013). Effects of concussion on attention and executive function in adolescents. *Medicine and Science in Sports and Exercise, 45,* 1030–1037. doi:10.1249/MSS.0b013e3182814595.

Iverson, G. L., Lange, R. T., Waljas, M., Liimatainen, S., Dastidar, P., Hartikainen, K. M., ... Ohman, J. (2012). Outcome from complicated versus uncomplicated mild traumatic brain injury. *Rehabilitation Research and Practice, 2012,* 415740. doi:10.1155/2012/415740.

Iverson, G. L., Lovell, M. R., & Collins, M. W. (2003). Interpreting change on ImPACT following sport concussion. *The Clinical Neuropsychologist, 17,* 460–467. doi:10.1076/clin.17.4.460.27934.

Iverson, G. L., Lovell, M. R., Smith, S., & Franzen, M. D. (2000). Prevalence of abnormal CT-scans following mild head injury. *Brain Injury, 14,* 1057–1061.

Kerr, Z. Y., Zuckerman, S. L., Wasserman, E. B., Covassin, T., Djoko, A., & Dompier, T. P. (2016). Concussion symptoms and return to play time in youth, high school, and college American football athletes. *JAMA Pediatrics, 170,* 647–653. doi:10.1001/jamapediatrics.2016.0073.

Killam, C., Cautin, R. L., & Santucci, A. C. (2005). Assessing the enduring residual neuropsychological effects of head trauma in college athletes who participate in contact sports. *Archives of Clinical Neuropsychology, 20,* 599–611. doi:10.1016/j. acn.2005.02.001.

Koerte, I. K., Mayinger, M., Muehlmann, M., Kaufmann, D., Lin, A. P., Steffinger, D., … Shenton, M. E. (2016). Cortical thinning in former professional soccer players. *Brain Imaging and Behavior, 10,* 792–798. doi:10.1007/s11682-015-9442-0.

Kraus, N., Lindley, T., Colegrove, D., Krizman, J., Otto-Meyer, S., Thompson, E. C., & White-Schwoch, T. (2017). The neural legacy of a single concussion. *Neuroscience Letters, 646,* 21–23. doi:10.1016/j.neulet.2017.03.008.

Louey, A. G., Cromer, J. A., Schembri, A. J., Darby, D. G., Maruff, P., Makdissi, M., & McCrory, P. (2014). Detecting cognitive impairment after concussion: Sensitivity of change from baseline and normative data methods using the CogSport/Axon cognitive test battery. *Archives of Clinical Neuropsychology, 29,* 432–441. doi:10.1093/arclin/acu020.

Makdissi, M., Davis, G., Jordan, B., Patricios, J., Purcell, L., & Putukian, M. (2013). Revisiting the modifiers: How should the evaluation and management of acute concussions differ in specific groups? *British Journal of Sports Medicine, 47,* 314–320. doi:10.1136/bjsports-2013-092256.

Manley, G., Gardner, A. J., Schneider, K. J., Guskiewicz, K. M., Bailes, J., Cantu, R. C., … Iverson, G. L. (2017). A systematic review of potential long-term effects of sport-related concussion. *British Journal of Sports Medicine, 51,* 969–977. doi:10.1136/bjsports-2017-097791.

McCrory, P., Meeuwisse, W., Dvorak, J., Aubry, M., Bailes, J., Broglio, S., … Vos, P. E. (2017). Consensus statement on concussion in sport—The 5th international conference on concussion in sport held in Berlin, October 2016. *British Journal of Sports Medicine, 51,* 838–847. doi:10.1136/bjsports-2017-097699.

McCrory, P., Meeuwisse, W., Johnston, K., Dvorak, J., Aubry, M., Molloy, M., & Cantu, R. (2009). Consensus statement on concussion in sport—The 3rd international conference on concussion in sport held in Zurich, November 2008. *PM & R: The Journal of Injury, Function, and Rehabilitation, 1,* 406–420. doi:10.1016/j.pmrj.2009.03.010.

Meier, T. B., Bellgowan, P. S., Singh, R., Kuplicki, R., Polanski, D. W., & Mayer, A. R. (2015). Recovery of cerebral blood flow following sports-related concussion. *JAMA Neurol, 72,* 530–538. doi:10.1001/jamaneurol.2014.4778.

Merz, Z. C., Perry, J. E., & Ross, M. J. (2018). The role of the clinical sport neuropsychologist: An introductory case example. *Case Studies in Sport and Exercise Psychology, 2,* 1–11.

Meythaler, J. M., Peduzzi, J. D., Eleftheriou, E., & Novack, T. A. (2001). Current concepts: Diffuse axonal injury-associated traumatic brain injury. *Archives of Physical Medicine and Rehabilitation, 82,* 1461–1471.

Miles, L., Grossman, R. I., Johnson, G., Babb, J. S., Diller, L., & Inglese, M. (2008). Short-term DTI predictors of cognitive dysfunction in mild traumatic brain injury. *Brain Injury, 22,* 115–122. doi:10.1080/02699050801888816.

Moore, D. R., Pindus, D. M., Raine, L. B., Drollette, E. S., Scudder, M. R., Ellemberg, D., & Hillman, C. H. (2015). The persistent influence of concussion on attention, executive control and neuroelectric function in preadolescent children. *International Journal of Psychophysiology, 99,* 85–95. doi:10.1016/j. ijpsycho.2015.11.010.

Moore, R. D., Lepine, J., & Ellemberg, D. (2017). The independent influence of concussive and sub-concussive impacts on soccer players' neurophysiological and neuropsychological function. *International Journal of Psychophysiology*, *112*, 22–30. doi:10.1016/j.ijpsycho.2016.11.011.

Moore, R. D., Pindus, D. M., Drolette, E. S., Scudder, M. R., Raine, L. B., & Hillman, C. H. (2015). The persistent influence of pediatric concussion on attention and cognitive control during flanker performance. *Biological Psychology*, *109*, 93–102. doi:10.1016/j.biopsycho.2015.04.008.

Morgan, C. D., Zuckerman, S. L., King, L. E., Beaird, S. E., Sills, A. K., & Solomon, G. S. (2015). Post-concussion syndrome (PCS) in a youth population: Defining the diagnostic value and cost-utility of brain imaging. *Child's Nervous System*, *31*, 2305–2309. doi:10.1007/s00381-015-2916-y.

Morgan, C. D., Zuckerman, S. L., Lee, Y. M., King, L., Beaird, S., Sills, A. K., & Solomon, G. S. (2015). Predictors of postconcussion syndrome after sports-related concussion in young athletes: A matched case-control study. *Journal of Neurosurgery. Pediatrics*, *15*, 589–598. doi:10.3171/2014.10.Peds14356.

Moser, R. S., Schatz, P., Neidzwski, K., & Ott, S. D. (2011). Group versus individual administration affects baseline neurocognitive test performance. *American Journal of Sports Medicine*, *39*, 2325–2330. doi:10.1177/0363546511417114.

Ott, S. D., Bailey, C. M., & Broshek, D. K. (2018). An interdisciplinary approach to sports concussion evaluation and management: The role of a neuropsychologist. *Archives of Clinical Neuropsychology*, *33*, 319–329. doi:10.1093/arclin/acx132.

Ozen, L. J., Itier, R. J., Preston, F. F., & Fernandes, M. A. (2013). Long-term working memory deficits after concussion: Electrophysiological evidence. *Brain Injury*, *27*, 1244–1255. doi:10.3109/02699052.2013.804207.

Radoi, A., Poca, M. A., Canas, V., Cevallos, J. M., Membrado, L., Saavedra, M. C., … Sahuquillo, J. (2018). Neuropsychological alterations and neuroradiological findings in patients with post-traumatic concussion: Results of a pilot study. *Neurologia*, *33*, 427–437. doi:10.1016/j.nrl.2016.10.003.

Raji, C. A., Tarzwell, R., Pavel, D., Schneider, H., Uszler, M., Thornton, J., … Henderson, T. (2014). Clinical utility of SPECT neuroimaging in the diagnosis and treatment of traumatic brain injury: A systematic review. *PLoS ONE*, *9*, e91088. doi:10.1371/journal.pone.0091088.

Randolph, C., Karantzoulis, S., & Guskiewicz, K. (2013). Prevalence and characterization of mild cognitive impairment in retired national football league players. *Journal of the International Neuropsychological Society*, *19*, 873–880. doi:10.1017/s1355617713000805.

Romero, K., Lobaugh, N. J., Black, S. E., Ehrlich, L., & Feinstein, A. (2015). Old wine in new bottles: Validating the clinical utility of SPECT in predicting cognitive performance in mild traumatic brain injury. *Psychiatry Research*, *231*, 15–24. doi:10.1016/j.pscychresns.2014.11.003.

Rose, S. C., Weber, K. D., Collen, J. B., & Heyer, G. L. (2015). The diagnosis and management of concussion in children and adolescents. *Pediatric Neurology*, *53*, 108–118. doi:10.1016/j.pediatrneurol.2015.04.003.

Ruff, R. M., Camenzuli, L., & Mueller, J. (1996). Miserable minority: Emotional risk factors that influence the outcome of a mild traumatic brain injury. *Brain Injury*, *10*, 551–565.

Sharp, D. J., & Ham, T. E. (2011). Investigating white matter injury after mild traumatic brain injury. *Current Opinion in Neurology*, *24*, 558–563. doi:10.1097/WCO.0b013e32834cd523.

Shenton, M. E., Hamoda, H. M., Schneiderman, J. S., Bouix, S., Pasternak, O., Rathi, Y., ... Zafonte, R. (2012). A review of magnetic resonance imaging and diffusion tensor imaging findings in mild traumatic brain injury. *Brain Imaging and Behavior, 6,* 137–192. doi:10.1007/s11682-012-9156-5.

Sicard, V., Moore, R. D., & Ellemberg, D. (2017). Sensitivity of the cogstate test battery for detecting prolonged cognitive alterations stemming from sport-related concussions. *Clinical Journal of Sport Medicine: Official Journal of the Canadian Academy of Sport Medicine.* Advance online publication. doi:10.1097/jsm.0000000000000492.

Sicard, V., Moore, R. D., & Ellemberg, D. (2018). Long-term cognitive outcomes in male and female athletes following sport-related concussions. *International Journal of Psychophysiology.* Advance online publication. doi:10.1016/j.ijpsycho.2018.03.011.

Slobounov, S., Gay, M., Johnson, B., & Zhang, K. (2012). Concussion in athletics: Ongoing clinical and brain imaging research controversies. *Brain Imaging and Behavior, 6,* 224–243. doi:10.1007/s11682-012-9167-2.

Sports Neuropsychology Society. (2017). Our Mission. Retrieved from www.sportsneuropsychologysociety.com/our-mission/.

Thatcher, R. W., North, D. M., Curtin, R. T., Walker, R. A., Biver, C. J., Gomez, J. F., & Salazar, A. M. (2001). An EEG severity index of traumatic brain injury. *Journal of Neuropsychiatry and Clinical Neurosciences, 13,* 77–87. doi:10.1176/jnp.13.1.77.

Thompson, J., Sebastianelli, W., & Slobounov, S. (2005). EEG and postural correlates of mild traumatic brain injury in athletes. *Neuroscience Letters, 377*(3), 158–163. doi:10.1016/j.neulet.2004.11.090.

Vagnozzi, R., Signoretti, S., Tavazzi, B., Floris, R., Ludovici, A., Marziali, S., ... Lazzarino, G. (2008). Temporal window of metabolic brain vulnerability to concussion: A pilot 1H-magnetic resonance spectroscopic study in concussed athletes-part III. *Neurosurgery, 62,* 1286–1295. doi:10.1227/01.neu.0000333300.34189.74.

Van Kampen, D. A., Lovell, M. R., Pardini, J. E., Collins, M. W., & Fu, F. H. (2006). The "value added" of neurocognitive testing after sports-related concussion. *American Journal of Sports Medicine, 34,* 1630–1635. doi:10.1177/0363546506288677.

Yeo, R. A., Phillips, J. P., Jung, R. E., Brown, A. J., Campbell, R. C., & Brooks, W. M. (2006). Magnetic resonance spectroscopy detects brain injury and predicts cognitive functioning in children with brain injuries. *Journal of Neurotrauma, 23,* 1427–1435. doi:10.1089/neu.2006.23.1427.

Zuckerman, S. L., Yengo-Kahn, A. M., Buckley, T. A., Solomon, G. S., Sills, A. K., & Kerr, Z. Y. (2016). Predictors of postconcussion syndrome in collegiate student-athletes. *Neurosurgical Focus, 40,* E13. doi:10.3171/2016.1.Focus15593.

4 Psychological outcomes associated with concussion

Anthony P. Kontos

Introduction

Many athletes experience psychological issues following concussion that might include anxiety, depression, and behavioral changes such as irritability and impulsivity. We found that 29% of athletes with this injury report at least one psychological symptom following a concussion (Kontos et al., 2012). In fact, psychological issues have become such a substantial and common feature of concussion that we recently added a psychiatrist to our concussion faculty at the University of Pittsburgh Medical Center (UPMC) Concussion Program to treat patients with psychological issues following this injury. Although these issues have been recognized by clinicians for some time, until recently, these issues received little attention in the literature. In 2017, I edited a special issue in the journal *Sport, Exercise, and Performance Psychology* that featured articles focusing on topics from the role of personality on concussion outcomes (Beidler et al., 2017; O'Rourke et al., 2017) to the psychological response following concussion (Andre-Morin, Caron, & Bloom 2017; Turner et al., 2017). One of the consistent threads throughout this special issue was the relative dearth of research regarding psychological issues associated with concussion. Therefore, the objective of this chapter is to examine psychological issues following concussion within an emerging, clinical profiles-based conceptual framework (Collins et al., 2016; Collins et al., 2014). In so doing, this chapter will examine different psychological responses to concussion and the factors that might influence those responses. Related issues including somatization, social support, and coping will also be discussed. Finally, approaches to managing and treating these issues will be described.

Clinical profiles approach to concussion

Concussion is a heterogeneous injury involving different symptoms (e.g., headache, dizziness, fatigue) and impairments (e.g., cognitive, vestibular, ocular). As such, no two concussions are exactly the same and therefore should not be conceptualized, assessed, or treated as such. Concussions should be assessed using a comprehensive, multidomain assessment (e.g., symptomns, cognitive, vestibular, ocular, balance, psychology) to capture this heterogeneity. However, concussions do share certain characteristics resulting in distinct subtypes or profiles. We (Collins et al., 2014; Kontos & Collins, 2018) have developed a model of concussion involving six clinical profiles: cognitive, ocular, vestibular, migraine, anxiety/mood, and cervical. This approach allows clinicians to identify an athlete's profile(s) following a concussion to inform more targeted management and treatment strategies to enhance recovery (Kontos & Collins, 2018). Clinical profiles are categorized as primary, secondary, or tertiary, with primary profiles being the predominate profile that warrants the focus of initial management and treatment interventions. However, clinical profiles are not mutually exclusive and often overlap, resulting in a more complex presentation and challenge for treating clinicians. For example, an athlete may have a primary migraine profile but also have concurrent secondary vestibular and anxiety/mood profiles. In contrast, another athlete may only have an ocular profile. One of the more challenging clinical profiles to evaluate and treat is the anxiety/mood profile. In the following sections I describe the charateristics of the anxiety/mood clinical profile, review data on its prevalence in a sports concussion clinic population, and discuss how profiles may overlap.

Anxiety/mood clinical profile

Each concussion clinical profile is characterized by specific symptoms, exam findings, and risk factors. The anxiety/mood clinical profile involves two sets of symptoms that may occur independently or together. The mood-related symptoms involve sadness/irritability, worry, anger, loss of motivation/interest, feelings of hopelessness, fatigue, and disrupted sleep, among others (Collins et al., 2014; Sandel et al., 2017). The anxiety-related symptoms involve nervousness, worry/fear, shakiness, sweating, dizziness, panic attacks, and nausea, among others (Collins et al., 2014; Sandel et al., 2017). In addition, athletes with this clinical profile may isolate themselves socially, have difficulty turning off their thoughts, ruminate about their injury, and be hyper-focused on their symptoms (Kontos & Collins, 2018). Risk factors for the anxiety/mood profiles include a personal or family history of psychiatric issues, comorbid migraine and sleep issues, and life stressors (Kontos & Collins, 2018). The characteristics of athletes with the anxiety/mood clinical profile are described in more detail by Sandel and colleagues (Sandel et al., 2017).

Prevalence of anxiety/mood clinical profile

As mentioned previously, anxiety and mood-related symptoms are common following concussion and often aggregate into an affective cluster, even in the first week following injury (Kontos et al., 2012). Females report higher levels of these affective symptoms following concussion than do males, but there do not appear to be age differences (Kontos et al., 2012). However, in the same study, females also report higher levels of affective symptoms at baseline, suggesting that gender differences in post-injury levels may not reflect the effects of the concussion itself. There are limited data on the prevalence of each concussion clinical profile. We recently conducted a retrospective chart review of 188 patients from a sport-concussion clinic within 90 days of injury and reported that the anxiety/mood profile was the most common primary profile among our patients (Kontos et al., in press). In fact, over 28% of patients were categorized with the anxiety/mood profile as their primary profile.

Overlap of clinical profiles

The anxiety/mood profile, like other profiles, does not typically occur in isolation (Kontos & Collins, 2018). As such, we were interested in which profiles were related to or co-occurred with the anxiety/mood profile. More specifically, my colleagues and I (Kontos et al., in press) found that when anxiety/mood was the primary profile, patients were 3.46 times (Chi square = 13.71, 95% CI = 1.82–6.61, p < 0.001) more likely to have a co-occurring secondary migraine profile. This finding is intuitive in that anxiety/mood disruptions have been reported to be associated with migraine symptoms (Formeister et al., 2018). Migraine headaches are often unpredictable and hard to prevent, which may also lead to anxiety and feelings of hopelessness associated with the anxiety/mood clinical profile following concussion. We also found that patients with a primary migraine clinical profile were 4.44 times (Chi square = 11.51, 95% CI = 1.89–10.43, p < 0.001) more likely to have a co-occurring vestibular clinical profile (Kontos et al., in press). This finding may reflect the fact that vestibular and anxiety/mood clinical profiles both may involve disruption of vestibular and limbic system components of the brain, which are linked via neuronal pathways, per Sufrinko et al. (2018).

The preceding findings were highlighted to demonstrate the interrelationships among the profiles and the potential to better understand a profile's origins based on other co-occurring profiles. In these cases, the evidence suggests that migraine and vestibular symptoms may underlie or drive some of the anxiety/mood issues in patients. However, the order of association is difficult to determine from these findings. As such, the anxiety/mood profile and associated symptoms may drive the development of secondary migraine and vestibular symptoms. Regardless, these findings emphasize the complex nature of both presentation and potential etiology of anxiety/mood and related clinical profiles and concomitant psychological issues following concussion.

Etiology of psychological issues following concussion

One of the challenges in assessing and treating psychological issues following concussion is to determine the etiology of the symptoms. Unfortunately, many clinicians assume that the presentation of symptoms alone are sufficient to diagnose and develop a treatment plan. However, in so doing, symptoms may persist if the underlying cause is not addressed. This concern is magnified by the fact that many symptoms of concussion overlap with symptoms of mood and anxiety related issues (see Table 4.1). In addition, other clinical profiles may be driving anxiety/mood or vice versa. For example, a patient may present with primarily anxiety symptoms, but upon further evaluation, they may also have vestibular symptoms such as vertigo, which could be precipitating the anxiety symptoms. Similarly, another patient may have primarily migraine symptoms, including headache, nausea, and sensitivity to light, which may result in anxiety associated with the unpredictability and intensity of the migraine headaches.

Psychological issues such as changes in behavior and mood following a concussion may emanate from micro-structural, connectivity, and metabolic changes to the brain following injury. In contrast, some patients may experience psychological responses to changes associated with their concussion such as disrupted schedules, social isolation, and frustration with longer than expected recovery (Kontos & Collins, 2018). Concussion may also "fight dirty" and magnify pre-existing psychological issues. For instance, a patient with a history of anxiety may experience anxious mood following their concussion, whereas a patient without a history of anxiety may not. In fact, researchers have reported that pre-existing psychological disorders are a strong predictor of prolonged symptoms and recovery following a concussion (Guerriero et al., 2018). Finally, patients may have unrelated, co-morbid, psychological issues that occur concurrently with their concussion but are not a result of the injury. For example, a patient may develop an adjustment disorder following a move to college that happened to coincide with the timing of their concussion. In this case, although the adjustment disorder may affect their recovery from concussion, it is not a result of the injury.

Table 4.1 Overlap of symptoms from anxiety, depression, and/or concussion

Anxiety	BOTH Anxiety and Concussion	Concussion	BOTH Concussion and Depression	Depression
Worry/fear	Headache	Vomiting	Fatigue	Guilt
Shortness of breath	Nervousness	Vision problems	Sadness	Amotivation
Body pain	Fatigue	Fogginess	Sleep problems	Weight gain/loss
Dry mouth	Numbness	Imbalance	Confusion	Anger
Sweating	Tingling	Sensitivity to light/noise	Difficulty concentrating	Self-criticism
Palpitations	Nausea		Trouble remembering	Indecision
Feeling of choking	Dizziness		Irritability	
Sleep problems			More emotional	

Theoretical framework for psychological responses to concussion

There are several well-established models of psychological responses to injury from the sport psychology literature, including the Stress Model of Injury in Sports proposed by Williams and Anderson (1998), and the Integrated Model of Response to Injury in Sport from Wiese-Bjornstal Smith, Schaffer, and Morrey (1998). The Stress Model focuses on factors that influence the likelihood of injury, whereas the Integrated Model emphasizes the psychological responses following injury. Although neither of these models was developed for concussion specifically, tenets from both models are applicable to understanding why an athlete may be at risk for a concussion or how they may respond psychologically following a concussion. For example, the components of the Stress Model include antecedents of injury that might influence concussion risk. Specifically, an athlete characterized by impulsivity (i.e., personality) or a recent demotion in team standing (i.e., history of stressors) may result in an attentional distraction during performance that could increase the likelihood of a concussion.

Following a concussion, the Integrated Model, and in particular, the behavioral and emotional response components, are germane to understanding athletes' psychological response to a concussion. For example, following a concussion, an athlete may have limited social support and engage in poor adherence to pre-scribed therapies (i.e., behavioral response), and be frustrated over the lack of control of recovery (i.e., emotional response). These characteristics may adversely affect the recovery process but help to identify athletes at risk for an anxiety/mood profile. Although there is limited empirical support for these models in concussion, researchers have begun adapting them to this injury (e.g., Wiese-Bjornstal et al., 2015), and it is recommended that researchers begin using them to better understand this complicated brain injury.

Specific psychological issues following concussion

Anxiety

Nearly one in five athletes reports some level of anxiety following a concussion (Kontos et al., 2012). Anxiety may emanate from worry and fear associated with an uncertain outcome or recovery or from the types of symptoms and clinical profiles that an athlete experiences following concussion (Kontos & Collins, 2018). For example, an athlete with a vestibular clinical profile, characterized by symptoms like dizziness or vertigo, may experience concomitant anxiety when these symptoms occur or in anticipation of the next time that they might occur. Similarly, an athlete with a migraine clinical profile following concussion may experience anxiety related to the uncontrollable and aversive headache, nausea, and light/noise sensitivity that characterize their migraine-like symptoms. Regardless of its cause, anxiety following a concussion is associated with prolonged symptoms (Grubenhoff et al., 2014) and depressed mood (Yang et al., 2015). However, anxiety does not seem to persist, with researchers reporting that at one year post-injury, anxiety was no different in individuals who had a concussion compared to those who had not (Theadom et al., 2016).

Depression

Estimates suggest that up to 6% of athletes experience clinical depression following a concussion (Jorge & Robinson, 2002). However, little is known about who is most at risk for developing depression following a concussion. It is generally thought that athletes that take longer to recover are more likely to experience anxiety/mood issues, including depression, following a concussion. It is important to note that most athletes will experience only mild, sub-clinical levels of depressed mood following a concussion that are transient in nature. Research suggests that sub-clinical increases in depressed mood persist out to 14 days post-concussion (Kontos et al., 2012; Mainwaring et al., 2010). However, our research (Covassin et al., 2012) on non-concussed athletes suggests that baseline levels of depressed mood must be considered to disentangle pre-existing from post-injury mood. Specifically, my colleagues and I reported that 2% of athletes reported high (moderate to severe) levels of depression on self-report measures (Covassin et al., 2012). As such, baseline measures of depression can help inform subsequent evaluations of mood following a concussion. Researchers suggest that persistent depressed mood may be associated with concussion history (Mrazik et al., 2016). However, further prospective research in this area is needed to better understand the long-term effects of concussion on depressed mood.

Sleep

Sleep difficulties may be a symptom of or result in psychological issues following concussion. As many as 80% of athletes may experience sleep difficulties following a concussion (Tkachenko et al., 2016). Among the common sleep disturbances are hypersomnia and insomnia, as well as circadian disruptions. Researchers suggest that sleep problems are common for athletes experiencing psychological issues following concussion, including anxiety, post-traumatic stress, and depression (Wickwire et al., 2016). Both too much and too little sleep following concussion in athletes can result in problems (Kostyun, Milewski, & Hafeez, 2015). In addition, athletes with pre-existing sleep difficulties may be at greater risk for prolonged post-concussion symptoms and impairment (Sufrinko et al., 2015).

Malingering

"Concussion is the new lower back pain" is a common refrain among clinicians and insurers. Concussion is hard to exclude as a diagnosis, difficult to objectively measure and track recovery, and based largely on self-reported symptoms; all of which make it ideal for malingering. With this statement as a backdrop, malingering, or the exaggeration or fabrication of symptoms for some external gain, may occur in athletes following a concussion. Most athletes are hyper-motivated to return to sport following a concussion and thus prefer to minimize or deny symptoms. However, some athletes may engage in malingering to avoid having to win back their spot in a starting line-up, continue to play a sport they no longer love, or to maintain a scholarship for a team on which they no longer want to be a part. Malingering has been documented following concussion in non-athletes, especially those with pending litigation (Feinstein et al., 2001). Unfortunately, there is a dearth of empirical data on malingering in athletes following concussion. Regardless, clinicians should be mindful of potential malingering, particularly in athletes who have experienced other psychological issues following their concussion.

Factors that influence psychological responses to concussion

Personality

As with any psychological issues, the personality of an athlete may play a role in determining an athlete's psychological response to concussion and increase or decrease the likelihood that they develop psychological issues following injury. While this statement is intuitive, there is limited empirical support for the association of personality to psychological issues following concussion in the literature. O'Rourke et al. (2017) reported that over 40% of the variability of concussion symptoms was attributable to a set of personality characteristics that included anxiety, athletic identity, and amotivation. Researchers have also reported that anxiety sensitivity, or fear associated with bodily sensations, is associated with higher post-concussion symptoms and psychological distress (Wood et al., 2014). This research may relate to the role of other personality factors, such as somatization, on psychological issues following concussion.

An emerging personality trait that may influence psychological responses to concussion and overall symptom burden following injury is somatization. Somatization is characterized by internal stress or other issues manifesting as somatic complaints (Postilnik et al., 2006). For example, a somaticizing athlete dealing with the stress of an upcoming championship match may experience stomach pain. Recently, we reported that high somatization scores were associated with longer recovery and higher symptoms in adolescents and children following a concussion (Root et al., 2016). In another study, researchers reported that high somatization was associated with state anxiety and may influence the development of anxiety/mood symptoms and clinical profiles (Grubenhoff et al., 2014).

Coping and social support

The role of coping, which can be positive (e.g., problem-solving) or negative (e.g., avoidance) and involve either emotion-focused (e.g., humor) or problem-focused (e.g., changing one's schedule) strategies, is not well understood in athletes following concussion. Woodrome et al. (2011) reported that emotion-focused coping was associated with higher symptoms following concussion.

We found that athletes engaged in very limited coping overall following a concussion, compared to after orthopedic injuries (Kontos et al., 2013). Research on social support in athletes following concussion is even more scarce than research for coping. Researchers have reported that social support following a concussion is similar for concussed and orthopedically injured athletes, but the former perceive less value from support than the latter (Covassin et al., 2014). Although both coping and social support likely influence psychological issues following concussion, more research in this area is needed to better understand the nature and effects of both factors.

Assessment of psychological symptoms and issues

Psychological screening following concussion

Most concussion symptom inventories such as the Post-Concussion Symptom Scale (PCSS: Lovell et al., 2006) include very few items that assess psychological symptoms such as anxiety, sadness, and irritability. As such, additional screening tools should be used to identify athletes with potential psychological issues or anxiety/mood clinical profiles. However, concussion symptom inventories like the PCSS can help identify athletes who score high in the affective (i.e., psychological, emotional) symptom cluster (Kontos et al., 2012). Athletes with this cluster of symptoms may warrant further evaluation for anxiety and mood-related issues. However, clinicians should not rely solely on concussion symptom scales to screen athletes for psychological issues following concussion. Additional screening tools that assess both anxiety and depressed mood should be employed to provide more in-depth information. Other measures that evaluate suicide and post-traumatic stress (PTS) may be warranted with certain at-risk athletes following concussion but are beyond the scope of the discussion in this brief review.

A good measure that covers anxiety, depression, and somatization (see Personality section) is the Behavioral Symptom Inventory 18-item (BSI-18; Derogatis, 2001). The BSI is a brief, self-report inventory that yields an overall symptom severity score, as well as subscale scores for anxiety, depression, and somatization. Among the screening tools specifically for anxiety is the Generalized Anxiety Disorder 7-item (GAD-7: Spitzer et al., 2006), which is a brief self-report of anxiety-related symptoms for high school-aged and older athletes. For depressed mood, the Patient Health Questionnaire 9-item (PHQ-9; Kroenke, Spitzer, & Williams, 2002) provides a brief assessment for older adolescents and adults. In children and younger adolescents, the Mood and Feeling Questionnaire (MFQ: Angold et al., 1987) is a good choice to evaluate depressed mood. Although the assessment of personality can be complicated and lengthy, a targeted approach focusing on somatization using the PHQ-15 (Kroenke, Spitzer, & Williams, 2001), a somatization measure, the Children's Somatization Inventory (CSI: Walker & Garber, 2003), or the somatization component of the BSI could be useful in identifying athletes at risk for anxiety/mood clinical profiles and other psychological issues following concussion.

Utility of baseline symptom assessments

While baseline neurocognitive and balance assessments are often conducted as part of athletes' pre-participation physical examinations at the beginning of the season, assessments of symptoms are less common. Baseline concussion and psychological or affective symptoms are important to understanding post-injury symptoms, as many athletes report high levels of baseline symptoms that might overlap with concussion and more specifically the anxiety/mood clinical profile (Iverson & Lange, 2003). We have reported previously that athletes with high levels of baseline symptoms often report the same levels of post-concussion symptoms (Custer et al., 2016). Without a baseline assessment, these athletes appear to be more severely symptomatic following injury when, in fact, they were high in symptoms prior to injury. It is also plausible that high scores on affective or psychological symptoms at baseline may help identify athletes at risk for anxiety/ mood clinical profiles following a concussion.

In another study we highlighted the benefits of assessing baseline depression symptoms specifically (using Beck's Depression Inventory-II [BDI-II]) in order to better understand changes in mood following injury in both high school and collegiate athletes (Kontos et al., 2012). Our findings demonstrated sub-clinical changes in depressed mood from baseline to 14 days post-injury. Moreover, we were able to identify several athletes who reported clinical levels of depression on the BDI-II that would have otherwise gone undetected without a baseline assessment of mood (Kontos et al., 2012). Whenever feasible, both baseline concussion and psychological symptom assessments should be employed as part of a pre-participation physical exam.

Preventing psychological responses with behavioral regulation

Much of the current approach to concussion clinical care involving psychological issues is reactive in that it focuses on treating these psychological symptoms once they are identified or diagnosed. A potentially more effective approach may revolve around preventing psychological issues following concussion from developing in the first place. Such an approach emphasizes early behavioral regulation strategies including sleep regulation, nutrition/hydration, physical activity, and stress management for use with all concussion patients (Collins et al., 2014). However, this approach is in contrast to the symptom-based approaches to activity and behavior following concussion outlined in the recent Concussion in Sport Group consensus statement (e.g., McCrory et al., 2017). These current approaches suggest only engaging in activities that do not provoke *any* symptoms at all. More recent approaches to actively treating concussion utilize an expose-recover model similar to that used in exercise, wherein some symptom provocation during or following activity is expected. The challenge, of course, is in balancing too little (i.e., rest)—per current consensus— with too much activity, as both could exacerbate symptoms and impairment following concussion.

Current approaches to treatment

There are relatively few empirically-supported therapeutic approaches to treating psychological issues following concussion. Cognitive behavioral therapy (CBT) is a treatment strategy that incorporates management and regulation of behavior together with changes in cognitive appraisals using talk therapy sessions. Al Sayegh, Sandford, and Carson (2010) reported a substantial effect for CBT over standard of care in improving psychological function. Another emerging approach for reducing symptoms following concussion involves mindfulness, which often combines physiological stress reduction (e.g., breathing, physical activity) with attentional and cognitive focused tasks. In a randomized controlled trial (RCT), Azulay et al. (2013) reported that mindfulness improved quality of life and self-efficacy in chronic patients with mTBI. It is important to note that the research on treatments for psychological issues following concussion has not focused on athletes and has not differentiated effects among patients with specific clinical profiles, such as anxiety/mood, from those with other profiles. As such, the treatment effects for these approaches may be more or less robust for athletes depending on their clinical profile(s).

Importance of referrals for psychological issues following concussion

Typically, athletes with persistent psychological issues following concussion are referred for specialty mental healthcare. These referrals are particularly important for a concussion clinician who may lack appropriate training in mental health/ psychology or who does not have sufficient time to devote to longer term psychological care of concussed athletes. In today's world of challenging insurance reimbursements and limitations on universal healthcare coverage for specialty healthcare, mental health/psychology referrals following concussion may be restricted or even not covered. In fact, in some of my recent outreach work in European countries with universal health insurance, I found that access to and coverage for concussion care was limited to an initial assessment visit. When referrals were covered, they were typically covered at a lower level of care. Therefore, referrals to licensed, master's-level mental health professionals including social workers, counselors, and other therapists—who may provide appropriate psychological treatment under the supervision of a coordinating psychologist or psychiatrist—may be ideal in these circumstances.

Although licensed mental health professionals, such as psychologists and social workers, often provide the bulk of psychological care for athletes following a concussion, psychiatrists may also serve as a referral. In fact, our sports concussion clinic at UPMC recently hired a psychiatrist for two days a week to see our patients who experience persistent (i.e., resistant to behavioral regulation strategies) psychological issues following concussion. We could easily fill our psychiatrist's clinic schedule with concussion patients for the entire week and still have some patients without appointments. A psychiatrist is able to conduct or manage patient behavioral and cognitive therapy sessions—often supervising master's-level therapists—and prescribe medications that may be needed in more intractable patients with psychological issues following concussion. Although patients needing medication represent a minority of total concussion patients, they often require multiple visits and present with complex symptoms and impairments. As such, in states, provinces, and countries without prescription privileges for psychologists, a psychiatrist can address both aspects of patient care. It is important to note that while psychiatrists are not typically trained in concussion, a specialized concussion training and mentoring program can address this limitation to their training. This fact, combined with the ability to manage both cognitive and behavioral therapy and medications, makes psychiatrists an ideal referral for concussion patients with psychological issues, especially those who may need medications or longer-term therapy following injury.

Interdisciplinary team approach to concussion

Psychological issues following concussion highlight the need for a team approach to assessing and treating athletes with this injury. As described in Kontos and Collins (2018), a team approach centers around a coordinating clinician. This individual can represent a variety of fields including psychology, neuropsychology, neurology, and primary care sports medicine among others. Ideally, a treatment team would cover specialty areas of assessment and therapy including psychological (i.e., psychology, psychiatry), vestibular (i.e., vestibular/neurophysical therapy), vision (i.e., neuro-optometry), exertion (i.e., physical therapy), cervical (i.e., physical medicine and rehabilitation), and medication management (i.e., primary care sports medicine). However, available resources may limit the scope and members of a team. Regardless, given the prevalence and challenges associated with psychological issues following concussion, a psychological/mental health professional is a key member of any concussion treatment team.

Conclusion

Psychological issues following concussion are common and can be conceptualized, assessed, and treated using a clinical profiles approach. Anxiety and depression are the most typical psychological responses following a concussion but may have different underlying etiologies. Among personality factors influencing psychological issues following concussion, somatization may have the largest effect. Both baseline (i.e., pre-participant physical examination) and post-concussion screening should be employed by clinicians to better understand the nature of psychological issues in athletes that can be attributed to the injury. Although treatments for psychological issues following concussion including CBT, and mindfulness can be effective, a general behavioral regulation approach to all athletes may help to prevent the development of many psychological issues following this injury. Finally, whenever feasible, an interdisciplinary, team-based approach to assessing and treating psychological issues—either in-house or through a referral network—is advocated.

References

Al Sayegh, A., Sandford, D., & Carson, A. J. (2010). Psychological approaches to treatment of postconcussion syndrome: a systematic review. *Journal of Neurology, Neurosurgery, & Psychiatry, 81,* 1128–1134.

Andre-Morin, D., Caron, J., & Bloom, G. (2017). Exploring the unique challenges faced by female university athletes experiencing prolonged concussion symptoms. *Sport, Exercise, & Performance Psychology, 6,* 289–303.

Angold, A., Weissman, M. M., John, K., Merikangas, K. R., Prusoff, B. A., Wickramaratne, P., … Warner, V. (1987). Parent and child reports of depressive symptoms in children at low and high risk of depression. *Journal of Child Psychology & Psychiatry, 28,* 901–915.

Azulay, J., Smart, C. M., Mott, T., & Cicerone, K. D. (2013). A pilot study examining the effect of mindfulness-based stress reduction on symptoms of chronic mild traumatic brain injury/postconcussive syndrome. *Journal of Head Trauma & Rehabilitation, 28,* 323–331.

Beidler, E., Donnellan, M. B., Covassin, T., Phelps, A., & Kontos, A. (2017). The association between personality traits and sport-related concussion history in collegiate student-athletes. *Sport, Exercise, & Performance Psychology, 6,* 252–261.

Collins, M. W., Kontos, A. P., Okonkwo, D., Almquist, J., Bailes, J., Barisa, M., … Cardenas, J. (2016). Statement from the Targeted Evaluation and Active Management (TEAM) Approaches to Treating Concussion Meeting in Pittsburgh, October 15–16, 2015. *Neurosurgery, 79,* 912–929.

Collins, M., Kontos, A., Reynolds, E., Murawski, C., & Fu, F. (2014). A comprehensive, targeted approach to the clinical care of athletes following sport-related concussion. *Knee Surgery, Sports Traumatology, Arthroscopy, 22,* 235–246.

Covassin, T., Crutcher, B., Bleecker, A., Heiden, E. O., Dailey, A., & Yang, J. (2014). Postinjury anxiety and social support among collegiate athletes: A comparison between orthopaedic injuries and concussions. *Journal of Athletic Training, 49,* 462–468.

Covassin, T., Elbin III, R. J., Larson, E., & Kontos, A. P. (2012). Sex and age differences in depression and baseline sport-related concussion neurocognitive performance and symptoms. *Clinical Journal of Sport Medicine, 22,* 98–104.

Custer, A., Sufrinko, A., Elbin, R., Covassin, T., Collins, M., & Kontos, A. (2016). High baseline postconcussion symptom scores and concussion outcomes in athletes. *Journal of Athletic Training, 51,* 136–141.

Derogatis, L. (2001). *Brief Symptom Inventory (BSI)-18: Administration, scoring and procedures manual.* Minneapolis, MN: NCS Pearson.

Feinstein, A., Ouchterlony, D., Somerville, J., & Jardine, A. (2001). The effects of litigation on symptom expression: A prospective study following mild traumatic brain injury. *Medicine, Science & Law, 41,* 116–121.

Formeister, E. J., Rizk, H. G., Kohn, M. A., & Sharon, J. D. (2018). The epidemiology of vestibular migraine: A population-based survey study. *Otology and Neurology, 39,* 1037–1044.

Grubenhoff, J. A., Deakyne, S. J., Brou, L., Bajaj, L., Comstock, R. D., & Kirkwood, M. W. (2014). Acute concussion symptom severity and delayed symptom resolution. *Pediatrics, 134,* 54–62.

Guerriero, R. M., Kuemmerle, K., Pepin, M. J., Tayler, A. M., Wolff, R. & Meehan, W. P. 3rd (2018). The association between premorbid conditions in school-aged children with prolonged concussion recovery. *Journal of Child Neurolology*, *33*, 168–173.

Iverson, G. L., & Lange, R. T. (2003). Examination of "postconcussion-like" symptoms in a healthy sample. *Applied Neuropsychology*, *10*, 137–144.

Jorge, R., & Robinson, R. G. (2002). Mood disorders following traumatic brain injury. *Neurological Rehabilitation*, *17*, 311–324.

Kontos, A. P., & Collins, M. W. (2018). *Concussion: A clinical profile approach to assessment and treatment*. American Psychological Association Books: Washington, DC.

Kontos, A. P., Collins, M. W., Holland, C. L., Reeves, V. L., Edelman, K., Benso, S., … Okonkwo, D. (2018). Preliminary evidence for improvement in symptoms, cognitive, vestibular, and oculomotor outcomes following targeted intervention with chronic mTBI patients. *Military Medicine*, *183*, 333–338.

Kontos, A. P., Covassin, T., Elbin, R., & Parker, T. (2012). Depression and neurocognitive performance after concussion among male and female high school and collegiate athletes. *Archives of Physical Medicine and Rehabilitation*, *93*, 1751–1756.

Kontos, A. P., Elbin, R., Lau, B., Simensky, S., Freund, B., French, J., & Collins, M. W. (2013). Posttraumatic migraine as a predictor of recovery and cognitive impairment after sport-related concussion. *The American Journal of Sports Medicine*, *41*, 1497–1504.

Kontos, A. P., Elbin, R., Schatz, P., Covassin, T., Henry, L., Pardini, J., & Collins, M. W. (2012). A revised factor structure for the post-concussion symptom scale baseline and postconcussion factors. *The American Journal of Sports Medicine*, *40*, 2375–2384.

Kontos, A. P., Sufrinko, A., Sandel, N., Emami, K., & Collins, M. W. (in press). Sport-related concussion clinical profiles: Clinical characteristics, targeted treatments, and preliminary evidence. *Current Sports Medicine Reports*.

Kostyun, R. O., Milewski, M. D., & Hafeez, I. (2015). Sleep disturbance and neurocognitive function during the recovery from a sport-related concussion in adolescents. *The American Journal of Sports Medicine*, *43*, 633–640.

Kroenke, K., Spitzer, R., & Williams, J. (2001). The PHQ-9: Validity of a brief depression severity measure. *Journal of General Internal Medicine*, *16*, 606–613.

Kroenke, K., Spitzer, R. L., & Williams, J. B. (2002). The PHQ-15: Validity of a new measure for evaluating the severity of somatic symptoms. *Psychosomatic Medicine*, *64*, 258–266.

Lovell, M. R., Iverson, G. L., Collins, M. W., Podell, K., Johnston, K. M., Pardini, D., … Maroon, J. C. (2006). Measurement of symptoms following sports-related concussion: Reliability and normative data for the post-concussion scale. *Applied Neuropsychology*, *13*, 166–174.

Mainwaring, L. M., Hutchison, M., Bisschop, S. M., Comper, P., & Richards, D. W. (2010). Emotional response to sport concussion compared to ACL injury. *Brain Injury*, *24*, 589–597.

McCrory, P., Meeuwisse, W., Dvorak, J., Aubry, M., Bailes, J., Broglio, S., … Davis, G. A. (2017). Consensus statement on concussion in sport—The 5th international conference on concussion in sport held in Berlin, October 2016. *British Journal of Sports Medicine, 51*, 838–847.

Mrazik, M., Brooks, B. L., Jubinville, A., Meeuwisse, W. H., & Emery, C. A. (2016). Psychosocial outcomes of sport concussions in youth hockey players. *Archives of Clinical Neuropsychology, 31*, 297–304.

O'Rourke, D., Smith, R., Punt, S., Coppel, D. B., & Breiger, D. (2017). Psychosocial correlates of young athletes' self-reported concussion symptoms during the course of recovery. *Sport, Exercise, & Performance Psychology, 6*, 262–276.

Postilnik, I., Eisman, H. D., Price, R., & Fogel, J. (2006). An algorithm for defining somatization in children. *Journal of the Canadian Academy of Child and Adolescent Psychiatry 15*, 64–74.

Root, J. M., Zuckerbraun, N., Brent, D., Kontos, A. P., & Hickey, R. (2016). History of somatization is associated with prolonged recovery from concussion. *Pediatrics, 174*, 39–44.

Sandel, N., Reynolds, E., Cohen, P. E., Gillie, B. L., & Kontos, A. P. (2017). Anxiety and mood clinical profile following sport-related concussion: From risk factors to treatment. *Sport, Exercise, & Performance Psychology, 6*, 304–323.

Spitzer, R. L., Krocnke, K., Williams, J. B., & Lowe, B. (2006). A brief measure for assessing generalized anxiety disorder: The GAD-7. *Archives of Internal Medicine, 166*, 1092–1097.

Sufrinko, A., McAllister-Deitrick, J., Elbin, R. J., Collins, M. W., & Kontos, A. P. (2018). Family history of migraine associated with posttraumatic migraine symptoms following sport-related concussion. *Journal of Head Trauma & Rehabilitation, 33*, 7–14.

Sufrinko, A., Pearce, K., Elbin, R., Covassin, T., Johnson, E., Collins, M., & Kontos, A. P. (2015). The effect of preinjury sleep difficulties on neurocognitive impairment and symptoms after sport-related concussion. *The American Journal of Sports Medicine, 43*, 3055–3061.

Theadom, A., Parag, V., Dowell, T., McPherson, K., Starkey, N., Barker-Collo, S., … Group, B. R. (2016). Persistent problems 1 year after mild traumatic brain injury: A longitudinal population study in New Zealand. *British Journal of General Practice, 66*, e16–23.

Tkachenko, N., Singh, K., Hasanaj, L., Serrano, L., & Kothare, S. V. (2016). Sleep disorders associated with mild traumatic brain injury using sport concussion assessment tool 3. *Pediatric Neurology, 57*, 46–50.

Turner, S., Langdon, J., Shaver, G., Graham, V., Naugle, K., & Buckley, T. (2017). Comparison of psychological response between concussion and musculoskeletal injury in collegiate athletes. *Sport, Exercise, & Performance Psychology, 6*, 277–288.

Walker, L. S., & Garber, J. (2003). *Manual for the children's somatization inventory.* Nashville, TN: Vanderbilt University Medical Center.

Wickwire, E. M., Williams, S. G., Roth, T., Capaldi, V. F., Jaffe, M., Moline, M., … Germain, A. (2016). Sleep, sleep disorders, and mild traumatic brain injury. What we know and what we need to know: Findings from a national working group. *Neurotherapeutics, 13*, 403–417.

Wiese-Bjornstal, D., Smith, A., Shaffer, S., & Morrey, M. (1998). An integrated model of response to sport injury: Psychological and sociological dynamics. *Journal of Applied Sport Psychology, 10*, 46–69.

Wiese-Bjornstal, D., White, A. C., Russell, H. C., & Smith A. M. (2015). Psychology of sport concusisons. *Kinesiology Review, 4*, 169–189.

Williams, J. M., & Anderson, M. B. (1998). Psychosocial antecedents of sport injury: Review and critique of the stress and injury model. *Journal of Applied Sport Psychology, 10,* 5–25.

Wood, R. L., O'Hagan, G., Williams, C., McCabe, M., & Chadwick N., (2014). Anxiety sensitivity and alexithymia as mediators of postconcussion syndromefollowing mild traumatic brain injury. *Journal of Head Trauma and Rehabilitation, 29,* E9–E17.

Woodrome, S. E., Yeates, K. O., Taylor, H. G., Rusin, J., Bangert, B., Dietrich, A., … Wright, M. (2011). Coping strategies as a predictor of post-concussive symptoms in children with mild traumatic brain injury versus mild orthopedic injury. *Journal of the International Neuropsychological Society, 17,* 317–326.

Yang, J., Peek-Asa, C., Covassin, T., & Torner, J. C. (2015). Post-concussion symptoms of depression and anxiety in Division I collegiate athletes. *Developmental Neuropsychology, 40,* 18–23.

5 Concussion education

Is it making a difference?

Jeffrey G. Caron

Introduction

Traumatic brain injuries (TBIs) are a global public health issue (Carroll & Rosner, 2012). An estimated 57 million people have been hospitalized worldwide with one or more TBI (Langlois, Rutland-Brown, & Wald, 2006). One type of TBI, concussion, is the most frequently occurring type of brain injury in sport and recreation. An estimated 1.6 to 3.8 million concussions occur annually in the United States (Langlois, Rutland-Brown, & Wald, 2006), however these statistics underestimate the true occurrence of sport-related concussions for a few reasons. First, obvious signs of injury are rarely present after acute concussive injury (McCrory et al., 2017), so many athletes are not evaluated for concussion by a health professional because the injury goes unrecognized by people in the sport environment (e.g., health professionals, teammates, coaches, and officials). Second, even when an athlete is identified as having potentially suffered a concussion, diagnosis relies on some degree of self-reporting of symptoms from the athlete (McCrory et al., 2017). This is problematic because 50–80% of athletes who think they suffered a concussion in the previous season did not report their symptoms to a health professional (e.g., Delaney et al., 2018; McCrea et al., 2004). Of particular relevance to this chapter, Dr. Scott Delaney and his colleagues conducted studies with collegiate (Delaney et al., 2015) and professional (Delaney et al., 2018) athletes to understand their reasons for not reporting symptoms of a concussion. In both studies, the most frequently reported reason was *"did not feel the concussion was serious/severe and felt you could still continue to play with little danger to yourself."* These findings indicate a need to educate athletes about concussions.

There have been dozens of scientific meetings on the topic of concussions since 2000. Likely the most well-known conference is the quadrennial meeting of the Concussion in Sport Group (CISG). The CISG is a multidisciplinary group of researchers, neurologists, neurosurgeons, neuropsychologists, primary care physicians, and sports medicine practitioners. Their meetings have taken place in Vienna (Aubry et al., 2002), Prague (McCrory et al., 2005), two in Zurich (McCrory et al., 2009; McCrory et al., 2013), and the most recent meeting was in Berlin (McCrory et al., 2017). Broadly speaking, the objective of these meetings is to identify effective ways to evaluate and manage concussions. Following each meeting, the CISG has produced recommendations that have largely shaped global best practices for managing sport-related concussions. The scientific impact of this conference can be evidenced by the number of citations (>100) and downloads (>90,000) of the Berlin consensus statement in less than 12 months (British Journal of Sports Medicine, 2018). Among their recommendations, the CISG has championed concussion education as a way to make sport safer and help prevent concussions (McCrory et al., 2017). From these meetings, researchers have gained an understanding of the type of information that should be included in concussion education, such as common signs and symptoms, safe management strategies, and long-term implications. However, researchers are still learning how concussion education efforts are reaching and impacting athletes and members of the sport community. In the remainder of this chapter, research on concussion education is highlighted, and implications for future research and practice are discussed.

Research on concussion education

To date, concussion education has primarily been disseminated using printed educational materials (e.g., pamphlets, posters, and handouts) and web-based platforms like websites and social networking sites (e.g., Facebook, YouTube). Canada's "ThinkFirst" (Parachute Canada, 2018) and the U.S. Centers for Disease Control and Prevention's "HEADS UP to concussions" (Sarmiento et al., 2014) are two North American examples of large-scale campaigns that have used printed educational materials in the past decade. Specific to the HEADS UP campaign, more than 6 million printed educational materials have been distributed to athletes, youth and high school coaches, health professionals, school professionals, and parents since the campaign began in the early 2000s (Sarmiento et al., 2014). Although the use of printed educational materials is relatively cost-effective and allows for information to be widely distributed to members of the sport community, evidence suggests that it may not be effective when used as a standalone strategy (e.g., Grudniewicz et al., 2015). Grudniewicz et al. (2015) conducted a systematic review and meta-analysis to examine the effectiveness of printed educational materials on physicians' ability to care for patients in healthcare settings. Forty studies were included in the study, and the authors concluded that printed educational materials were not effective at improving physicians' knowledge, behavior, or patient outcomes (Grudniewicz et al., 2015). At this time, there have not been any similar large-scale evaluations of the effectiveness of printed educational materials in the area of sport-related concussions (e.g., ThinkFirst, HEADS UP). Nonetheless, if we interpret the findings from Grudniewicz and colleagues' meta-analysis alongside the fact that printed education materials have been the most commonly-used strategy to disseminate concussion education, it should not be surprising to learn that the general public's knowledge of concussions remains "substantially inaccurate" (McKinlay, Bishop, & McLellan, 2011) or, at best, "modest" (Gardner et al., 2017).

Web-based platforms such as websites and social networking sites have also been used to disseminate concussion education. Given the prominence of web-based platforms, they offer researchers an opportunity to reach a wide audience within the sport community (e.g., coaches, athletes, parents, sport administrators) and provide them with concussion education. Our understanding of the effectiveness of web-based platforms in relation to concussion education is largely owed to work conducted by Dr. Osman Ahmed and his colleagues. Specific to websites, Ahmed et al. (2012) reviewed the quality of 43 concussion-related websites to see if they: (a) adhered to international quality standards for health websites (i.e., HONcode accreditation), (b) contained content that was in line with expert guidelines (e.g., CISG consensus statement), and (c) were comprehensible at a grade six reading level.[1] The results revealed that 70% (30/43) of the websites were not HONcode accredited and, on average, the content displayed on the websites was readable at a grade 11 level. The authors also found a large discrepancy with respect to adherence to expert guidelines, and that 40% (17/43) of the websites contained elements of incorrect information (see Table 5 in their article for specific examples). As for social networking sites, Ahmed and colleagues investigated how concussion images and content were being shared on social networking sites like Instagram (Ahmed, Lee, & Struik, 2016), Facebook (Ahmed et al., 2010), and YouTube (Williams et al., 2014). YouTube is one of the most widely used social networking sites, and it allows users to share videos and post comments about the videos. Among the findings from Williams and colleagues' (2014) review, they found that more than half (51%) of the videos originated from news and media organizations, whereas only 5% (5/98) were uploaded by concussion advocacy groups, government agencies, medical centers, or professional associations. Given that the content of YouTube videos is not regulated (Williams et al., 2014), it increases the possibility that incorrect information, or information that is not aligned with current best practices (e.g., CISG), can be distributed (and redistributed) to members of the sport community.

Mrazik et al. (2015) conducted an extensive review of concussion education efforts, including the use of websites and social networking sites. Among their findings, the authors noted there has been an ever-growing number of websites, smartphone/tablet applications, and social media sites dedicated to the topic of concussions. The problem, as the authors note, is that there have been too few evidence-based reviews of these sources of information (Mrazik et al., 2015).[2] In sum, web-based platforms like websites and social networking sites are an intriguing way to disseminate concussion information. However, there are still some challenges that must be addressed to improve web-based platforms as a strategy to educate members of the sport community about concussions.

Concussion education interventions

Caron et al. (2015) conducted a scoping review that focused exclusively on concussion education interventions that went beyond the use of passive strategies like printed educational materials and websites. The research questions that guided the review were: What populations have been included in concussion education interventions? What types of education interventions have been developed to disseminate concussion information? What is the content of concussion education interventions? What are the outcomes of these interventions? What instruments have been used to assess concussion education interventions? Out of 5,938 records identified, nine studies matched the criteria for inclusion.[3] The nine concussion education interventions included in the review were designed and implemented for athletes, high school students, university students, and coaches. The interventions consisted of four interactive oral presentations, two educational videos, and three computer-based learning programs. Although the content varied greatly, the most popular content was: symptomatology, management strategies, long-term sequelae, and return to play schedules. Each of these interventions were delivered at one time-point only, and only one study explicitly noted that their content was based on peer-reviewed expert guidelines. The instruments used to assess the interventions were primarily quantitative, most often using questionnaires and surveys (e.g., Rosenbaum Concussion Knowledge and Attitudes Survey; Rosenbaum & Arnett, 2010) and quizzes (e.g., true/false, multiple choice) to assess outcomes. The majority of the included studies reported short-term improvements in concussion knowledge after the interventions, however long-term improvements (i.e., three to six months) in knowledge, behaviors, and attitudes of concussions were less clear.

The cut-off date for inclusion in the Caron et al. (2015) review was February 21, 2014. Since then, researchers have continued to investigate concussion education interventions. A Google Scholar search was conducted prior to writing this chapter, using similar keywords to update the database of articles included in the 2015 review. Three studies were found to match the original inclusion criteria and are described in Table 5.1.[4] Overall, these interventions were in many ways similar to the studies included in the previous review. Two of the interventions were designed for high school athletes and one for high-performance ice hockey players aged 16–20. Two of the interventions were interactive oral presentations and one primarily used educational videos. Two of the three studies explicitly identified the content of their inventions. The interventions were primarily assessed using quantitative self-report measures and reported short-term improvements in knowledge but limited impact with respect to attitudes and behaviors.

The Caron et al. (2018) study addressed at least three gaps in the literature that have been identified in previous reviews (Caron et al., 2015; Mrazik et al., 2015; Provvidenza et al., 2013). First, principles of knowledge translation (KT) have rarely been adopted by researchers to inform concussion education interventions (e.g., Provvidenza et al., 2013). Caron et al. (2018) framed their study using the

Table 5.1 Examples of concussion education interventions published since February 2014

Studies	Methodology	Participants	Program	Instruments	Main Outcomes
Caron et al. (2018)	Mixed-method, non-randomized, pre-post study with a two-month follow-up. No control group.	35 male student-athletes aged 15–18 ($M_{age} = 15.94$, $SD = 0.34$).	*Content:* Developed in line with principles of knowledge translation (Graham et al., 2006), expert guidelines (McCrory et al., 2013), and a scoping review of concussion education interventions (Caron et al., 2015). Content focused on signs and symptoms, RTP, role of equipment, risk compensation, underreporting, long-term consequences, psychology of concussions, and how to create a safe and healthy sport environment. *Delivery:* Four 30-minute audiovisual presentations. Each consisted of slideshows, videos, pictures and animations, case studies, and group discussions.	*Quantitative:* The Rosenbaum Concussion Knowledge and Attitudes Survey-Student (RoCKAS-ST; Rosenbaum & Arnett, 2010) was used. It contains 55 items that assess concussion knowledge (CK) and concussion attitude (CA). RoCKAS-ST was completed at three time points: pre-, immediately post-, and two-months post-intervention. *Qualitative:* Focus Group interviews conducted two weeks after the intervention.	*Quantitative:* A one-way repeated measures ANOVA indicated CK scores (but not CA) were significantly different across time $F(2, 68) = 19.079$, $p < 0.001$, $\eta^2_p = 0.359$. For CK, pre- and immediately post-intervention scores ($t = -2.000$, $p < 0.001$, $d = -0.884$) and pre-intervention and two-months post-intervention scores ($t = -1.971$, $p < 0.001$, $d = -0.831$) were significantly different. No difference was found between post- and two-months post-intervention ($t = 0.029$, $p = 0.931$, $d = 0.014$). *Qualitative:* Participants said they acquired CK about the role of protective equipment and symptom variability. Some also reported intending to avoid dangerous in-game collisions in the future. (*Continued*)

Table 5.1 Continued

Studies	Methodology	Participants	Program	Instruments	Main Outcomes
Kroshus et al. (2015)	Randomized, controlled, pre-post study with one-month follow-up.	12 teams competing in men's Tier III junior ice hockey. Of the 256 athletes ($M_{age} = 19.15$, $SD = 0.85$) who were eligible, 102 participants (40%) completed measures at three time points.	*Content*: Not explicitly articulated. *Delivery*: Control group (four teams) received CDC's "Heads Up" fact sheet only. One arm of the intervention group (four teams) received the "Heads up" fact sheet AND a 12-minute video called "Concussions in Ice Hockey." Another arm of the intervention group (four teams) received the "Heads up" fact sheet AND watched a 90-minute video called "Head Games."	A 57-item questionnaire was compiled based on previous studies to assess attitude, reporting self-efficacy, and reporting intention (Kroshus, Baugh, Daneshvar, & Viswanath, 2014); knowledge and subjective norms (Rosenbaum & Arnett, 2010); and symptoms and behavior (Kaut et al., 2003).	Players in the "Concussions in Ice Hockey" condition reported increased perceptions that their teammates and most other athletes would engage in unsafe reporting behaviors. At one month post-intervention, there were no lasting changes in any of the three groups related to concussion reporting behavior or in any of the constructs (knowledge, reporting outcomes, self-efficacy, reporting intention).
Kurowski et al. (2015)	Randomized, pre-post study with a control group. Post-season data on behaviors were also collected.	Intervention group was 234 student-athletes ($M_{age} = 15.38$, 82.91% male), and the control group included 262 student-athletes ($M_{age} = 15.46$, 75.52% male). Sports included football, soccer, basketball, and wrestling.	*Content*: Developed based on expert guidelines (Herring et al., 2011; McCrory et al., 2009). Information included signs and symptoms, second impact syndrome, and potential chronic problems that could develop after concussion. *Delivery*: 20-minute audiovisual presentation with opportunities for participant questions.	36-item questionnaire modified from previous studies (Bramley et al., 2012; Sarmiento et al., 2010). Developed to assess athletes' knowledge of attitudes/behaviors towards concussion. 25 knowledge-based questions, and 11 focused on attitudes and behaviors.	For the intervention group, knowledge and attitudes/behaviors scores increased immediately post-education and then dissipated over time. Specific to attitudes/behaviors, 31/43 (72%) of athletes in the intervention group and 68/77 (88%) of athletes in the control group reported they continued playing with concussion symptoms. Additionally, 3/11 (27%) intervention and 3/13 (23%) control group participants indicated they returned to play before their symptoms had resolved.

knowledge to action cycle (cf. Graham et al., 2006), a KT framework that was designed to close the knowledge gap between researchers and knowledge users by appropriately adapting the content and delivery of interventions. Consistent with the knowledge to action cycle, the Caron et al. (2018) intervention was informed by a review of concussion education interventions, peer-reviewed articles, the most recent CISG consensus statement, and research with athletes and coaches at the high school. These steps were undertaken to ensure the content and delivery of the intervention were appropriately adapted for study participants.

A second gap in the literature has been the lack of qualitative research methodologies used to evaluate concussion education interventions (Caron et al., 2015; Mrazik et al., 2015). This is unfortunate because qualitative research methodologies have been a recommended strategy to evaluate KT interventions (Straus et al., 2013). Focus group interviews, one method of qualitative data collection, were used to evaluate the Caron et al. (2018) intervention to gain a more detailed understanding of the types of knowledge participants acquired and their overall perceptions of the intervention. One example of the type of knowledge that participants said they acquired from the intervention was that helmets and mouth guards were not designed to prevent concussions. Participants also said they enjoyed the interactive nature of the presentations, including the use of case study exemplars[5] and the opportunity to ask questions and engage in discussions. The use focus group interviews gave participants an opportunity to use their own words to describe their perspectives, which allowed for a deeper understanding of the impact of the intervention, especially when interpreted alongside the quantitative data that were collected (Caron et al., 2018).

A third gap is that the majority of concussion education interventions have been disseminated at one time-point only (Caron et al., 2015). Given that most concussion education interventions are 20–30 min in length (Caron et al., 2015), researchers have had to carefully consider the type of content that would be included in their interventions. Caron et al. (2018) delivered their intervention over the course of four interactive oral presentations. This allowed participants to be exposed to "classic" content (e.g., common symptoms, management strategies, long-term sequelae, and return to play schedules), as well as "novel" content about social-psychological aspects of concussions and creating a safe sporting environment. The use of multiple education sessions could be a beneficial strategy to help reduce feelings of being overwhelmed with content, which may occur in single-session interventions. However, more research is needed before more conclusive statements can be made about the effectiveness of multiple education sessions with respect to changes in concussion knowledge, attitudes, and behaviors.

In sum, most concussion education has been disseminated in the form of printed educational materials, websites, and social networking sites. Evidence about the effectiveness of these modalities is currently either inconclusive or has suggested that they may not be effective when used as a standalone educational strategy. Interventions have also been used to disseminate concussion education. Most of these interventions have educated members of the sport community using interactive oral presentations—typically at one time point only. Overall, concussion education interventions have demonstrated short-term improvements in knowledge, however their impact beyond three months on knowledge, attitudes, and behaviors remains uncertain at this time.

Implications for future research and practice

Although it could be argued that the reach of concussion education has improved general awareness of the injury (Gardner et al., 2017), the long-term impact of these efforts on the sport community is still largely unknown. As a result, researchers must continue to investigate strategies that will improve the impact of interventions to help prevent concussions and to make sport safer. This section offers some suggestions based on previous research, as well as other avenues that could be explored to improve concussion education efforts.

Although the intervention from Caron and colleagues (2018) was created to address previous gaps in the literature, limitations still existed. In particular, the sample was all male and there was no control condition. Additionally, the four interactive oral presentations were delivered over the course of one month. Mrazik et al. (2015) noted that KT should be viewed as an ongoing process and involve continued dialogue between researchers and knowledge users (Mrazik et al., 2015). As such, future concussion education interventions using KT frameworks should be implemented and assessed over longer periods of time (e.g., 12 or 24 months), and researchers should report how the content and delivery of interventions are refined over time.

Concussion education interventions have not impacted participants' knowledge beyond three months (Caron et al., 2015; Mrazik et al., 2015). One interpretation of this finding could be that more longitudinal designs are needed to make a greater impact on athletes' knowledge. However, another way to interpret the finding is that researchers should think more deeply about the ultimate goal of improving athletes' knowledge of concussions. Is the assumption that athletes will behave more safely, or that sport administrators will enact policies designed to make sport safer once equipped with adequate knowledge of concussions? There is ample evidence to suggest that concussion knowledge alone will be insufficient to prevent concussions and encourage people to make safer decisions (e.g., Chrisman, Quitiquit, & Rivara, 2013; Delaney et al., 2018). For example, Chrisman, Quitiquit, & Rivera (2013) noted that although the adolescent athletes in their study recognized concussions as being a serious injury, some said they would likely continue playing with a suspected concussion because, as one football athlete noted, "You don't want to look like a baby" (p. 333). Additionally, many sports around the world still permit unsafe practices that are known to cause concussions. Sports like American football and rugby still permit tackling among children and young adolescents, and ice hockey continues to tolerate fighting (i.e., on-ice altercations). And of course, there remain gladiatorial sports like mixed martial arts and boxing, where victory is often achieved through the delivery of multiple concussive or subconcussive blows to an opponent.

Although knowledge should continue to be an important part of interventions, researchers should be aware that improvements in knowledge alone are unlikely to result in meaningful changes to athletes' concussion-related attitudes and behaviors.

Indeed, a focus of future research and intervention in this domain should be on changing concussion-related behaviors such as risky tackling/body checking and reporting a possible concussion. Behavior change has received a great deal of attention in relation to other health-related topics like smoking, physical activity, and diet, to name a few (Conner & Norman, 2017; Kelly & Barker, 2016). Although there is evidence that interventions have had some impact on changing individual's behaviors (Conner & Norman, 2017), researchers have noted more work is needed to improve the impact of behavior change interventions (Kelly & Barker, 2016). To date, there have not been any interventions developed with the expressed intent of changing concussion-related behaviors. This is not surprising given that the study of concussions is relatively new when compared to other health topics (e.g., smoking). As such, there is a great opportunity for researchers to begin developing behavior change interventions—either as part of concussion education or separately. Behavior change is discussed in more detail in another chapter in this book, including how researchers can learn from behavior change research in other domains to develop these types of interventions for concussions (see Chapter 6 in this book).

Researchers have also suggested that the use of technology could be useful in improving concussion education interventions (Mrazik et al., 2015). Although concussion education interventions have yet to be delivered primarily through social networking sites, this is an exciting area for future research given the prevalence of social networking sites and the broad use of smartphones devices among members of the sport community. Additionally, limited attention has been paid to the use of educational video games for improving concussion-related behaviors. This is unfortunate given that 97% of adolescents age 12–17 play computer, web, portable, or console video games (Lenhart et al., 2008). Video games that have rules, goals, and a stated purpose beyond pure entertainment are called "serious games." There is quite an extensive body of literature that has looked at the use and effectiveness of serious games as a health education intervention (e.g., Hieftje et al., 2013). Serious games have been developed to address health conditions such as HIV/AIDS, cancer, and diabetes, to name a few (Fiellin, Heiftje, & Duncan, 2014). There is evidence that playing serious games allows users to acquire new information and skills in a virtual environment that can be transferred into meaningful real-life changes in knowledge and behaviors (Bainbridge, 2007). Taken together, researchers are encouraged to investigate how technologies, like social networking sites and serious games, could be used as interventions to produce meaningful changes in athletes' knowledge, attitudes, and behaviors of concussions.

Up to this point, the chapter has focused on a number of issues facing concussion education in the present and in the future. However, we have yet to discuss "who" should disseminate concussion education, which is a critical practical consideration. This is a particularly important point to address because there have been an increasing number of "concussion experts" and "concussion clinics" appearing all over the world. Ellis and colleagues (2017) conducted a Google search to investigate the provision of concussion healthcare in Canada. Their study revealed a few areas of concern. In particular, the authors found that two companies have created "training and certification programs" that have been delivered to more than 100 healthcare providers across Canada. This type of training, although permissible by law, is *not* synonymous with nationally licensed clinical training (e.g., Royal College of Physicians and Surgeons of Canada). Although it is beyond the scope of this chapter to comment on the competency and training of health professionals to evaluate and manage concussions, here are some questions to consider when seeking an expert to disseminate concussion education to your team, group, or sport organization:

• What is their educational background?
• Has the majority of their training dealt with sport-related concussions?
• What are the key meetings/documents that inform their research and/or professional practice related to concussions?
• What is their experience working in sport?

Some of the most common educational backgrounds among individuals working within the area of sport-related concussions include sports medicine, neuropsychology, physiotherapy, and athletic therapy/training (Ellis et al., 2017). Indeed, facilitators of concussion education should have acquired knowledge and expertise through one of the medical or health degrees above, or a master's or doctoral degree in a health-related field (e.g., Kinesiology; Caron et al., 2018). Researchers have also suggested that sport psychology professionals could be an ideal member of the sports medicine team to deliver concussion education (Caron et al., 2018; Kontos, Collins, & Russo, 2004). Sport psychology professionals often conduct educational interventions with individuals and teams about psychological and social aspects of injury recovery (Schwab Reese, Pittsinger, & Yang, 2012) and issues related to well-being, such as doping, drug abuse, and mental health (Williams, 2010). Further, McCrory et al. (2005) discussed the role of sport psychology with concussed athletes at the 2nd CISG conference in Prague. As a result, it seems reasonable for sport psychology professionals to become more involved in delivering concussion education interventions.

Conclusions

Research on concussion education is still in its early stages of development. To date, concussion education has been disseminated using printed educational materials, web-based platforms (websites, social networking sites), and, to a lesser extent, targeted interventions. So far, these initiatives have reported short-term improvements in knowledge, but the long-term benefits on knowledge, attitudes, and behaviors are less clear. To address these shortcomings, there is a need to develop interventions in line with principles of KT and ensure that messaging around concussion knowledge is supplemented with strategies to change/modify concussion-related attitudes and behaviors. Indeed, targeted behavior change interventions are needed to prevent or reduce risky/aggressive behaviors that result in concussions. Technologies such as social networking sites and serious games are interesting platforms that could be used to deliver future interventions, especially when considering the prevalence of these technologies among adolescents and young adults.

In reading this chapter, it should be evident that there are a multitude of factors that should be considered when developing and implementing concussion education interventions. Can it be concluded that concussion education is making a difference? Concussion education has certainly improved general awareness of the injury, but more work is needed to make a profound impact on the health and safety of the sport community. The hope is that the information and resources provided can be useful in developing more effective concussion education interventions now and in the future. It is imperative that researchers continue investigating the best ways to educate athletes about concussions to prevent the injury and preserve athletes' short- and long-term health.

Acknowledgment

I would like to thank Dr. Les Podlog for his insightful comments and suggestions on earlier drafts of this chapter.

Notes

1 It is recommended that health information be written at or below a grade 6 level so it can be understood by the general public (Hersh, Salzman, & Snyderman, 2015).
2 See Table 2 in the Mrazik et al. (2015) article for reviews on web-based concussion resources.
3 See Table 1 from Caron et al. (2015) for a detailed description of the findings from the included studies.
4 It is important to note that the review was not exhaustive. The intent was to provide examples of some of the research that has been conducted since the 2015 review.
5 See the supplemental online material in Caron et al. (2018) for quotes from the participants.

References

Ahmed, O. H., Lee, H., & Struik, L. L. (2016). A picture tells a thousand words: A content analysis of concussion-related images online. *Physical Therapy in Sport, 21*, 82–86. doi:10.1016/j.ptsp.2016.03.001.
Ahmed, O. H., Sullivan, S. J., Schneiders, A. G., & McCrory, P. (2010). iSupport: Do social networking sites have a role to play in concussion awareness? *Disability and Rehabilitation, 32*, 1877–1883. doi:10.3109/09638281003734409.

Ahmed, O. H., Sullivan, S. J., Schneiders, A. G., & McCrory, P. R. (2012). Concussion information online: Evaluation of information quality, content and readability of concussion-related websites. *British Journal of Sports Medicine, 46*, 675–683. doi:10.1136/bjsm.2010.081620.

Aubry, M., Cantu, R., Dvorak, J., Graf-Baumann, T., Johnston, K. M., Kelley, J., ... & Schamasch, P. (2002). Summary and agreement statement of the 1st international symposium on concussion in sport, Vienna 2001. *Clinical Journal of Sports Medicine, 12*, 6–11. doi:10.1136/bjsm.36.1.6.

Bainbridge, W. S. (2007). The scientific research potential of virtual worlds. *Science, 317*, 472–476. doi:10.1126/science.1146930.

British Journal of Sports Medicine. (2018, January 8). Usage statistics of the Concussion in Sport group 2017 consensus statement. Retrieved from: http://bjsm.bmj.com/content/early/2017/04/26/bjsports-2017-097699. altmetrics#.

Caron, J. G., Rathwell, S., Delaney, J. S., Johnston, K. M., Ptito, A., & Bloom, G. A. (2018). Development, implementation and assessment of a concussion education programme for high school student-athletes. *Journal of Sports Sciences, 36*, 48–55. doi:10.1080/02640414.2017.1280180.

Caron, J. G., Bloom, G. A., Falcão, W. R., & Sweet, S. N. (2015). An examination of concussion education programmes: A scoping review methodology. *Injury Prevention, 21*, 301–308. doi:10.1136/injuryprev-2014-041479.

Carroll, L., & Rosner, D. (2012). *The concussion crisis: Anatomy of a silent epidemic.* New York: Simon & Schuster.

Chrisman, S. P., Quitiquit, C., & Rivara, F. P. (2013). Qualitative study of barriers to concussive symptom reporting in high school athletics. *Journal of Adolescent Health, 52*, 330–335. doi:10.1016.j.jadohealth.2012.10.271.

Conner, M., & Norman, P. (2017). Health behaviour: Current issues and challenges. *Psychology & Health, 32*(8), 895–906. doi:10.1080/08870446.20 17.1336240.

Delaney, J. S., Caron, J. G., Correa, J. A., & Bloom, G. A. (2018). Why professional football players chose not to reveal their concussion symptoms during a practice or game. *Clinical Journal of Sports Medicine, 28*, 1–12. doi:10.1097/ JSM.0000000000000495.

Delaney, J. S., Lamfookon, C., Bloom, G. A., Al-Kashmiri, A., & Correa, J. A. (2015). Why university athletes choose not to reveal their concussion symptoms during a practice or game. *Clinical Journal of Sports Medicine, 25*, 113–125. doi:10.1097/ JSM.0000000000000112.

Ellis, M. J., Ritchie, L., Selci, E., Chu, S., McDonald, P., & Russell, K. (2017). Googling concussion care: A critical appraisal of online concussion healthcare providers and practices in Canada. *Clinical Journal of Sport Medicine, 27*, 179–182. doi:10.1097/JSM.0000000000000305.

Fiellin, L. E., Hieftje, K. D., & Duncan, L. D. (2014). Videogames, here for good. *Pediatrics, 134*, 849–851. doi:10.1542/peds.2014-0941.

Gardner, A. J., Kay-Lambkin, F., Shultz, S. R., & Iverson, G. L. (2017). Level of knowledge and attitude towards sport-related concussion among the general public. *British Journal of Sports Medicine, 51*, A68–A68.

Graham, I. D., Logan, J., Harrison, M. B., Straus, S. E., Tetroe, J., Caswell, W., & Robinson, N. (2006). Lost in knowledge translation: Time for a map? *Journal of Continuing Education in the Health Professions, 26*, 13–24. doi:10.1002/ chp.47.

Grudniewicz, A., Kealy, R., Rodseth, R. N., Hamid, J., Rudoler, D., & Straus, S. E. (2015). What is the effectiveness of printed educational materials on primary care physician knowledge, behaviour, and patient outcomes: A systematic review and meta-analyses. *Implementation Science*, *10*, 164.

Herring, S. A., Cantu, R. C., Guskiewicz, K. M., Putukian, M., Kibler, W. B., Bergfeld, J. A., ... & Indelicato, P. A. (2011). Concussion (mild traumatic brain injury) and the team physician: A consensus statement—2011 update. *Medicine and Science in Sports and Exercise*, *43*(12), 2412–2422.

Hersh, L., Salzman, B., & Snyderman, D. (2015). Health literacy in primary care practice. *American Family Physician*, *92*, 118–124.

Hieftje, K., Edelman, E. J., Camenga, D. R., & Fiellin, L. E. (2013). Electronic media-based health interventions promoting behavior change in youth: A systematic review. *JAMA Pediatrics*, *167*, 574–580. doi:10.1001/jamapediatrics.2013.1095.

Kaut, K. P., DePompei, R., Kerr, J., & Congeni, J. (2003). Reports of head injury and symptom knowledge among college athletes: Implications for assessment and educational intervention. *Clinical Journal of Sport Medicine*, *13*(4), 213–221.

Kelly, M. P., & Barker, M. (2016). Why is changing health-related behaviour so difficult? *Public Health*, *136*, 109–116. doi: 10.1016/j.puhe.2016.03.030.

Kontos, A. P., Collins, M., & Russo, S. A. (2004). An introduction to sports concussion for the sport psychology consultant. *Journal of Applied Sport Psychology*, *16*, 220–235. doi:10.1080/10413200490485568.

Kroshus, E., Baugh, C. M., Daneshvar, D. H., & Viswanath, K. (2014). Understanding concussion reporting using a model based on the theory of planned behavior. *Journal of Adolescent Health*, *54*(3), 269–274.

Kroshus, E., Baugh, C. M., Hawrilenko, M., & Daneshvar, D. H. (2015). Pilot randomized evaluation of publicly available concussion education materials: Evidence of a possible negative effect. *Health Education & Behavior*, *42*, 153–162. doi:10.1177/1090198114543011.

Kurowski, B. G., Pomerantz, W. J., Schaiper, C., Ho, M., & Gittelman, M. A. (2015). Impact of preseason concussion education on knowledge, attitudes, and behaviors of high school athletes. *The Journal of Trauma and Acute Care Surgery*, *79*, S21–S28. doi:10.1097/TA.0000000000000675.

Langlois, J. A., Rutland-Brown, W., & Wald, M. M. (2006). The epidemiology and impact of traumatic brain injury: A brief overview. *The Journal of Head Trauma Rehabilitation*, *21*, 375–378.

Lenhart, A., Kahne, J., Middaugh, E., Macgill, A. R., Evans, C., & Vitak, J. (2008). Teens, video games, and civics: Teens' gaming experiences are diverse and include significant social interaction and civic engagement. *Pew Internet & American Life Project*. Retrieved from: https://files.eric.ed.gov/fulltext/ED525058.pdf.

McCrea, M., Hammeke, T., Olsen, G., Leo, P., & Guskiewicz, K. (2004). Unreported concussion in high school football players: Implications for prevention. *Clinical Journal of Sport Medicine*, *14*, 13–17.

McCrory, P., Johnston, K., Meeuwisse, W., Aubry, M., Cantu, R., Dvorak, J., ... & Schamasch, P. (2005). Summary and agreement statement of the 2nd international conference on concussion in sport, Prague 2004. *British Journal of Sports Medicine*, *39*, 196–204. doi:10.1136/bjsm.2005.018614.

McCrory, P., Meeuwisse, W. H., Aubry, M., Cantu, B., Dvorak, J., Echemendia, R. J., ... & Turner, M. (2013). Consensus statement on concussion in sport: The 4th International conference on concussion in sport held in Zurich,

November 2012. *British Journal of Sports Medicine*, *47*, 250–258. doi:10.1136/bjsports-2013-092313.

McCrory, P., Meeuwisse, W., Dvorak, J., Aubry, M., Bailes, J., Broglio, S., ... & Davis, G. A. (2017). Consensus statement on concussion in sport—The 5th international conference on concussion in sport held in Berlin, October 2016. *British Journal of Sports Medicine*, *51*, 838–847. doi:10.1136/bjsports-2017-097699.

McCrory, P., Meeuwisse, W., Johnston, K., Dvorak, J., Aubry, M., Molloy, M., & Cantu, R. (2009). Consensus statement on concussion in sport: The 3rd international conference on concussion in sport held in Zurich, November 2008. *British Journal of Sports Medicine*, *43*, 76–84. doi:10.1136/bjsm.2009.058248.

McKinlay, A., Bishop, A., & McLellan, T. (2011). Public knowledge of "concussion" and the different terminology used to communicate about mild traumatic brain injury (MTBI). *Brain Injury*, *25*, 761–766. doi:10.3109/02699052.2011.579935.

Mrazik, M., Dennison, C. R., Brooks, B. L., Yeates, K. O., Babul, S., & Naidu, D. (2015). A qualitative review of sports concussion education: Prime time for evidence-based knowledge translation. *British Journal of Sports Medicine*, *49*, 1548–1553. doi:10.1136/bjsports-2015-094848.

Parachute Canada. (2018, January 8). *Concussion awareness initiative*. Retrieved from: www.parachutecanada.org/thinkfirstcanada.

Provvidenza, C., Engebretsen, L., Tator, C., Kissick, J., McCrory, P., Sills, A., & Johnston, K. M. (2013). From consensus to action: knowledge transfer, education and influencing policy on sports concussion. *British Journal of Sports Medicine*, *47*, 332–338. doi:10.1136/bjsports-2012-092099.

Rosenbaum, A. M., & Arnett, P. A. (2010). The development of a survey to examine knowledge about and attitudes toward concussion in high-school students. *Journal of Clinical and Experimental Neuropsychology*, *32*, 44–55. doi:10.1080/13803390902806535.

Sarmiento, K., Mitchko, J., Klein, C., & Wong, S. (2010). Evaluation of the Centers for Disease Control and Prevention's concussion initiative for high school coaches: "Heads up: Concussion in high school sports". *Journal of School Health*, *80*(3), 112–118.

Sarmiento, K., Hoffman, R., Dmitrovski, Z., & Lee, R. (2014). A 10-year review of the Centers for Disease Control and Prevention's *Heads Up* initiatives: Bringing concussion awareness to the forefront. *Journal of Safety Research*, *50*, 143–147. doi:10.1016/j.jsr.2014.05.003.

Schwab Reese, L. M., Pittsinger, R., & Yang, J. (2012). Effectiveness of psychological intervention following sport injury. *Journal of Sport and Health Science*, *1*, 71–79. doi:10.1016/j.jshs.2012.06.003.

Straus, S. E., Tetroe, J., Bhattacharyya, O., Zwarenstein, M., & Graham, I. D. (2013). Monitoring knowledge use and evaluating outcomes. In S. E. Straus, J. Tetroe, & I. D. Graham (Eds.), *Knowledge Translation in health care: Moving from evidence to practice* (2nd ed., pp. 227–236). West Sussex, UK: Wiley & Sons.

Williams, J. M. (Ed.). (2010). *Applied sport psychology: Personal growth to peak performance* (6th ed.). New York: McGraw-Hill.

Williams, D., Sullivan, S. J., Schneiders, A. G., Ahmed, O. H., Lee, H., Balasundaram, A. P., & McCrory, P. R. (2014). Big hits on the small screen: An evaluation of concussion-related videos on YouTube. *British Journal of Sports Medicine*, *48*, 107–111 doi:10.1136/bjsports-2012-091853.

6 Theoretical implications and applications for understanding and changing concussion-related behaviors

Emilie Michalovic, Jeffrey G. Caron, and Shane N. Sweet

Introduction

Changing health behaviors is difficult, as evidenced by the general public's non-compliance to various health behavior guidelines. For instance, only one-third of individuals follow 50% of the recommended nutrition guidelines (de Ridder et al., 2017), and just 15% of Canadians are currently meeting the physical activity recommendations (Colley et al., 2011). Concussion-related behaviors are not immune to these challenges. A recent study found that more than 80% of professional players in the Canadian Football League did not seek medical attention after suffering a suspected concussion, despite being aware of the adverse short- and long-term health implications associated with the injury (Delaney et al., 2018). Therefore, understanding concussion-related behaviors is important in making sports safer and reducing the rates of concussions. However, we have learned from other health fields that understanding (and changing) behavior is complex.

Attempts to change health behaviors have mostly been unsuccessful because many interventions focus solely on providing knowledge, which assumes that people will act rationally once they are made aware of the negative implications of continuing to engage in unhealthy behaviors (Kelly & Barker, 2016). A recent special issue in *Psychology & Health* featured reviews of intervention studies conducted on changing behaviors related to (a) smoking, (b) physical activity, (c) binge drinking, and (d) diet. Overall, these interventions had only a small effect on changing behaviors (Conner & Norman, 2017). The common theme from these reviews was that the researchers could not explain why their interventions were only marginally effective. Unfortunately, current health behavior interventions are typically only *inspired* by theory and not truly *grounded* in theory (Conner & Norman, 2017). Researchers have noted that testing interventions that are grounded in theory will be important to move the field of health behavior change forward (Kelly & Barker, 2016; Conner & Norman, 2017). Researchers using theory to study concussions can (and should) learn from these reviews. Grounding concussion research and interventions in theory may provide researchers with insight into the key ingredients to understand and change concussion-related behaviors.

Theories that have been applied to concussion research

A theory consists of a set of interrelated constructs or variables that aim to explain the *why*, *when*, and *how* of a behavior. A strong theory should also be testable, falsifiable, and refutable (Popper, 1962). Theories provide a common language of the factors that explain a behavior. As such, theories provide a roadmap for understanding a behavior by outlining and hypothesizing the relationship between a set of variables and the behavior (Michie, Atkins, & West, 2014). When applied to the study of concussions, theories can help us understand the variables that predict concussion-related behaviors. Concussion-related behaviors include concussion reporting (e.g., Register-Mihalik et al., 2013), help-seeking (e.g., Kroshus et al., 2016), and adherence to physician-administered rehabilitation (e.g., Moor et al., 2015). Once behaviors are understood, they can be measured in targeted interventions. As a result, grounding interventions in theory allows researchers to test the effects of an intervention on the psychosocial variables (or intervention ingredients) and, in turn, determine if these variables explain the effect of the intervention. This section will review two theories that have been used to study concussions to date. For these two theories, we provide an overview of the theoretical tenets and empirical examples of how they have been used in concussion research.

Theory of planned behavior

Theoretical tenets

In the theory of planned behavior (TPB; Ajzen, 1991), attitudes (i.e., beliefs about affective or cognitive consequences of a behavior), subjective norms (i.e., perceptions of social pressures to perform a behavior), and perceived behavioral control (i.e., perceptions of personal control over a behavior) are determinants of intentions (i.e., willingness to do a behavior). A person's intention to engage in a behavior is theorized to be the best predictor of that behavior. Additionally, a person's perceived behavioral control is directly linked to behavior. See Ajzen (1991) for a visual depiction of TPB.

Empirical examples

TBP is the most popular theory used in concussion research (e.g., Kroshus et al., 2014; Newton et al., 2014; Register-Mihalik et al., 2013; Rigby, Vela, & Housman, 2013). Concussion researchers have used TPB to investigate athletes' intentions to report concussions to predict actual concussion-reporting behaviors (Kroshus et al., 2014; Register-Mihalik et al., 2013). Register-Mihalik et al. (2013) used TPB to investigate concussion-reporting intentions and recalled concussion-reporting behaviors[1] among a sample of 167 high school athletes. The findings indicated that TPB explained 58% of the variance in athletes' intentions to report concussions, but intentions to report injuries were not significantly associated with reporting recalled concussion events (i.e., their actual behaviors). Kroshus et al. (2014) also sought to determine whether TPB could predict athletes' retrospective concussion-reporting behaviors. The sample consisted of 256 male ice hockey athletes 18 to 21 years of age. In this study, all relationships testing TPB were significant. Specifically, TPB variables explained 22% and 10% of the variance of intentions and concussion-reporting behavior, respectively. In sum, there is support for TPB for understanding athletes' intentions to report suspected concussions; however, there is mixed evidence regarding whether intentions are associated with reporting behaviors.

Social cognitive theory

Theoretical tenets

In social cognitive theory (SCT; Bandura, 2004), personal (cognitive, affective, biological), behavioral, and environmental factors are interconnected concepts that explain human actions. The central premise of the theory is that all three are reciprocally related and important for understanding behavior. In 2004, Bandura outlined a SCT model that can be utilized for health behaviors. In this model, health behaviors are influenced by personal factors, namely self-efficacy, outcome expectancies, goals, and sociostructural factors (i.e., environment). There is a direct relationship between self-efficacy beliefs and behavior and an indirect relationship between self-efficacy beliefs and behavior through outcome expectancies, goals, and sociostructural factors. See Bandura (2004) for a visual depiction of SCT.

Empirical examples

There is some emerging concussion research that has used SCT or SCT constructs to understand concussion-related behaviors (e.g., Hunt, Harris, & Way, 2017; Kroshus et al., 2015). For example, Kroshus et al. (2015) focused on the interplay between behavioral and environmental factors of SCT. Specifically, they investigated the extent to which pressure from teammates, coaches, parents, and fans (i.e., sociostructural factors) was associated with athletes' intentions to report suspected concussion events (as a proxy to concussion-reporting behavior). Participants were 328 male and female U.S. collegiate athletes from a variety of contact and collision sports (e.g., soccer, lacrosse, basketball). Results indicated that pressure from teammates, parents, and fans (but not coaches) was associated with lower intentions to report a concussion. Thus, there is some preliminary evidence to suggest that SCT (as per the environmental dimension) provides a framework for understanding the social variables involved in athletes reporting possible concussions (Hunt et al., 2017; Kroshus et al., 2015).

Theories that could be applied to concussion research

In this section, we describe four theories that could assist with understanding and changing concussion-related behaviors. Understandably, it is beyond the scope of this chapter to provide a description of all potential theories that can be applied to concussion research. Nonetheless, the four theories we outline below have been supported in other health-related contexts (e.g., exercise: Sniehotta, Scholz, & Schwarzer, 2005; physical activity: Fortier et al., 2012; condom use: Larios et al., 2009; smoking cessation: Fulton et al., 2016) and may be of interest to researchers who want to understand and change concussion-related behaviors. For more information about theories that have been used to study human behavior, please consult Michie and colleagues' (2014) comprehensive book: *ABC of Behaviour Change Theories* (www.behaviourchangetheories.com/).

For each of the four theories below, we explain the theoretical tenets, provide empirical examples of how the theory has been used with other health behaviors, and postulate how concussion researchers might use these theories. Our description of the *theoretical tenets* is meant to provide an overview and should not be considered a substitute for reading the original articles. In the *empirical examples* sections, we provide evidence of how the theories have been used to both understand and change behavior. The examples in the *application to concussion research* sections are meant to provide a snapshot of theory-guided concussion research rather than detailing an entire research study. As such, we kept these examples brief and focused only on certain parts of a theory. Researchers who are planning to conduct theory-based research should consider all components of a theory.

Health action process approach

Theoretical tenets

The health action process approach (HAPA) model is comprised of two main phases: motivational and volitional (Schwarzer, 2008). In the motivational phase, outcome expectations, action self-efficacy, and risk perception are predictors of intentions. In the volitional phase, action planning, coping planning, maintenance self-efficacy, and recovery self-efficacy are determinants of behavior. One benefit of HAPA is that it was designed to overcome the intention-behavior gap (Schwarzer, 2008). Specifically, action and coping planning are hypothesized to help individuals translate their *intentions* to perform a behavior into *actually performing* a behavior. Action planning is the process of creating a specific plan that details *when* a person will perform a certain behavior, *where* they will perform the behavior, *what* they will do, and for *how long*. Coping planning involves creating specific plans to overcome foreseeable barriers to performing the behavior (see the examples in Figure 6.1).

Empirical examples to understand behavior

Studies grounded in HAPA have shown support for this framework across health behaviors (e.g., Ernsting et al., 2013). For example, in a sample of cardiac

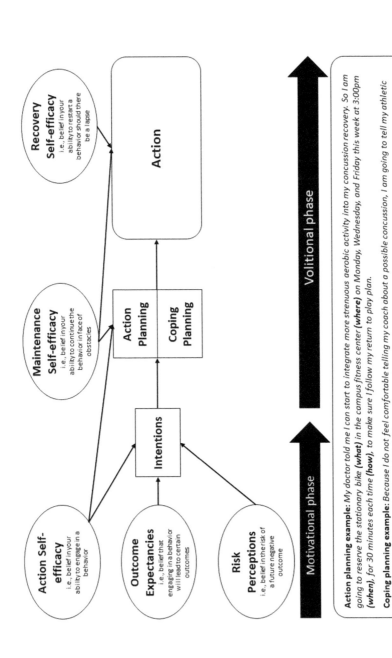

The figure shows the Health Action Process Approach model with the following elements:

Action Self-efficacy — i.e., belief in your ability to engage in a behavior

Outcome Expectancies — i.e., belief that engaging in a behavior will lead to certain outcomes

Risk Perceptions — i.e., belief in the risk of a future negative outcome

Maintenance Self-efficacy — i.e., belief in your ability to continue the behavior in face of obstacles

Recovery Self-efficacy — i.e., belief in your ability to restart a behavior should there be a lapse

Intentions

Action Planning / Coping Planning

Action

Motivational phase → Volitional phase

Action planning example: My doctor told me I can start to integrate more strenuous aerobic activity into my concussion recovery. So I am going to reserve the stationary bike (**what**) in the campus fitness center (**where**) on Monday, Wednesday, and Friday this week at 3:00pm (**when**), for 30 minutes each time (**how**), to make sure I follow my return to play plan.

Coping planning example: Because I do not feel comfortable telling my coach about a possible concussion, I am going to tell my athletic therapist about my symptoms if ever I think I have a concussion.

Figure 6.1 Health action process approach.

Note: Adapted from Schwarzer, R. (2014, October 13). Health Action Process Approach. Retrieved January 29, 2018, from www.hapa-model.de/.

rehabilitation participants, outcome expectations, action self-efficacy, and risk perceptions significantly predicted 69% of the variance in intention, while action planning and maintenance self-efficacy predicted 24% of the variance in exercise two months later (Sniehotta, Scholz, & Schwarzer, 2005). Support for the HAPA model has also been found in other health behaviors, such as condom use (Teng & Mak, 2011) and smoking cessation (Radtke et al., 2012).

Empirical examples to change behavior

Interventions have also integrated action and coping planning to promote various health behaviors. In a meta-analysis of action and coping planning, Carraro and Gaudreau (2013) found that intentions to be physically active predicted action and coping planning. Both forms of planning also significantly predicted physical activity. Action and coping planning were also found to be effective processes in translating people's intentions to engage in physical activity into actually engaging in physical activity (Carraro & Gaudreau, 2013; Rhodes & Pfaeffli, 2010).

Application to concussion research

HAPA can be utilized to understand and change concussion-related behaviors. For instance, the HAPA variables of risk perceptions, outcome expectancies, and action self-efficacy could be used to understand coaches' intentions towards promoting safe play among their athletes (see example in Figure 6.1). Further, action and coping planning and maintenance self-efficacy could be measured to understand how coaches promote safe play. HAPA could also be used to develop concussion behavior change interventions. For example, researchers could have athletes create coping plans to report a concussion (for themselves and for teammates) as part of a pre-season concussion education session and measure concussion-reporting behaviors throughout a season.

Self-determination theory

Theoretical tenets

Self-determination theory (SDT) is a meta-theory of motivation and personality that is comprised of six mini-theories (Ryan & Deci, 2017). Similar to HAPA and TPB, SDT examines an individual's personal factors for engaging in behaviors. SDT diverges from HAPA and TPB because it also considers a person's environment. In SDT, the environment can positively or negatively influence a person's three basic psychological needs of autonomy, competence, and relatedness. If these three psychological needs are satisfied, a person's motivation to engage in a behavior will be more autonomous; whereas, controlled motivation is more likely to occur when the three basic psychological needs are being thwarted.[2] Having a more autonomous form of motivation is associated with increased positive affective, behavioral, and cognitive outcomes (Ryan & Deci, 2017; see Figure 6.2).

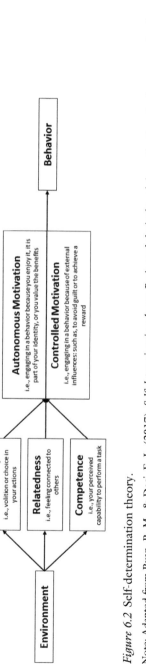

Figure 6.2 Self-determination theory.

Note: Adapted from Ryan, R. M., & Deci, E. L. (2017). *Self-determination theory: Basic psychological needs in motivation, development, and wellness.* New York, NY: The Guilford Press.

Empirical examples to understand behavior

SDT has been tested and supported across health behaviors and populations (Phillips & Guarnaccia, 2017). In a physical activity setting, autonomous motivation was found to be consistently and positively related with physical activity participation; whereas, controlled motivation had no relationship (Teixeira et al., 2012). Other studies have also supported the relationship between the basic psychological needs and autonomous motivation within a physical activity context (Barbeau, Sweet, & Fortier, 2010; McEwan & Sweet, 2012; Saebu, Sørensen, & Halvari, 2013).

Empirical examples to change behavior

SDT-based interventions have also been tested. For example, Silva and colleagues (2010) demonstrated that participants who were exposed to an SDT-based intervention had greater increases in physical activity and improvements in body composition when compared to a control group. Specifically, participants were provided with autonomy support during the intervention sessions and given techniques to promote competence towards maintaining their physical activity and weight loss goals. Intervention participants also had higher autonomous motivation than the control group (Silva et al., 2010). The intervention from Silva et al. is but one example of an intervention that demonstrates how researchers can promote autonomous motivation, which translates to the uptake of positive health behaviors. See Fortier et al. (2012) for a review of physical activity interventions grounded in SDT.

Application to concussion research

SDT can provide researchers with a lens to conceptualize and identify the environmental factors related to athletes' basic psychological needs and autonomous motivation. For instance, researchers could aim to understand how teammates', coaches', or parents' interpersonal interactions with the athletes are associated with athletes' basic psychological needs during concussion recovery. SDT-based interventions could also be designed to teach coaches how to interact with their athletes to foster athletes' autonomous motivation to engage in safe play or concussion-reporting.

Social ecological model

Theoretical tenets

The social ecological model (SEM) of human development is a framework for understanding the interactions between different systems of society. SEM extends from solely understanding (or changing) behavior at the individual or interpersonal levels, by also considering the role of society and social structures. There are five systems of the ecological environment and each of the systems influence behavior change in a different way (Brofenbrenner, 1977).

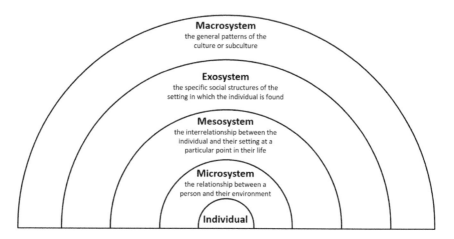

Figure 6.3 The social ecological model.

Note: Adapted from Brofenbrenner, U. (1977). Toward an experimental ecology of human development. *American Psychologist, 32,* 513–531. doi:10.1037/0003-066X.32.7.513.

To summarize briefly, the five systems are: (a) the individual; (b) the microsystem; (c) the mesosystem; (d) the exosystem; and (e) the macrosystem (see Figure 6.3, which provides definitions of the systems). According to SEM, all aspects of a person's environment are important for behavior change, and the interaction of these systems is necessary for understanding human behavior (Brofenbrenner, 1977; see Figure 6.3).

Empirical examples to understand behavior

Researchers have used SEM to help explain health-related behaviors. For example, Thornton et al. (2016) found that participants' demographic (i.e., being non-Hispanic white ethnicity), psychological (i.e., increased social support), and environmental (i.e., proximity to a park) factors were positively related to participation in moderate-to-vigorous physical activity. Thus, physical activity participation was influenced across three of SEM's systems: by (a) the individual (i.e., being non-Hispanic), (b) their microsystem (i.e., proximity to a park), and (c) their exosystem (i.e., increased social support).

SEM has also been used to explain condom use in female sex workers. Larios et al. (2009) found that the social structures that supported access to condoms (i.e., the exosystem) were negatively related to having unprotected sex. Whereas, working in a setting where female sex workers were provided with monetary incentives for unprotected sex was positively related to unprotected sex. Therefore, in this context, the social structures of sex workers (i.e., the exosystem) and the relationship between the sex worker and their setting (i.e., mesosystem) were essential in understanding female sex workers' condom-use behavior. As such,

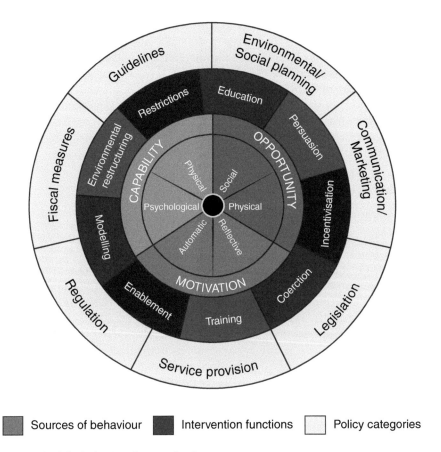

Sources of behaviour   Intervention functions   Policy categories

Figure 6.4 The behavior change wheel.

Note: From Michie, S., van Stralen, M. M., & West, R. (2011). The behaviour change wheel: A new method for characterising and designing behaviour change interventions. *Implementation Science*, 6, 42. doi:10.1186/1748-5908-6-42. Originally published by BioMed Central, open access under Creative Commons Attribution (CC-BY) license.

SEM allows researchers to understand the broader social contexts alongside the individual factors that predict behaviors.

Application to concussion research

SEM may also be pertinent for concussion research given that concussion-related behaviors are embedded within larger social structures that include teams, parents, fans, and media. To date, no research has used SEM to understand concussion-related behaviors. However, Kerr et al. (2014) conducted a systematic review on concussion disclosure and framed their findings in the structures of SEM. In their review, they found that the majority of the published articles

(n = 20) explored the individual reasons for not disclosing a concussion; whereas, only three articles examined policy level (macrosystem) reasons for the lack on concussion disclosure.

Other applications of SEM in concussion research could involve exploring the interactions between each of the five systems of SEM and concussion-reporting. For instance, an athlete's intentions to report a concussion could result more so from the effects of their macrosystem (i.e., the social construction of toughness in sport) than from their individual characteristics (i.e., their own beliefs about concussion-reporting). Once these systems are better understood, interventions targeting athletes' behaviors or policies/protocols could be developed.

The behavior change wheel

Theoretical tenets

The behavior change wheel (BCW) is a guide to designing and evaluating behavior change interventions and is composed of three layers (Michie, van Stralen, & West, 2011). The first layer is known as COM-B: that Capability, Opportunity, and Motivation are the key ingredients to performing a Behavior (Michie et al., 2011). The second layer provides nine intervention functions that can be used to target individuals' capability, opportunity, and motivation. The third layer identifies seven different types of policies that can be used to deliver the intervention functions. It is important to note that not all intervention functions target all COM-B variables and vice versa. The process through which researchers identify which policy and intervention functions they want to use to change a person's capability, opportunity, or motivation is called conducting a behavioral analysis. Performing a behavioral analysis prior to designing an intervention is a strength of the BCW.

Empirical examples to change behavior

The BCW is a relatively new framework and, as a result, the associated research is limited. In one example, researchers used the BCW to understand how to increase attendance at smoking cessation services (Fulton et al., 2016). Results from Fulton and colleagues' (2016) behavioral analysis indicated that the intervention functions that were most applicable to their intervention were: education, persuasion, modeling, incentivization, environmental restructuring, and enablement (Fulton et al., 2016). Thus, the findings from their study (i.e., the behavioral analysis) informed the ingredients that would be necessary for intervention.

Application to concussion research

There are a number of applications of COM-B for understanding and changing concussion-related behaviors. Specific to adherence to concussion rehabilitation, the COM-B model could be used to understand athletes' perceptions of how adhering to concussion rehabilitation is related to their short- and long-term health (i.e., capability) and how support from others (i.e., opportunity) is associated with adherence. In turn, once these factors were understood (i.e., the behavior analysis), researchers could design an intervention aimed at improving athletes' adherence to rehabilitation.

In sum, we have presented and explained four theories that we feel could be applied to understand and change concussion-related behaviors in the future. Below we provide some lessons learned from other fields when applying and testing theory to health behavior change, as well as discuss the implications of theory on future research in the field of concussions.

Implications for future research

The use of theory in concussion research is still in its early stages of development. As a result, a recommendation for concussion researchers is to learn from theory-driven research conducted in other health-related domains. Researchers using theory to understand or change concussion-related behaviors should be explicit and identify their frameworks at the forefront of the design of a research project. In doing so, researchers will have to identify and select the theoretical variables they plan on testing and the analyses they plan on running to ensure proper theory and hypothesis testing. Researchers who are unsure whether their study or intervention is theory-based should consult the Theory Coding Scheme (Michie & Prestwich, 2010). This tool was primarily designed to evaluate the use of theories in interventions, but it can also be used when designing a behavior change intervention (see Sweet et al., 2017 as an example).

How to use theory to inform research

Although it may seem intuitive, the first step in building a theory-based study or intervention is taking the time to decide which behavior(s) you would like to understand or change. The behavior you select must be something that can be measured by strong, validated tools. Once the behavior is identified, you can make an informed decision about the theory you should use. Identifying the behavior will also enable you to select the proper measures for the theory you selected. As well, to maximize the impact of a theory-based intervention, ensure that the ingredients of the intervention are directly aimed at changing the theoretical variables and the behavior selected.

Second, if testing a theory, it is critical that you test the entire theory rather than "cherry-picking" variables of the theory (Prestwich et al., 2014). As highlighted in Prestwich et al.'s (2014) meta-analysis, few interventions targeted all theoretical constructs from a specific theory. Similarly, Painter et al. (2008) reported that only 7% of studies that used a theory tested at least half of its constructs. These findings are concerning when considering that theories are conceptualized as interrelated constructs, but these interrelationships are not being properly tested in health behavior research. Therefore, we urge concussion researchers to include all of the variables of a theory when trying to understand or change concussion-related behaviors.

Third, Michie and Pretwich's (2010) Theory Coding Scheme is an excellent resource for researchers to consult when designing a theory-based intervention to ensure they account for all dimensions of a theory in their intervention. As Prestwich et al. (2014) found in their meta-analysis, health behavior interventions have rarely aligned components of their interventions with theoretical constructs. To determine the effectiveness of a theory-based intervention, it is critical that each intervention component is connected to the theoretical constructs you are aiming to foster. A few resources are available to help first classify the components of an intervention. For example, Michie and colleagues' (2011) taxonomy of behavior change techniques is a comprehensive list and definition of 93 possible intervention techniques (see the supplementary material of Michie et al., 2011). There is also a training course available for individuals who are interested in learning to code behavior change techniques in current interventions (www.bct-taxonomy.com/). For researchers conducting interventions that involve interactions between two or more individuals, it is important to use tools that take into account interpersonal techniques of the intervention. Researchers have previously noted that interpersonal techniques are missing from the Michie and colleagues' (2011) taxonomy of behavior change techniques (Hardcastle & Hagger, 2016). If relevant, researchers could look into the list of relational techniques reported in Hardcastle and colleagues' (2017) article or in the Motivational Interviewing Treatment Integrity tool (Moyers et al., 2016). Examples of intervention studies that linked intervention components to theoretical variables can be found in the literature; such as, interventions grounded in SDT (Fortier et al., 2007; Sweet et al., 2017).

Fourth, health behavior change researchers have recently criticized the continued use of TPB, and some have even called for its "retirement" (Sniehotta, Presseau, & Araújo-Soares, 2014). The reliance of observational designs and lack of experimental evidence (e.g., Rhodes & Dickau, 2012) provide a rationale for this "retirement," as does the growing awareness of the gap between intentions and behaviors (Sheeran & Webb, 2016). More explicit efforts are needed to examine the intention-behavior relationship, as multiple variables could explain this relationship (Sheeran & Webb, 2016). HAPA, which was explained earlier, suggests action and coping planning as variables that can bridge the intention to behavior gap. These variables, and others, could be utilized in concussion research to further understand the relationship between intentions and behavior (see Sheeran & Webb, 2016 for a review). In sum, we recommend that concussion researchers do not take for granted that intentions to engage in a behavior automatically lead to a change in behavior. Researchers are encouraged to find the appropriate theoretical framework or approach that can enhance that relationship in their study.

Conclusions

The recommendations presented in this chapter are in line with current available evidence and were presented with the intent of maximizing the use of theory in concussion research. We feel that concussion researchers are in a good position to continue using theory to understand and change concussion-related behaviors. Selecting, applying, and properly testing theory will help bring a deeper understanding of the psychosocial variables of concussion-related behaviors. Our hope is that this information will be of use to concussion researchers and help them avoid some of the same pitfalls experienced by researchers in other health-related domains.

Notes

1 Retrospective account of concussions occurred during their own athletic careers.
2 In this chapter, we have chosen to focus only on autonomous and controlled motivation. However, motivation, as per SDT, is much more complex than the description provided in this chapter. We encourage readers to consult Ryan and Deci (2017) for a more detailed description.

References

Ajzen, I. (1991). The theory of planned behavior. *Organizational Behavior and Human Decision Processes*, *50*, 179—211. doi:10.1016/0749-5978(91)90020-T.

Bandura, A. (2004). Health promotion by social cognitive means. *Health Education & Behavior*, *31*, 143–164. doi:10.1177/1090198104263660.

Barbeau, A., Sweet, S. N., & Fortier, M. S (2010). A path-analytic model of self-determination theory in a physical activity context. *Journal of Applied Biobehavioral Research,14*(3),103–118.doi:10.1111/j.1751-9861.2009.00043.x.

Brofenbrenner, U. (1977). Toward an experimental ecology of human development. *American Psychologist*, *32*, 513–531. doi:10.1037/0003-066X.32.7.513.

Carraro, N., & Gaudreau, P. (2013). Spontaneous and experimentally induced action planning and coping planning for physical activity: A meta-analysis. *Psychology of Sport and Exercise*, *14*, 228–248. doi:10.1016/j.psychsport.2012.10.004.

Colley, R. C., Garriguet, D., Janssen, I., Craig, C. L., Clarke, J., & Tremblay, M. S. (2011). Physical activity of Canadian adults: Accelerometer results from the 2007 to 2009 Canadian Health Measures Survey. *Health Reports*, *22*, 7–14.

Conner, M., & Norman, P. (2017). Health behaviour: Current issues and challenges. *Psychology & Health*, *32*(8), 895–906. doi: 10.1080/08870446.2017.1336240.

Delaney, J. S., Caron, J. G., Correa, J. A., & Bloom, G. A. (2018). Why professional football players chose not to reveal their concussion symptoms during a practice or game. *Clinical Journal of Sport Medicine*, *28*, 1–12. doi:10.1097/JSM.0000000000000495.

de Ridder, D., Kroese, F., Evers, C., Adriaanse, M., & Gillebaart, M. (2017). Healthy diet: Health impact, prevalence, correlates, and interventions. *Psychology & Health*, *32*, 907–941. doi:10.1080/08870446.2017.1316849.

Ernsting, A., Gellert, P., Schneider, M., & Lippke, S. (2013). A mediator model to predict workplace influenza vaccination behaviour: An application of the health action process approach. *Psychology & Health*, *28*, 579–592. doi:10.1080/08870446.2012.753072.

Fortier, M. S., Duda, J. L., Guerin, E., & Teixeira, P. J. (2012). Promoting physical activity: Development and testing of self-determination theory-based interventions. *International Journal of Behavioral Nutrition and Physical Activity*, *9*, 20–34. doi:10.1186/1479-5868-9-20.

Fortier, M. S., Sweet, S. N., O'Sullivan, T. L., & Williams, G. C. (2007). A self-determination process model of physical activity adoption in the context of a randomized controlled trial. *Psychology of Sport and Exercise, 8*, 741–757. doi:10.1016/j.psychsport.2006.10.006.

Fulton, E. A., Brown, K. E., Kwah, K. L., & Wild, S. (2016). StopApp: Using the behaviour change wheel to develop an app to increase uptake and attendance at NHS Stop Smoking Services. *Healthcare, 4*, 31–46. doi:10.3390/healthcare4020031.

Hardcastle, S. J., Fortier, M., Blake, N., & Hagger, M. S. (2017). Identifying content-based and relational techniques to change behaviour in motivational interviewing. *Health Psychology Review, 11*, 1–16. doi:10.1080/17437199.2016.1190659.

Hardcastle, S. J., & Hagger, M. S. (2016). Psychographic profiling for effective health behavior change interventions. *Frontiers in Psychology, 6*, 1–2. doi:10.3389/fpsyg.2015.01988.

Hunt, T. N., Harris, L., & Way, D. (2017). The impact of concussion education on the knowledge and perceived expertise of novice health care professionals. *Athletic Training Education Journal, 12*, 26–38. doi: 10.4085/120126.

Kelly, M. P., & Barker, M. (2016). Why is changing health-related behaviour so difficult? *Public Health, 136*, 109–116. doi:10.1016/j.puhe.2016.03.030.

Kerr, Z. Y., Register-Mihalik, J. K., Marshall, S. W., Evenson, K. R., Mihalik, J. P., & Guskiewicz, K. M. (2014). Disclosure and non-disclosure of concussion and concussion symptoms in athletes: Review and application of the socio-ecological framework. *Brain Injury, 28*, 1009–1021. doi:10.3109/02699052.2014.904049.

Kroshus, E., Baugh, C. M., Daneshvar, D. H., & Viswanath, K. (2014). Understanding concussion reporting using a model based on the theory of planned behavior. *Journal of Adolescent Health, 54*, 269–274. doi:10.1016/j.jadohealth.2013.11.011.

Kroshus, E., Garnett, B., Hawrilenko, M., Baugh, C. M., & Calzo, J. P. (2015). Concussion under-reporting and pressure from coaches, teammates, fans, and parents. *Social Science & Medicine, 134*, 66–75. doi:10.1016/j.socscimed.2015.04.011.

Kroshus, E., Garnett, B. R., Baugh, C. M., & Calzo, J. P. (2016). Engaging teammates in the promotion of concussion help seeking. *Health Education & Behavior, 43*, 442–451. doi:10.1177/1090198115602676.

Larios, S. E., Lozada, R., Strathdee, S. A., Semple, S. J., Roesch, S., Staines, H., ... Magis-Rodriguez, C. (2009). An exploration of contextual factors that influence HIV risk in female sex workers in Mexico: The social ecological model applied to HIV risk behaviors. *AIDS Care, 21*, 1335–1342. doi:10.1080/09540120902803190.

McEwan, D., & Sweet, S. N. (2012). Needs satisfaction, self-determined motivation and health-enhancing physical activity. *Health and Fitness Journal of Canada, 5*, 3–17.

Michie, S., & Prestwich, A. (2010). Are interventions theory-based? Development of a theory coding scheme. *Health Psychology, 29*, 1–8. doi:10.1037/a0016939.

Michie, S., van Stralen, M. M., & West, R. (2011). The behaviour change wheel: A new method for characterising and designing behaviour change interventions. *Implementation Science, 6*, 42. doi:10.1186/1748-5908-6-42.

Michie, S., Atkins, L., & West, R. (2014). *The behaviour change wheel: A guide to designing interventions*. Great Britain: Silverback publishing.

Michie, S. F., West, R., Campbell, R., Brown, J., & Gainforth, H. (2014). *ABC of behaviour change theories*. Great Britain: Silverback Publishing.

Moor, H. M., Eisenhauer, R. C., Killian, K. D., Proudfoot, N., Henriques, A. A., Congeni, J. A., & Reneker, J. C. (2015). The relationship between adherence behaviors and recovery time in adolescents after a sports-related concussion: An observational study. *International Journal of Sports Physical Therapy, 10*, 225–233.

Moyers, T. B., Rowell, L. N., Manuel, J. K., Ernst, D., & Houck, J. M. (2016). The motivational interviewing treatment integrity code (MITI 4): Rationale, preliminary reliability and validity. *Journal of Substance Abuse Treatment, 65*, 36–42. doi:10.1016/j.jsat.2016.01.001.

Newton, J. D., White, P. E., Ewing, M. T., Makdissi, M., Davis, G. A., Donaldson, A., ... & Finch, C. F. (2014). Intention to use sport concussion guidelines among community-level coaches and sports trainers. *Journal of Science and Medicine in Sport, 17*, 469–473. doi: 10.1016/j.jsams.2013.10.240.

Painter, J. E., Borba, C. P., Hynes, M., Mays, D., & Glanz, K. (2008). The use of theory in health behavior research from 2000 to 2005: A systematic review. *Annals of Behavioral Medicine, 35*, 358–362. doi:10.1007/s12160-008-9042-y.

Phillips, A. S., & Guarnaccia, C. A. (2017). Self-determination theory and motivational interviewing interventions for type 2 diabetes prevention and treatment: A systematic review. *Journal of Health Psychology*, Advanced Online Publication. doi:10.1177/1359105317737606.

Popper, K. R. (1962). On the sources of knowledge and of ignorance. *Philosophy and Phenomenological Research, 23*, 292–293. doi:10.2307/2104935.

Prestwich, A., Sniehotta, F. F., Whittington, C., Dombrowski, S. U., Rogers, L., & Michie, S. (2014). Does theory influence the effectiveness of health behavior interventions? Meta-analysis. *Health Psychology, 33*, 465–474. doi:10.1037/a0032853.

Radtke, T., Scholz, U., Keller, R., & Hornung, R. (2012). Smoking is ok as long as I eat healthily: Compensatory health beliefs and their role for intentions and smoking within the Health Action Process Approach. *Psychology & Health, 27*, 91–107. doi:10.1080/08870446.2011.603422.

Register-Mihalik, J. K., Linnan, L. A., Marshall, S. W., McLeod, T. C. V., Mueller, F. O., & Guskiewicz, K. M. (2013). Using theory to understand high school aged athletes' intentions to report sport-related concussion: Implications for concussion education initiatives. *Brain Injury, 27*, 878–886. doi:10.3109/02699052.2013.775508.

Rhodes, R. E., & Dickau, L. (2012). Experimental evidence for the intention-behavior relationship in the physical activity domains: A meta-analysis. *Health Psychology, 31*(6), 724–727. doi: 10.1037/a0027290.

Rhodes, R. E., & Pfaeffli, L. A. (2010). Mediators of physical activity behaviour change among adult non-clinical populations: A review update. *International Journal of Behavioral Nutrition and Physical Activity, 7*(1), 37–48. doi: 10.1186/1479-5868-7-37.

Rigby, J., Vela, L., & Housman, J. (2013). Understanding athletic trainers' beliefs toward a multifaceted sport-related concussion approach: Application of the theory of planned behavior. *Journal of Athletic Training, 48*, 636–644. doi: 10.4085/1062-6050-48.3.10.

Ryan, R. M., & Deci, E. L. (2017). *Self-Determination Theory: Basic Psychological Needs in Motivation, Development, and Wellness.* New York, NY: The Guilford Press.

Saebu, M., Sørensen, M., & Halvari, H. (2013). Motivation for physical activity in young adults with physical disabilities during a rehabilitation stay: A longitudinal test of self-determination theory. *Journal of Applied Social Psychology, 43*, 612–625. doi:10.1111/j.1559-1816.2013.01042.x.

Schwarzer, R. (2008). Modeling health behavior change: How to predict and modify the adoption and maintenance of health behaviors. *Applied Psychology, 57*, 1–29. doi:10.1111/j.1464-0597.2007.00325.x.

Schwarzer, R. (2014, October 13). Health Action Process Approach. Retrieved January 29, 2018, from www.hapa-model.de/.

Sheeran P., & Webb, T. L. (2016). The intention-behavior gap. *Social and Personality Psychology Compass, 10*, 503–518. doi:10.1111/spc3.12265.

Silva, M. N., Vieira, P. N., Coutinho, S. R., Minderico, C. S., Matos, M. G., Sardinha, L. B., & Teixeira, P. J. (2010). Using self-determination theory to promote physical activity and weight control: A randomized controlled trial in women. *Journal of Behavioural Medicine, 33*, 110–122. doi:10.1007/s10865-009-9239-y.

Sniehotta, F. F., Scholz, U., & Schwarzer, R. (2005). Bridging the intention-behaviour gap: Planning, self-efficacy, and action control in the adoption and maintenance of physical exercise. *Psychology & Health, 20*, 143–160. doi:10.1080/08870440512331317670.

Sniehotta, F. F., Presseau, J., & Araújo-Soares, V. (2014). Time to retire the theory of planned behaviour. *Health Psychology Review, 8*, 1–7. doi:10.1080/17437199.2013.869710.

Sweet, S. N., Rocchi, M., Arbour-Nicitopoulos, K., Kairy, D., & Fillion, B. (2017). A telerehabilitation approach to enhance quality of life through exercise among adults with paraplegia: Study protocol. *JMIR Research Protocols, 6*, e202. doi:10.2196/resprot.8047.

Teixeira, P. J., Carraça, E. V, Markland, D., Silva, M. N., & Ryan, R. M. (2012). Exercise, physical activity, and self-determination theory: A systematic review. *International Journal of Behavioral Nutrition and Physical Activity, 9*, 78–108. doi:10.1186/1479-5868-9-78.

Teng, Y., & Mak, W. W. S. (2011). The role of planning and self-efficacy in condom use among men who have sex with men: An application of the Health Action Process Approach model. *Health Psychology, 30*, 119–128. doi:10.1037/a0022023

Thornton, C. M., Kerr, J., Conway, T. L., Saelens, B. E., Sallis, J. F., Ahn, D. K., … King, A. C. (2016). Physical activity in older adults: An ecological approach. *Annals of Behavioral Medicine, 51*(2), 119–128.

7 A psychological skills training program for concussed athletes

Cassandra M. Seguin and Natalie Durand-Bush

Introduction

> There's one thing that I wouldn't wish on my worst enemy. It's not the head shot I took. I can barely remember that part. It's not even the pain and anxiety that I went through after the hit. The thing that I wouldn't wish on my worst enemy is the moment when you know that it's all over. Everything you've worked for since you were a kid … it's really over, and you can't fool yourself anymore.
>
> (Former National Hockey League player Marc Savard, *Players' Tribune*, May 16, 2017)

Concussions have become a high priority in the last 20 years, particularly in sport (Daneshvar et al., 2011). Courageous athletes like Canadian professional hockey player Marc Savard, New Zealand All Blacks rugby player Ben Afeaki, and U.S. bobsledder Elana Meyers Taylor have recounted their difficult experiences with concussions in the media in the hopes of raising awareness and providing assistance to athletes facing similar challenges. Advocates and sport organizations have also been conducting work to prevent and reduce these types of brain injuries in sport, as they can have serious long-lasting implications for the physical and mental health of athletes. For example, Hockey Hall of Fame goaltender Ken Dryden has been pressuring the National Hockey League to penalize any play involving intentional head contact. His new book titled *Game Change: The Life and Death of Steve Montador and the Future of Hockey* (Dryden, 2017) sheds light on the urgency to keep athletes safer in sport.

Despite this ongoing work, injuries remain a common occurrence in sport. Interestingly, studies have shown that psychological skills are important for the rehabilitation of injured athletes (Arvinen-Barrow et al., 2015; Clement, Granquist, & Arvinen-Barrow, 2013; Hamson-Utley, Martin, & Walters, 2008; I. Yoon & Y-J. Yoon, 2014). For instance, Arvinen-Barrow and colleagues (2015) reported that goal setting, imagery, positive self-talk, and relaxation are key in athletes' recovery from sport injuries. I. Yoon & Y-J. Yoon (2014) stated that the implementation of a PST program with an injured professional soccer player that targeted goal-setting, anxiety reduction, concentration, and confidence led to decreases in anxiety, depression, tension, and fatigue, as well as increases in concentration, confidence, and vigor.

Based on the aforementioned findings, one could argue that such psychological skills may be valuable for the specific rehabilitation of concussion injuries. The integration of such skills could ultimately support pre-existing multi-faceted concussion treatment plans. These treatment approaches often include prescribed exercise, pharmacological interventions, vestibular therapy, oculomotor and vision therapies, and cognitive therapy interventions (Elbin, Schatz, Lowder, & Kontos, 2014). However, they do not focus on psychological skills training. Thus, specific and accessible psychological skills programs or interventions to guide this aspect of the recovery of concussed athletes remain limited.

The following chapter introduces a Psychological Skills Training (PST) program that we designed to assist athletes in their post-concussion rehabilitation process. The program was developed based on the literature on concussions and sport psychology, as well as Zimmerman's (2000) model of self-regulated learning and performance. The six week program fosters athletes' learning and application of self-regulation, goal-setting, relaxation, and imagery skills to improve self-control and symptom experience. We first provide a definition of concussions and briefly review common symptoms and treatment options. We then address how the PST program was developed, describe the sections of the program, and provide concrete strategies to implement it. Finally, we share recommendations for future research and practice.

Definition and symptoms of concussions

Researchers have had difficulties agreeing upon a definition for concussions (e.g. Helmy, Agarwal, & Hutchinson, 2013; McCrea et al., 2012), the signs and symptoms of concussions (e.g. Chiang et al., 2016; King, 2014), and the effective management of post-concussion rehabilitation (Terrell et al., 2014; Thomas et al., 2017). Recently, McCrory and colleagues (2017) published the *5th Consensus statement on concussion in sport*, in which they defined concussions as "a traumatic brain injury induced by biomechanical forces" (McCrory et al., 2017, p. 839). The impact created by these forces causes brain tissues to deform due to increased intracranial pressure (Ruhe, Gansslen, & Klein, 2013). According to Gay (2016), such impacts from biomechanical forces and intracranial pressure can lead to metabolic dysregulation, oxidative damage and apoptosis, and a variety of other molecular impacts and conditions. Despite the recent increase in sport-related concussion awareness and the acknowledgment of the unique and individual nature of the concussion experience (Gay, 2016; Stoler & Hill, 2013), serious gaps pertaining to the management of concussions remain (Government of Canada, 2018).

Concussions, in general, are difficult injuries to study due to variation in the experience of impact, degree of severity, and resulting symptoms (Stoler & Hill, 2013). Symptoms can affect individuals not only physically (e.g., headaches; Jordan 2013) but also psychologically (e.g., anxiety; Caron et al., 2013), behaviorally (impulsiveness; e.g., Lynch et al., 2015), emotionally (e.g., depression; Caron et al., 2013), and socially (e.g., social isolation; Delaney et al., 2015). According to McCrory and colleagues (2017), *post-concussion syndrome* or *persistent post-concussive symptoms* involve "symptoms that persist beyond expected time frames (i.e., < 10–14 days in adults and < 4 weeks in children)" (p. 842). Given the range of concussion symptoms and experiences, person-centered approaches encompassing different intervention techniques are required to best meet the needs of athletes recovering from concussions.

Treatment of concussions

Due to the lack of research specifically focusing on *sport-related* concussion rehabilitation measures, general rehabilitation practices introduced as "concussion" and "mild TBI" treatment strategies are presented. Complete rest has traditionally been recommended during the recovery process until all symptoms have been alleviated (Anderson, 2012; Moran et al., 2015). More recently, nutritional supplements (Ashbaugh & McGrew, 2016), pharmaceutical treatments, such as amitriptyline (Burke et al., 2015; Moran et al., 2015), massage techniques (Burns, 2015), progressive exercise (Broglio et al., 2014; Moran et al., 2015), and targeted breathing (Burns, 2015) have emerged as possible treatment modalities. Other researchers have focused on psychosocial components of symptom management, for example, psychoeducation programs (Caron et al., 2015; Davies, 2016), cognitive behavioral treatment (Kjeldgaard et al., 2014; Sayegh, Sandford, & Carson, 2010), social engagement (Snell et al., 2015), and client-centered counseling approaches (Rees & Bellon, 2007). However, there has been little discussion of the use of PST programs for concussion rehabilitation.

Only in recent years has psychological skills training been considered as a management strategy for concussion injuries. For example, Bloom et al. (2004) suggested the following:

> The use of sport psychology techniques in the management of concussion may assist in solving some of the real and very practical problems facing clinicians, namely certain aspects of the post-concussive syndrome and the influence of anxiety and other adverse psychological states, which in turn may impact on injury outcome.
>
> (p. 520)

To our knowledge, this information has not been applied, and researchers have yet to develop multi-faceted psychological approaches for the management of concussion symptoms in athletes. This area of research remains in its infancy, and a need has been expressed for the development of PST programs to assist individuals who are recovering from sport-related concussions (Kontos, Byrd, & Cormier, 2017).

While research on the use of psychological skills for the rehabilitation of concussed athletes is practically non-existent, some researchers have shed light on potential psychological skills training methods through which athletes' concussion symptoms could be supported. According to Waid-Ebbs and colleagues (2014), goal-management training may be useful to address executive function deficits, such as difficulties completing tasks that involve planning, decision-making, and information processing. In their study, this form of training included defining goals, listing steps required for goal achievement, and regularly revisiting goals to ensure barriers were addressed and adjustments were made as needed. Results revealed significant performance improvements across executive functions on the implemented computerized task, although the researchers noted a lack of generalizability across populations (Waid-Ebbs et al., 2014).

In another study, a ten-week mindfulness-based, stress-reduction training was delivered to individuals suffering from chronic mild TBIs and post-concussive syndrome (Azulay et al., 2013). Specifically, the program was based on what Kabat-Zinn (1982) identified as regular mindfulness meditation, which includes body scans, mindfulness breath, and a variety of yoga exercises. Azulay and colleagues (2013) altered this program to address the TBI population by reducing group sizes, increasing explanation and practice times, and adding several repetition opportunities to each homework assignment. Engagement in these activities increased participants' quality of life, self-efficacy, awareness, and TBI symptoms. Furthermore, Azulay and colleagues (2013) noted an important connection to attention and self-regulation training, which they suggested should be further investigated within the TBI population. Additionally, Schwab Reese, Pittsinger, and Yang (2012) found that imagery and relaxation training were successful in reducing concussion symptoms (e.g., anxiety) and increasing psychological coping skills (e.g., emotion regulation) in injured competitive and recreational athletes aged 17 and older.

Mental performance consultants (MPCs),[1] who are psychological skills training specialists, can play a vital role in the rehabilitation of concussed athletes. MPCs work primarily in sport and exercise contexts to help athletes develop psychosocial competencies to strengthen their athletic performance and well-being. MPCs support athletes' goals and efforts to optimize their functioning and cope with daily stressors associated with their sport and general life (Canadian Sport Psychology Association, 2018; Association for Applied Sport Psychology, 2018). However, while MPCs have knowledge and training in sport sciences, counseling, and psychology, many are not trained as clinical psychologists and cannot diagnose and treat mental disorders. Nonetheless, they play an important role as a member of athletes' integrated support teams and can contribute to the management of concussion symptoms (Covassin et al., 2013). Since athletes may experience clinical symptoms and develop a mental illness as a result of a concussion (Caron et al., 2013), MPCs who are not clinically trained should refer athletes to a registered psychologist if they observe such symptoms.

In sum, goal-setting, self-regulated practice, imagery, and relaxation appear to be valuable psychological skills that could be included in a structured program designed to assist athletes in the management of their concussion symptoms. MPCs could feasibly integrate these skills into a self-regulation framework to empower individuals to take charge of their recovery through planning, self-monitoring, and self-reflection (Durand-Bush, McNeill, & Collins, 2015; Zimmerman, 2000). Concussed athletes could then exert some self-control in identifying, monitoring, and evaluating symptoms and goals throughout their rehabilitation process.

A psychological skills training program for concussed athletes

Development of the PST program

The PST program for concussed athletes was developed as a tool that MPCs can implement with athletes who have sustained a concussion. It is based on the literature and a mental skills workbook that has been successfully used with healthy and injured athletes (Durand-Bush, 2016). The goal of this program is to help athletes during their post-concussion recovery process by implementing psychological skills to improve their overall functioning and their physical, cognitive, emotional, behavioral, and/or social concussion symptoms. It is not meant to replace concussion rehabilitative practices, but rather to support athletes through the use of psychological skills and strategies. The program itself is composed of four psychological skills training sections, each including a variety of exercises that can be geared toward the athletes' personal experience. The content of each section will be illustrated in subsequent tables. The general sequence of the program is as follows: (1) Intake and Self-Regulation, (2) Goal-Setting and Goal-Management, (3) Relaxation, (4) Imagery, and (5) Wrap-Up and Future Plans. However, sections can be re-ordered based on preference and symptom priority.

This program should be implemented relatively early in the recovery process (e.g., as early as 48–72 hours post-injury; McCrory et al., 2017) so that athletes can begin to manage their injury as soon as possible. Ideally, MPCs should introduce one section of the PST program each week of the six-week program so that athletes can learn and implement mental skills on a gradual and consistent basis and avoid symptom thresholds. However, the program and individual sessions should be tailored to athletes' needs (Koehn, Morris, & Watt, 2014) and take into consideration the severity and frequency of their symptoms and overall mental state (Venville et al., 2015). For instance, if athletes are experiencing severe symptoms, it may be necessary to have sessions every two weeks or to have shorter sessions. On the other hand, athletes with mild symptoms may be able to tolerate two sessions per week to get through the program more quickly. While it is recommended to introduce all four sections, some programs may be condensed to only address a few select skills based on athletes' preferences and recommendations from medical staff. Irrespective of the length of athletes' rehabilitation process and severity of concussion symptoms, MPCs should always work in collaboration with the other members of athletes' integrated support teams (e.g., physician, concussion specialist, athletic therapist, strength and conditioning coach) to optimize the recovery process (Johnston et al., 2004).

MPCs should exercise caution in their selection of consulting techniques when working with concussed athletes. For example, although person-centered approaches are ideal to address the subjective nature of athletes' experience, they can place too much cognitive demand on the athletes. Thus, more directive, concrete, and/or behavioral approaches are appropriate when individuals' cognitive abilities are impaired (Miltenberger, 2012; Wilson, 2011). Additionally, concussion injuries require great understanding and control of symptom thresholds (e.g., athletes should stop an activity if symptoms arise or persist; McCrory et al., 2017). However, as seen in high-performance sport, athletes train to continually surpass pain and performance thresholds (Astokorki & Mauger, 2016), an aspect that may become integral to their athletic and personal identities (Martin, Fogarty, & Albion, 2014). Yet, this is typically counterintuitive to recommended approaches for concussion recovery (McCrory et al., 2017), and as such, athletes may be required to adjust their expectations and goals during their rehabilitation process. MPCs can help athletes by promoting threshold understanding, tolerance, and acceptance throughout the PST program. McCrory and colleagues (2017) make this explicit in their discussion of rest and recovery:

> After a brief period of rest during the acute phase (24–48 hours) after injury, patients can be encouraged to become gradually and progressively more active while staying below their cognitive and physical symptom-exacerbation thresholds (i.e., activity level should not bring on or worsen their symptoms).
>
> (p. 842)

It is important to recognize that the effects of the PST program may not be immediate, thus delayed gratification must be expected. Moreover, as with any intervention program, athletes must be committed to the process and try, to the best of their abilities, to complete the exercises that are offered. Athletes must also be honest with themselves and the MPC. Should any of the exercises negatively impact the athletes' recovery, they should be modified or terminated.

Illustration of the PST program

Section 1: Intake and self-regulation

The first section of the PST program focuses on assessment and self-regulation. The intake process involves collecting athletes' basic demographic information (e.g., name, address, age, sport, competition level, date, and types of injuries, etc.) and major areas of concern and interest (e.g., anxiety, self-confidence, fear of re-injury, performance slump, etc.) using a standard intake form or an interview guide. It is recommended to ask athletes if they prefer to provide the information verbally or in writing, given that writing may be too taxing on them. Written or verbal tasks may also be broken down into smaller increments (e.g., 10–15 minutes) to make them more manageable. The intake process is meant to give MPCs insight into the athletes' injury, concerns/issues, and mental skills that would be important to address in the PST program.

The self-regulation component is informed by Zimmerman's (2000) work. Self-regulation involves the effective management of one's inner states (i.e., thoughts, emotions, physiology), behaviors, and environment. It is cyclical in nature because feedback is continuously used to make adjustments from past to present self-regulatory efforts. Adjustments are necessary because "personal, behavioral, and environmental factors are constantly changing during the course of learning and performance, and must be observed or monitored" (Zimmerman, 2000, p. 14). In the case of concussions, this is particularly important since athletes' experiences are unique; athletes must be aware of their symptoms and progress through ongoing self-monitoring during the recovery process and after they return to play.

To facilitate this, MPCs may begin by going through a checklist of symptoms with athletes and ask them to note the severity and frequency of these symptoms (see Table 7.1). Athletes should also note symptom triggers as well as conditions that intensify or minimize their symptom experience. Self-regulation can then be enacted to avoid symptom triggers and increase exposure to stimuli leading to progress. Through self-awareness, athletes can learn to regulate their behaviors to respect their needs during recovery. MPCs using this tool should specify that it is intended to help athletes better understand their unique concussion experience and promote self-monitoring. This checklist is not meant to replace neuropsychological and other forms of medical symptom evaluation, nor to evaluate symptoms for any type of return to learn or return to play decisions.

Positive and negative triggers for symptom management

The following self-monitoring exercise is designed to assist athletes in tracking specific behaviors and factors that can positively or negatively impact the severity and frequency of their symptoms. By keeping a log of daily activities, sleep, nutrition, hydration, and interactions, athletes can become more aware of what helps or hinders their symptom experience. This log should be kept in whatever form works best for them; for example, if athletes find writing challenging, they can use an audio log. They will likely have a good idea of what influences their symptoms, but it is important to provide the clearest picture possible to inform their future self-regulatory efforts.

MPCs can invite athletes to keep a log of the following components over the course of the following week (see Table 7.2):

- Sleep (number of hours, naps, sleep latency and disturbances, fatigue during day/night; e.g., took an hour to fall asleep)
- Nutrition (type, amount, and time of meals, vitamins, supplements; e.g., omega-3, magnesium)
- Hydration (type, amount, and time of fluid consumption; e.g., water, coffee)
- Activities (type, frequency, and time of activities; e.g., homework, meetings)
- Interactions (type, frequency, and impact of interactions; e.g., in person, phone, email, text, positive/negative)
- Mood and energy (morning, afternoon, evening; e.g., positive mood, medium energy throughout morning)

Table 7.1 Concussion symptom checklist

Concussion Symptom Checklist. Note the symptoms you are currently experiencing by placing a checkmark in all boxes that apply. Indicate the severity and frequency of your symptoms and which ones are a priority for you.

Physical Symptoms

☐ Concussive Convulsions
☐ (Excessive) Fatigue
☐ Hand Tremors
☐ Headaches
☐ Impact Seizures
☐ Leg Tremors

☐ Nausea
☐ Neck Pain
☐ Sexual Dysfunction
☐ Stationary Loss of Balance
☐ Vomiting
☐ Unsteadiness While Walking

Comments

Cognitive Symptoms

☐ Amnesia/Other Memory Impairments
☐ Blurred Vision
☐ Confusion
☐ Decreased Speed of
   Information Processing
☐ Difficulty Concentrating
☐ Disorientation
☐ Dizziness
☐ Easily Distracted

☐ Feeling in a Fog
☐ Loss of Smell
☐ Loss of Taste
☐ Nightmares (Beyond Usual
   Frequency)
☐ Not Feeling Present (Aware)
☐ Sensitivity to Light (Photophobia)
☐ Sensitivity to Sound (Hyperacusis)
☐ Vertigo

Comments

Emotional Symptoms

☐ Anger
☐ Anxiety
☐ Depression
☐ Helplessness

☐ Mood Swings
☐ Nervousness
☐ Unusual Frustration
☐ Fear

Comments

Behavioral Symptoms

☐ Decreased Reaction Time
☐ Difficulty Falling Asleep
☐ Impulsive
☐ Impaired Performance
   (if returned to play)

☐ Impaired Coordination
☐ Abnormal Decisions (making
   choices you would not normally
   make)
☐ Staring Off into Space

Comments

Social Symptoms

☐ Decreased Desire to Engage in Social
   Activities
☐ Difficulty Finding Words

☐ Difficulty Speaking
☐ Feeling Socially Isolated

Comments

Table 7.2 Log of daily activities

Log of Daily Activities. For the next week, keep a record of your daily activities so you can track what helps and what hinders your recovery process. Make copies of the sheet below and note your responses for each day of the week.

Date _____

Sleep
How did I sleep last night, and for how long? Did I have a hard time falling asleep? Was I able to stay asleep? Did I have any nightmares? Did I feel rested when I woke up this morning? Did I nap during the day?

Food & Hydration
What and when did I eat/drink today? Did I take any vitamins/supplements? Did this have a positive, negative, or no impact?

Breakfast	Time of day _____
Lunch	Time of day _____
Dinner	Time of day _____
Snacks	Time of day _____
Fluids	Time of day _____
Vitamins/Supplements	Time of day _____

Activities
What did I do today and when/for how long? Was I effective or not?

Social Interactions
Did I talk to/do things with people today, and if so, when and for how long? Were these interactions positive, negative, or neutral?

Mood
How was my mood today? Was it consistent throughout the day? If not, how often did it fluctuate? What triggered my mood changes?

Energy
How was my energy today? Was it consistent throughout the day? At what point of the day was I most energized and most tired?

After completing the log for a week, MPCs should help athletes identify patterns in symptom experience in relation to the different components they tracked and integrate this information in the following goal-setting/goal-management section. Athletes should be invited to discuss any self-management skills and strategies they are currently using to (1) avoid stimuli that worsen symptoms and (2) seek stimuli that promote healing. From this point on, athletes should do regular check-ins throughout the day to reflect on their physical, cognitive, behavioral, emotional, and social symptoms and regularly note in their log how they are progressing throughout the PST program. Sharing their observations with trustworthy friends or family members promotes positive social interactions and support, which are vital for self-regulation and recovery (Covassin et al., 2014).

Section 2: Goal-setting and goal-management

The second section of the PST program focuses on goal-setting and goal-management. According to a systematic review conducted by Heaney et al. (2015), goal-setting is one of the most important psychological skills employed in sport injury rehabilitation. Brett, Skykes, and Pires-Yfantouda (2017) reiterated this point in their own review, indicating that goal-setting "is widely considered to be best practice in facilitating client involvement and engagement with rehabilitation" (p. 960).

This section of the program is therefore designed to help athletes set weekly and daily goals using the SMARTEST principle (Durand-Bush, 2016) and integrates goals of self-acceptance (Orlick, 2015). Due to the nature of concussions, recovery can be a difficult process requiring constant adjustment. Setting and managing goals is therefore an important step in the athletes' recovery, as goals direct athletes' self-regulatory efforts (Zimmerman, 2000).

Athletes are typically familiar with goal-setting, however it is important that this skill be properly explained in line with concussion rehabilitation. With physical injuries, rehabilitation and progress are often easy to track; for example, athletes can do physiotherapy and *see* improvements in strength, range of motion, and movement control. Part of what makes concussions challenging for athletes is that they cannot always see and feel progress. Furthermore, if athletes overly focus on long-term recovery, a lack of perceivable progress could potentially hinder their motivation and self-efficacy; hence, the value of discussing delay of gratification during the goal achievement process (Zimmerman, 2000). Setting short-term and daily goals and respecting the SMARTEST principle helps to provide purpose and meaning and increase perceived control and success during the athletes' demanding journey.

SMARTEST goals

SMARTEST goals (Specific, Measurable, Action-Based, Realistic, Time-Based, Elastic, Sensation-Matched, and Trustworthy) enable athletes to establish concrete and measurable targets to attain, while enacting a feasible action plan allowing them to stay focused on the present. SMARTEST goals also help athletes to sufficiently stretch their goals to achieve success and work within a self-determined time frame to remain motivated. Finally, SMARTEST goals allow athletes to stay in tune with their emotions and bodily sensations and strive to feel the way they want while accomplishing their goals, which fosters motivation and self-efficacy. Equally, by integrating a period to repeat the achievement of goals, athletes learn the importance of deliberate practice and maintenance in order to optimize learning and refrain from setting new targets too quickly, which can set them up for failure. Within the PST program, MPCs should help athletes set SMARTEST goals at the beginning of each week, which can be complemented by daily goals and goals of self-acceptance (see Table 7.3).

Goals of self-acceptance

Goals of self-acceptance are designed to help athletes to be kind to themselves and to be patient, particularly if they do not recover as smoothly and as quickly as desired. Some questions that may be considered when designing these goals are listed below.

- How can I be okay with myself when I am not participating in my sport?
- If I am not able to reach one or some of my short-term goals, how can I help myself stay motivated?
- Which resources are available to me through this process (e.g., support staff, family, personal skills, education/knowledge)?
- How can I stay committed to myself and remember that I am a worthy human being, even when things do not go as planned?

Weekly, daily, and self-acceptance goals should be kept in a visible place to serve as a reminder when athletes need it. These goals should be monitored by both athletes and MPCs and revised as necessary through effective goal management (e.g., regular check-ins). For instance, if symptoms worsen as a result of a particular goal, this goal should be adapted or discontinued. As previously mentioned, focusing on more immediate goals is strongly encouraged. If athletes digress to more long-term objectives, MPCs can gently bring them back to short-term goals that are within their control. Once symptoms have been alleviated, long-term goals (e.g., return to play) may be easier to envision.

Section 3: Relaxation

Concussions are often stressful for athletes, particularly if their future in sport is unknown. Based on the symptoms identified in Section 1 and the goals set in Section 2, relaxation can be introduced as a valuable psychological skill in this third component of the PST program. Relaxation is a technique that can help athletes to counter the stress response and decrease their arousal to an optimal level for different tasks they need to perform (Arvinen-Barrow et al., 2015;

Table 7.3 SMARTEST goals

Specific	Formulate your goal in a clear, detailed, positive manner based on what you want to accomplish or improve.
	ex. Improve the length of time I exercise on my stationary bike.
Measurable	Quantify your goal to be able to measure what you accomplish or improve and compare your current and desired target.
	ex. Improve the length of time I exercise on my stationary bike from 15 to 20 minutes.
Action-Based	Identify the actions required to reach your goal in order to guide your efforts and focus on appropriate elements or steps.
	ex. Exercise when I get up in the morning since I have more energy then. Prepare my water bottle to stay hydrated while I exercise. Listen to music while exercising to stay motivated. Talk to myself positively to remain confident in my abilities. Congratulate myself for every 5-minute target I complete.
Realistic	Set a goal that is challenging but attainable based on your current skills and the resources you have. If in doubt, check with your medical team.
	ex. I have time to exercise for 20 minutes in the morning. My level of energy and focus are sufficient enough to do this. If I have to, I will increase my time by one minute each time I exercise this week to make it easier to go from 15 to 20 minutes.
Time-Based	Set a deadline by which you want to reach your goal based on your current skills and the resources you have. Adapt the deadline as necessary.
	ex. I want to be able to exercise for 20 minutes by March 31st.
Elastic	Create a window of opportunity (acceptable achievement zone) to increase your chances of success, reduce excessive pressure, and even possibly surpass your anticipated target or result.
	ex. I will be happy if I can exercise anywhere from 18 to 22 minutes by the end of this week.
Sensation-Matched	Match your goal with the sensations you want to experience while trying to achieve it in order to optimize effort, passion, and resilience. Feeling "on" (i.e., the way you want) on a regular basis will strengthen your self-efficacy and motivation. Feeling "off" on a regular basis may signify that you should revisit your goal.
	ex. I want to feel confident, in control, challenged, and in tune with my body while improving the time I exercise on the stationary bike.
Trustworthy	Identify a reasonable timeframe to repeat your goal achievement so that you fully trust that you can consistently attain it before increasing the difficulty of your goal or setting a new one.
	ex. I will maintain this 20-minute target for at least two weeks before increasing my time to 25 minutes.

My weekly goal. Identify a weekly goal for your recovery, taking into consideration the different skills and resources you have at the moment and the concussion symptoms you want to improve. Set a goal that is within your control and a goal of self-acceptance to ensure you remain compassionate toward yourself as you experience both success and setbacks in this process. Respect the SMARTEST principle when setting your weekly goal.

S

M

A

R

T

E

S

T

My daily goals. Identify daily goals, taking into consideration the process on which you must focus to achieve your weekly goal. Identify controllable, concrete actions or steps that will allow you to stay in the "here-and-now" and execute your tasks with high quality and efficiency. Choose actions that will lead you to learn and improve on a daily basis. Consider the actions you identified above while addressing the "A" (Action-based) in your SMARTEST weekly goal.

My goal of self-acceptance. Identify a goal that will allow you to accept and appreciate yourself, regardless of your progress this week; *ex. I will feel good about the effort I invest in my healing process this week, regardless of how big or small it is and regardless if I can see progress or not.*

Pelka & Kellman, 2017). It can help them to remain focused, calm, and in control, and to accept with confidence the challenges they face. From a physiological standpoint, relaxation allows athletes to breathe slower and conserve energy by pumping blood at a slower rate. It also helps them to stay loose and increase movement fluidity by reducing muscle tension (Pineschi & Di Pietro, 2013).

This relaxation section includes different scripts that can be used to improve symptoms such as sleep disturbance, fatigue, tension, tremors, and heightened emotions. These scripts focus on deep breathing (see Table 7.4), active progressive relaxation (see Table 7.5), and passive progressive relaxation (see Table 7.6). They were created based on the work of Durand-Bush (2016), Gurr (2015), and Baird and Sands (2004), as well as a relaxation workshop developed by Seguin and D'Angelo (2016).

The scripts should initially be used in-session and subsequently made available for athletes' independent use outside the sessions, based on the format that is most appealing to them (e.g., written or audio recording of script). The more frequently athletes engage in relaxation, the more benefits they are likely to derive. MPCs should strive to individualize the scripts by integrating relevant information that takes into account the athletes' unique concussion experience, concerns, and feedback. It is useful to ask athletes what words, images, and self-affirmations come to mind when they attempt to relax and to incorporate these aspects in their personalized scripts. Tables 7.4, 7.5, and 7.6 are examples of three different scripts that can be used as they appear or adapted based on athletes' symptoms and preferences. It is important to keep in mind that what works for one athlete may not work for another one.

Deep breathing

Breathing is a fundamental component of relaxation. Although it is automatically regulated by the autonomic nervous system, athletes can learn how to override this system in order to control their breathing and initiate the relaxation response. When athletes experience stress while recovering from their concussion, they can take charge of their breathing, allowing them to stay calm and composed and release any unnecessary muscle tension.

Active progressive relaxation

Active progressive relaxation is another valuable technique to develop, particularly if athletes have never done relaxation before. It involves consciously contracting and relaxing all the major muscles of the body, which helps athletes to become aware of the difference between being tense and being relaxed.

Passive progressive relaxation

Passive progressive relaxation is similar to active progressive relaxation, however it does not involve the active contraction and relaxation of muscles. It focuses on generating the relaxation response primarily through imagery and self-affirmations. It is therefore not surprising that this type of relaxation is frequently used in conjunction with or as a precursor to structured imagery exercises.

Table 7.4 Deep breathing

Deep breathing script. This relaxation script is designed to help you learn controlled breathing in moments of stress and heightened emotional states. For example, the exercise can be used in times of high distractibility, impulsivity, irritability, anger, anxiety, helplessness, frustration, and nervousness. Allocate five to ten minutes to complete the exercise and note how you feel before, during, and after it.

Find a comfortable position to do this focused breathing exercise.

Keep your eyes open and breathe in … and out … feel your belly gently rise … and fall …

Choose an object on which you can focus … Focus on that object for the next ten seconds while you continue breathing in and out … 1, 2, 3, 4, 5, 6, 7, 8, 9, 10.

Stay focused on this object, and with each breath you take … notice how your lungs fill with air, much like a bottle fills up from the bottom up … Inhale as long as you can, hold your breath for a moment, and then slowly and fully release the air from your lungs … That's good … When you are ready, close your eyes.

Remember to breathe from your diaphragm, the muscle in your belly that makes it rise and fall … If you can, breathe in through your nose and exhale through your mouth … If you are unable to do so, just breathe naturally while taking deep breaths in … and out … Feel your body relax with each breath.

Now, I will help you count from five to zero, and with each count, you will sink deeper and deeper into a state of relaxation … If you become distracted, just refocus on your breathing.

Repeat the number five to yourself, and take a full, slow breath in … As you focus on the number five … exhale slowly and completely … allowing the last little bit of air to escape gently from your lungs …

Say the number four to yourself, and as you take a full and slow breath in … focus on the number four … As you exhale, say to yourself: "I am more relaxed now than I was at number five." Exhale completely …

Now, repeat the number three to yourself, and take a full, slow breath in … When you are ready, exhale slowly and completely, saying to yourself: "I am more relaxed now than I was at number four."

Say the number two to yourself, and as you take a full and slow breath in … focus on the number two … As you exhale, say to yourself: "I am more relaxed now than I was at number three."

Now, repeat the number one to yourself, and take a full, slow breath in … as you focus on the number one … exhale slowly and completely, saying to yourself: "I am more relaxed now than I was at number two."

Say the number zero to yourself, and as you take a full and slow breath in … focus on the number zero … As you exhale, say to yourself: "I am more relaxed now than I was at number one." Allow yourself to exhale fully, and completely.

Notice your body … how you feel completely relaxed and free … Enjoy this sensation and know that you can recall it whenever you want simply by inhaling and exhaling.

Stay in this relaxed state as long as you want … When you are ready, open your eyes and move around a bit … feel how grounded and awake you are … feel how confident you are to tackle any situation … Be grateful and use your breathing to overcome the daily challenging situations you face.

Table 7.5 Active progressive relaxation

Active progressive relaxation script. The following relaxation script is designed to help you manage stress during the day and/or to fall asleep at night. The exercise can be used to improve fatigue, sleep disturbances (e.g., difficulties falling asleep, getting back to sleep after nightmares), and difficulties winding down due to increased muscle tension. Allocate 15 to 20 minutes to complete the exercise and note how you feel before, during, and after it.

Option 1. Begin by making yourself comfortable. Option 2. Find a relaxed position in which you can safely and comfortably fall asleep.

Allow your body to start relaxing.

Breathe in ... and out ... Breathe in relaxation ... and breathe out tension ... Breathe in calm ... and breathe out discomfort ...

Continue to take slow and relaxing breaths ... Feeling your lungs fill gently with air as you inhale ... and feeling your body warm itself as you exhale ...

Now, focus on your toes by clenching them tightly. Feel the tension in each curled toe as you continue to squeeze, squeeze, squeeze. Continue to activate this tension ... and then slowly release your toes ... Feel a warm sensation spreading through each toe and into the balls of your feet ... embrace the relaxation that is coming over them ...

Now, draw your attention to your ankles and arches by extending your toes away from your body and creating a distinct arch with your extended feet ... Try to extend your toes as far away as you can from your body, feeling your tendons and muscles stretching through this movement ... Squeeze your calf muscles tightly to do so, activating this powerful muscle group ... Continue extending your feet as powerfully as you can ... And then slowly relax your feet, feeling the relaxation stem up through your toes, through the balls of your feet, along your arches, up to your ankles, and through your calves ... Enjoy the relaxation as it spreads through your feet and lower legs ...

Next, focus on your shins by pointing your toes up toward your shins and knees. Activate your shin muscles, drawing all your energy toward that area ... Continue to focus on activating those muscles, squeezing them tightly, tightly, tightly ... And then slowly relax them. Feel your feet and legs relax gently as the muscles release any remaining tension. Notice the relaxation spread through your shins, calves, ankles, arches, and toes.

Now, bring your attention to your thighs. Begin activating your quad muscles, feeling strength and tension in the front of your upper legs as you squeeze, squeeze, squeeze. Continue squeezing your quads tightly, noticing the power and strength in your body as you do so ... and then allow your muscles to relax ... Feel the weight of your upper legs and let them sink into the chair or bed. Notice a warm sensation spreading through your upper legs, lower legs, through your ankles, feet, and toes. Enjoy this wonderful feeling of relaxation as you continue to breathe in ... and out ...

Bring your focus toward your glutes or buttocks. Squeeze them tightly, tightly, tightly with as much power as you can muster ... and then slowly begin to relax them ... Notice how the relaxation spreads through your glutes, quads, hamstrings, calves, shins, ankles, arches, and toes. Notice how comfortable you feel, as you relax more deeply.

(Continued)

Table 7.5 Continued

Now, draw your attention toward your core muscles ... imagine that these muscles are hugging your spine. Begin squeezing your abdominals and back muscles inward. Feel the strength of your core muscles as they squeeze, squeeze, squeeze. Continue to fully tighten your core muscles ... and then gradually relax them. Feel the relaxation come through your abs, stomach, and back ... down through your glutes, upper and lower legs, into your feet, and down through your toes. Enjoy the sensation as you continue to relax further.

Next, notice your shoulders and upper back. Start activating your rhomboids and traps as you squeeze your shoulder blades together. Continue to squeeze tightly, tightly, tightly, as you activate these strong muscles in your body. Feel the tension and strength of your muscles as you continue to squeeze ... and then allow these muscles to relax and sink heavily into the bed or chair. Notice the relaxation spreading through your upper and lower back, through your core and glutes, down through your thighs, calves, and shins, and finally through your feet and toes. Continue to take slow and deep breaths as you enjoy the feeling of relaxation spreading throughout your body.

Now, move your focus toward your arms. Make a fist with each hand ... and activate your forearm muscles, squeezing your fists tightly. Now pull your fists toward your shoulders to also activate your biceps. Feel the strength in your arms as you squeeze these muscles tighter and tighter ... Continue to hold this tension ... keep squeezing ... and then relax your arms and hands gently and completely, letting them rest on each side. Feel the relaxed sensation spread through your fingers ... your arms ... your upper back ... your lower back ... your abs ... your glutes ... quads ... hamstrings ... shins ... calves ... ankles ... arches ... and toes ...

Enjoy the warmth and heaviness of your body in this relaxed state ... Your breathing is slow and relaxed, your muscles are loose and free ... any tension you were feeling in your body has slipped away. Scan your body from head to toe one last time, and if you notice any tightness, let it go gently ... let it leave your body like a passing cloud in the sky, noticing it only for a moment before returning to your comfortable, relaxed state ... Enjoy this feeling as long as you want.

Option 1 – When you are ready, come back to your normal state of being. Take your time. Start by moving your fingers and toes. Then open your eyes, slowly stand up, and move around to get the blood circulating throughout your body. Take a few energizing breaths before you move on to another activity. Notice how content and rejuvenated you feel.

Option 2 – When you are ready, slowly allow yourself to drift into a deep sleep and let your body rejuvenate itself overnight so that you feel content and energized in the morning.

Section 4: Imagery

The final skill introduced in this PST program is imagery. Imagery is the ability to integrate the five senses (i.e., see, feel, hear, smell, and taste) to reproduce different experiences in the mind. It is a powerful skill that can positively influence athletes' Feelings, Actions, Thoughts, and Sensations (i.e., FAST). Imagery is particularly useful if athletes are injured and cannot physically train. They can use

Table 7.6 Passive progressive relaxation

Passive progressive relaxation script. This relaxation script is designed to help you take control of your thoughts and body in order to direct and inspire healing through imagery and positive self-affirmations. The exercise can be used when you experience blurred vision, dizziness, vertigo, headaches, loss of smell and/or taste, and photophobia (i.e., sensitivity to light), to give a few examples. However, it is not limited to these symptoms. Allocate 10 to 15 minutes to complete the exercise and note how you feel before, during, and after it.

Begin by finding a comfortable and relaxed position.

Allow your body to relax and refuel in the next little while.

Focus on your breathing ... breathe in ... and breathe out ...

Take a deep cleansing breath in ... and breathe out any tension and undesired thoughts and feelings you might have at the moment ...

Continue to breathe slowly and intentionally as you inhale relaxation ... and exhale physical and cognitive tension ...

Feel the relaxation emerge at the bottom of your feet ... as if you were stepping into a warm bath ... See and sense this warm and pleasant feeling of relaxation spread through your feet and up your ankles ... Notice the relaxation calmly rising above your ankles, flowing up your lower legs ... to your knees ... continuing up to your upper legs ...

Now, allow this relaxation to continue to spread throughout your body, rising now to your pelvic area and hips ... up your belly and your chest ... now your lower back and upper back ...

You can relax even further by letting your spine unwind ... starting where the top of your spine meets your head ... Feel the relaxation glide down your spine ... feel the muscles giving up their hold and giving in to the relaxing feeling ... Now, let this pleasant feeling of relaxation run back up your spine and let go of any tension that remains ...

Next, let your upper arms relax ... your elbows ... let the relaxation spread to your lower arms ... your wrists ... feel it spread to your hands ... down the back of your hands ... allowing the palms of your hands to feel heavy with the relaxation ... down each finger and thumb ... Notice how your hands feel pleasantly warm, heavy, and relaxed ...

See and feel your body relaxing further as your collarbone begins to widen and relax ... allow your shoulders to ease back slightly and gently ... your neck ... Allow all of your upper back to relax ...

Feel the relaxation spreading to your chin ... your mouth ... your cheeks ... your nose ... and eyes ... Notice how your eyelids are heavy ... and relaxed ... Notice your eyebrows relaxing ... your ears ... your forehead ... Your forehead feels cool and relaxed ...

Let the relaxation spread to the top and back of your head ... allowing all of your head to be completely relaxed ...

Your entire body now is calm and relaxed ... Feel the relaxation flowing freely throughout your body, from your head all the way down to your toes ...

(Continued)

Table 7.6 Continued

Now take some time to imagine a place where you feel calm and safe … a place that allows you to stay grounded, to be kind to yourself, and to care for yourself. See, hear, feel, smell, and taste everything that is helpful in this place. Your senses are there to help you to stay in tune with your body and your surroundings. Use them to your advantage …

Notice how much strength and resilience you have in this place … use this strength and resilience to address any concern you have regarding your concussion … your recovery process … your return to play. Accept the concussion symptoms you have instead of fighting them … Know that your body is strong and is working hard to overcome them. Trust the healing process … see and feel your body heal itself … one cell at time … with the nutrients and care you are giving it … See and feel yourself getting better and achieving small daily goals. Imagine getting healthier each day … overcoming symptoms … taking ownership of your recovery … getting back to leading a full, rich, and meaningful life.

Enjoy the feeling of being in this place … appreciate the energy, motivation, and confidence you get from it … Capture this feeling as best as you can … package it … and store it somewhere in your body so that you can access it anytime you need it. Whenever you face difficult challenges, know that you can access this feeling … this inner resilience to get you through challenges.

When you are ready, open your eyes … be grateful for this moment … feel at peace knowing that each day is a new one … trust your recovery and look forward to the next goal you will achieve.

imagery to create or recreate vivid and controlled experiences that facilitate skill maintenance, resilience, and recovery. In fact, studies have shown that imagery can enhance injured athletes' coping skills and adherence to their rehabilitation program (Cupal & Brewer, 2001; Wesch et al., 2011). In particular, imagery can help athletes rehearse rehabilitation exercises, visualize physiological processes involved in healing, set goals, manage emotions and pain, as well as increase self-efficacy (Cupal & Brewer, 2001; Driediger, Hall, & Callow, 2006).

In order to get insight into athletes' imagery skills, MPCs can guide them through the exercise in Table 7.7, which was adapted from Durand-Bush (2016). It is important to know which senses the athletes are comfortable using when engaging in imagery. Given that concussions can affect some of their senses (e.g., sight, sound, smell, taste; Headway, 2013; Littleton & Guskiewicz, 2013), imagery scripts should be adapted to best meet the needs of athletes. As symptoms improve, these scripts can be modified to progressively integrate all of the senses.

Following this assessment, MPCs can help athletes develop an imagery script to foster healing and recovery. The script provided in Table 7.8 serves as an example and can be used in conjunction with any of the relaxation scripts in the previous section. The content was developed based on the work of Durand-Bush (2016) and the Association of Applied Sport Psychology (2016). This script should be tailored to athletes' imagery skills and concussion symptoms and should be implemented regularly or as necessary in order to derive the most benefits.

Table 7.7 Imagery scan

Imagery scan. This exercise is meant to help you understand how skilled you are at engaging in imagery. It will allow you to assess your use of different senses (i.e., sight, sound, touch, smell, taste) and your ability to rehearse or reproduce movement in your mind. Be honest, as your responses will help tailor your imagery script. You can start by building on the senses you can comfortably use at the moment, and as symptoms improve, you can integrate other senses and movements that are relevant to you in order to create or recreate experiences that are as vivid and real as possible.

Look around you and notice as many things as possible. Now close your eyes and imagine yourself in this room.

How do you see yourself in this room? Are you seeing yourself from inside or outside your own body?

Do you see any colors? If so, which ones? How vivid or vague are these colors?

Do you hear any sounds? If so, which ones? How loud or soft are these sounds?

Do you smell any scents? If so, which ones? How strong or weak are these scents?

Do you taste any flavors? If so, which ones? How strong or weak are these flavors?

Do you feel any sensations when you touch things around you? If so, what sensations do you feel? How strong or weak are these sensations?

Do you feel and control your movements when you imagine yourself walking around in the room? If so, what do you feel when you move, and how ample or limited is your control?

Overall, how easy or difficult is it to imagine yourself in this room? What senses can you best use? To what extent can you imagine yourself moving in this room?

Section 5: Wrap-up and future plans

The final section of the PST program involves reviewing the materials covered in each section, assessing concussion symptom progress, re-evaluating goals, and establishing plans for the future. Self-reflection is a fundamental component of self-regulation (Zimmerman, 2000), and it is important that athletes reflect on their learning and experiences throughout the PST program. The exercise in Table 7.9 will help athletes assess the skills and strategies they used during their recovery, which will be helpful to determine the effect of the PST program as well as next steps. The content was informed by the work of Durand-Bush and colleagues (2015).

MPCs should debrief responses from the exercise in Table 7.9 with the athletes. It is important to recognize that athletes' recovery from their concussion may still be ongoing at this point in time. It is also possible that athletes may be unable to return to sport if they have sustained a serious concussion. As such,

Table 7.8 Healing imagery

Healing imagery script. This exercise was designed to help you imagine yourself recovering from your concussion. The script can be used by itself or it can be introduced after one of the relaxation scripts from the previous section, as these can help you get into the proper mindset to engage in imagery. The script allows you to focus on the area of your body that requires the most healing (e.g., brain, neck, spine, eyes) based on your current symptoms. Listen to your body as you perform the exercise and stop at any point in time if it is too difficult. As your symptoms improve, progressively set goals to increase the length of the imagery exercise. By doing so, you will also improve your focusing skills.

As you sit or lie comfortably, focus on your body and think about the healing that will take place ...

Imagine your current state of being and the concussion symptoms and concerns that you have ... It might be pain, tension, or worry, or other consequences of your concussion ... Whatever it is that you would like to heal, imagine this concern in your mind right now ...

Focus on the specific area in your body where your concern is present. Perhaps there are many areas that you would like to address ... But for now, choose the area that troubles you the most, and direct your focus to that area ...

As you imagine this area, picture a light that begins to purify and heal it ... This powerful light can be any color that is soothing ... see it engulf the area and spread through other nearby parts of your body ... This light contains all of the energy and nutrients required to heal the area ... Imagine this energy and these nutrients at work to restore the area ...

Your body has many ways of healing itself. Imagine your powerful immune system working in synch with all of your organs to alleviate your concussion symptoms ... promoting strength ... promoting growth of healthy tissue ... removing unhealthy matter from your body ... removing toxins, bacteria, or waste ... cleaning up and purifying your body ...

As you breathe in, imagine the healing light flowing, swirling, and touching all aspects of your body requiring healing ... As you breathe out, allow all unnecessary matter and waste to leave your body ...

Breathe in health, healing, and strength ...

Breathe out tension, worry, and weakness ...

See and feel the healing light progressively reducing the problem area ... see it getting smaller and smaller as your body recovers and carries away anything that is not good for you ...

Appreciate that your immune system is working to heal your concussion symptoms ... picture healthy cells, blood flow, and nutrients going to the places they need to go ... working as needed to heal your body ... Picture injured body tissues repairing themselves, as you bring healing awareness toward them ...

Your body is healing. Feel it ... be grateful for it ...

Take a few last moments to appreciate and support this healing process going on inside your body ... trust your body's ability to heal itself ... feel rejuvenated, calm, and at peace as you go about the rest of your day.

Table 7.9 PST program evaluation

PST program evaluation. Take a moment to evaluate your experience throughout this program. Consider the skills you learned and applied (i.e., self-regulation, goal-setting/goal-management, relaxation, imagery) and the strategies and tools you used (e.g., checklist, log, SMARTEST principle, scripts, scan) to facilitate your recovery. Also reflect on the external support you had (e.g., family, friends, teammates, medical staff), as this will help you moving forward. Write as much as you want in the space below and use the self-rating scales to determine the extent of your learning and the impact of the PST program.

What are the most valuable lessons of this PST program?

By completing the concussion checklist in Section 1 again and by comparing my symptoms at the beginning and the end of the program, which symptoms improved, worsened, and stayed the same?

Did I achieve the goals I set during the PST program? If so, what skills and/or strategies were the most useful to achieve these goals?

On a scale of one to five, to what extent did I improve the following skills targeted in the PST program (1 = little to no improvement and 5 = huge improvement)? Am I satisfied with this?

Self-regulation	1 2 3 4 5
Goal-setting/goal-management	1 2 3 4 5
Relaxation	1 2 3 4 5
Imagery	1 2 3 4 5

Did I have adequate external support and resources during this PST program? If so, which ones must I continue to rely on after this program?

Based on what I have learned and experienced in this PST program, what valuable next steps can I put in place to continue or maintain my recovery? Is there anything I should change? Is there anything new I should try?

MPCs must offer appropriate support following recommendations from medical staff and help athletes determine feasible next steps. As previously mentioned, this PST program is meant to *complement* athletes' rehabilitation process and provide them with skills and strategies to manage their concussion symptoms and consequences of their injury. Through increased control and self-regulation capacity, the PST program serves to help athletes maintain their motivation and self-efficacy required to adhere to recovery protocols, persevere through challenges and setbacks, and preserve their mental health.

Concluding remarks

> Are head shots a serious problem? Absolutely. They can be life-changing, and they should be out of the game. More important, all levels of hockey should have a system that prioritizes mental health resources for players who are suffering from postconcussion syndrome.
>
> (NHL player Marc Savard, *Players' Tribune*,
> May 16, 2017)

The aforesaid quote from Marc Savard, whose concussion ended his ice hockey career, illustrates the potential devastating outcome of this brain injury and the need for more mental health resources for concussed athletes. We hope that this chapter serves as an impetus to further develop PST resources for this population. Other valuable psychological skills, such as attentional control, emotion regulation, and self-talk could be included in concussed-centered PST programs. Concepts such as mindfulness and resilience could also be feasibly integrated, as they have been shown to be important in the rehabilitation of concussions. All in all, MPCs have multiple skills, techniques, and counseling approaches in their repertoire to assist concussed athletes in their recovery. Additional resources and research will facilitate the development of specialized approaches to optimize their work with this population.

Note

1 *Mental performance consultant (MPC)* and *Certified Mental Performance Consultant (CMPC)* are the terms used by the Canadian Sport Psychology Association (CSPA) and the Association for Applied Sport Psychology (AASP), respectively, to recognize practitioners who meet requirements to practice in the area of mental performance, mental training, and/or sport psychology in these countries.

References

Anderson, D. L. (2012). Finding stillness within the shaken brain. *Canadian Medical Association Journal*, *184*, 1816–1817. doi:10.1503/cmaj.120074.

Arvinen-Barrow, M., Clement, D., Hamson-Utley, J. J., Zakrajsek, R. A., Sae-Mi, L., Kamphoff, C., & Martin, S. B. (2015). Athletes' use of mental skills during sport injury rehabilitation. *Journal of Sport Rehabilitation*, 24, 189–197. doi:10.1123/jsr.2013-0148.

Ashbaugh, A., & McGrew, C. (2016). The role of nutritional supplements in sports concussion treatment. *Current Sports Medicine Reports*, 15, 16–19. doi:10.1249/JSR.0000000000000219.

Association for Applied Sport Psychology. (2016). Using the mind to heal the body: Imagery for injury rehabilitation. Retrieved from www.appliedsportpsych.org/resources/injury-rehabilitation/using-the-mind-to-heal-the-body-imagery-for-injury-rehabilitation/.

Association for Applied Sport Psychology. (2018). Ethics Code: AASP Ethical Principles and Standards. *About AASP*. Retrieved from www.appliedsportpsych.org/about/ethics/ethics-code/.

Astokorki, A. H. Y., & Mauger, A. R. (2016). Tolerance of exercise-induced pain at a fixed rating of perceived exertion predicts time trial cycling performance. *Scandinavian Journal of Medicine and Science in Sports*, 27, 309–317. doi.org/10.1111/sms.12659.

Azulay, J., Smart, C. M., Mott, T., & Cicerone, K. D. (2013). A pilot study examining the effect of mindfulness-based stress reduction on symptoms of chronic mild traumatic brain injury/postconcussive syndrome. *The Journal of Head Trauma Rehabilitation*, 28, 323–331. doi:10.1097/HTR.0b013e318250ebda.

Baird, C. L., & Sands, L. (2004). A pilot study of the effectiveness of guided imagery with progressive muscle relaxation to reduce chronic pain and mobility difficulties of osteoarthritis. *Pain Management Nursing*, 5, 97–104. doi:10.1016/j.pmn.2004.01.003.

Bloom, G. A., Horton, A. S., McCrory, P., & Johnston, K. M. (2004). Sport psychology and concussion: New impacts to explore. *British Journal of Sports Medicine*, 6, 1–2. doi:10.1136/bjsm.2004.011999.

Brett, C. E., Sykes, C., & Pires-Yfantouda, R. (2017). Interventions to increase engagement with rehabilitation in adults with acquired brain injury: A systematic review. *Neuropsychological Rehabilitation*, 27, 959–982. doi:10.1080/09602011.2015.1090459.

Broglio, S. P, Cantu, R. C., Gioia, G. A., Guskiewicz, K. M., Kutcher, J., Palm, M., & Valvovich McLeod, T. C. (2014). National athletic trainers' association position statement: Management of sport concussion. *Journal of Athletic Training*, 49, 245–265. doi:10.4085/1062-6050-49.1.07.

Burke, M. J., Fralick, M., Nejatbakhsh, N., Tartaglia, M. C., & Tator, C. H. (2015). In search of evidence-based treatment for concussion: Characteristics of current clinical trials. *Brain Injury*, 29, 300–305. doi:10.3109/02699052.2014.974673.

Burns, S. L. (2015). Concussion treatment using massage techniques: A case study. *International Journal of Therapeutic Massage and Bodywork*, 8, 12–17. Retrieved from www.ncbi.nlm.nih.gov/pmc/articles/PMC4455610/.

Canadian Sport Psychology Association. (2018). CSPA Code of Ethics. *Ethics*. Retrieved from www.cspa-acps.com/ethics.

Caron, J. G., Bloom, G. A., Falcão, W. R., & Sweet, S. N. (2015). An examination of concussion education programmes: A scoping review methodology. *Injury Prevention*, 21, 301–308. doi:org/10.1136/injuryprev-2014-041479.

Caron, J. G., Bloom, G. A., Johnston, K. M., & Sabiston, C. M. (2013). Effects of multiple concussions on retired national hockey league players. *Journal of Sport & Exercise Psychology*, 35, 168–179. doi:10.1123/jsep.35.2.168.

Chiang, C. C., Guo, S. E., Huang, K. C., & Lee, B. O. (2016). Trajectories and associated factors of quality of life, global outcome, and post-concussion symptoms in the first year following mild traumatic brain injury. *Quality of Life Research, 25*, 2009–2019. doi:10.1007/s11136-015-1215-0.

Clement, D., Granquist, M., & Arvinen-Barrow, M. (2013). Psychological aspects of athletic injuries as perceived by athletic trainers. *Journal of Athletic Training, 48*, 512–521. doi:10.1123/tsp.10.1.37.

Covassin, T., Crutcher, B., Bleecker, A., Heiden, E. O., Dailey, A., & Yang, J. (2014). Postinjury anxiety and social support among collegiate athletes: A comparison between orthopaedic injuries and concussions. *Journal of Athletic Training, 49*, 462–468. doi:10.4085/1062-6059-49.2.03.

Covassin, T., Elbin, R. J., Crutcher, B., Burkhart, S., & Kontos, A. (2013). The relationship between coping, neurocognitive performance, and concussion symptoms in high school and collegiate athletes. *The Sport Psychologist, 27*, 372–379. doi:10.1123/tsp.27.4.372.

Cupal, D. D., & Brewer, B. W. (2001). Effects of relaxation and guided imagery on knee strength, re-injury anxiety, and pain following anterior cruciate ligament reconstruction. *Rehabilitation Psychology, 46*, 28–43. Retrieved from http://psycnet.apa.org/buy/2001-14028-002.

Daneshvar, D. H., Nowinski, C. J., McKee, A. C., & Cantu, R. C. (2011). The epidemiology of sport-related concussion. *Clinical Journal of Sports Medicine, 30*, 1–17. doi:10.1016/j.csm.2010.08.006.

Davies, S. C. (2016). School-based traumatic brain injury and concussion management program. *Psychology in the Schools, 53*, 567–582. doi:10.1002/pits.21927.

Delaney, J. S., Lamfookon C., Bloom, G. A., Al-Kashmiri, A., & Correa, J. A. (2015). Why university athletes choose not to reveal their concussion symptoms during a practice or game. *Clinical Journal of Sport Medicine, 25*, 113–125. doi:10.1097/JSM.0000000000000112.

Driediger M., Hall C., & Callow N. (2006). Imagery use by injured athletes: A qualitative analysis. *Journal of Sport Sciences, 24*, 261–272. doi:10.1080/02640410500128221.

Durand-Bush, N. (2016). *Getting mentally fit for sport and life: A workbook to optimize performance and well-being*. Unpublished manuscript.

Durand-Bush, N., McNeill, K., & Collins, J. (2015). The self-regulation of sport coaches: How coaches can become masters of their own destiny. In P. Davis (Ed.), *The psychology of effective coaching and management* (pp. 217–265). Hauppauge, NY: Nova Publishers.

Dryden, K. (2017). *Game change: The life and death of Steve Montador and the future of hockey*. Toronto, ON: McClelland & Stewart.

Elbin, R. J., Schatz, P., Lowder, H. B., & Kontos, A. P. (2014). An empirical review of treatment and rehabilitation approaches used in the acute, sub-acute, and chronic phases of recovery following sports-related concussion. *Current Treatment Options in Neurology, 16*, 320–331. doi:10.1007/s11940-014-0320-7.

Gay, M. (2016). Treatment perspectives based on our current understanding of concussion. *Sports Medicine and Arthroscopy Review, 24*, 134–141. doi:10.1097/JSA.0000000000000124.

Government of Canada. (2018). Concussions in sport. Retrieved from www.canada.ca/en/canadian-heritage/services/concussions.html.

Gurr, B. (2015). *Headaches and brain injury from a biopsychosocial perspective: A practical psychotherapy guide*. London, UK: Karnac Books Ltd.

Hamson-Utley, J., Martin, S., & Walters, J. (2008). Athletic trainers' and physical therapists' perceptions of the effectiveness of psychological skills within sport injury rehabilitation programs. *Journal of Athletic Training, 43*, 258–264. Retrieved from www.natajournals.org/doi/pdf/10.4085/1062-6050-43.3.258.

Headway: The Brain Injury Association. (2013). Factsheet: Loss of taste and smell after brain injury. Retrieved from www.headway.org.uk/about-brain-injury/individuals/information-library/.

Heaney, C. A., Walker, N. C., Green, A. J. K., & Rostron, C. L. (2015). Sport psychology education for sport injury rehabilitation professionals: A systematic review. *Physical Therapy in Sport, 16*, 72–79. doi:10.1016/j.ptsp.2014.04.001.

Helmy, A., Agarwal, M., & Hutchinson, P. J. (2013). Concussion and sport. *British Journal of Sports Medicine, 347*, f5748. doi:10.1136/bmj.f5748.

Johnston, K. M., Bloom, G. A., Ramsay, J., Kissick, J., Montgomery, D., Foley, D., ... & Ptito, A. (2004). Current concepts in concussion rehabilitation. *Current Sports Medicine Reports, 3*, 316–323. doi:10.1007/s11932-996-0006-3

Jordan, B. D. (2013). The clinical spectrum of sport-related traumatic brain injury. *Nature Reviews Neurology, 9*, 222–230. doi:10.1038/nrneurol.2013.33.

Kabat-Zinn, J. (1982). An outpatient program in behavioral medicine for chronic pain patients based on the practice of mindfulness meditation: Theoretical considerations and preliminary results. *General Hospital Psychiatry, 4*, 33–47. doi:10.1016/0163-8343(82)90026-3.

King, N. S. (2014). Permanent post-concussion symptoms after mild head injury: A systematic review of age and gender factors. *NeuoroRehabilitation, 34*, 741–748. doi:10.3233/NRE-141072.

Kjeldgaard, D., Forchhammer, H. B., Teasdale, T. W., & Jensen, R. H. (2014). Cognitive behavioural treatment for the chronic post-traumatic headache patient: A randomized controlled trial. *The Journal of Headache and Pain, 15*, 81–91. doi:10.1186/1129-2377-15-81.

Koehn, S., Morris, T., & Watt, A. P. (2014). Imagery intervention to increase flow state and performance in competition. *Sport Psychologist, 28*, 48–59. doi:10.1123/tsp.2012-0106.

Kontos, A., Byrd, M., & Cormier, M. (2017, October). *The role of sport psychology in the treatment and rehabilitation of concussion.* Paper presented at 32nd Annual Conference of the Association for Applied Sport Psychology, Orlando, Florida, USA.

Kontos, A. P., Collins, M., & Russo, S. A. (2004). An introduction to sports concussion for the sport psychology consultant. *Journal of Applied Sport Psychology, 16*, 220–235. doi:10.1080/10413200490485568.

Littleton, A., & Guskiewicz, K. (2013). Current concepts in sport concussion management: A multifaceted approach. *Journal of Sport and Health Science, 2*, 227–235. doi:org/10.1016/j.jshs.2013.04.003.

Lynch, J. M., Anderson, M., Benton, B., & Green, S. S. (2015). The gaming of concussions: A unique intervention in postconcussion syndrome. *Journal of Athletic Training, 59*, 270–276. doi:10.4085/1062-6050-49.3.78.

Martin, L. A., Fogarty, G. J., & Albion, M. J. (2014). Changes in athletic identity and life satisfaction of elite athletes as a function of retirement status. *Journal of Applied Sport Psychology, 26*, 96–110. doi:10.1080/10413200.2013.798371.

McCrea, H. J., Perrine, K., Niogi, S., & Härtl, R. (2012). Concussion in sports. *Sports Health, 5*, 160–164. doi:10.1177/1941738112462203.

McCrory, P., Meeuwisse, W., Dvorak, J., Aubry, M., Bailes, J., Broglio, S., … Vos, P. E. (2017). Consensus statement on concussion in sport—The 5th international conference on concussion in sport held in Berlin, October 2016. *British Journal of Sport Medicine, 51*, 838–847. doi:10.1136/bjsports-2017-097699.

Miltenberger, R. G. (2012). *Behavior modification: Principles and procedures* (5th ed.). Belmont, CA: Brookes/Cole, Cengage Learning.

Moran, B., Tadikonda, P., Sneed, K. B., Hummel, M., Guiteau, S., & Coris, E. E. (2015). Postconcussive syndrome following sports-related concussion: A treatment overview for primary care physicians. *Southern Medical Journal, 108*, 553–558. doi:10.14423/SMJ.0000000000000340.

Orlick, T. (2015). *In pursuit of excellence: How to win in sport and life through mental training* (5th ed.). Champaign, IL: Human Kinetics.

Pelka, M., & Kellman, M. (2017). Relaxation and recovery in sport and performance. In *Oxford Research Encyclopedia of Psychology*. doi:10.1093/acrefore/9780190236557.013.153.

Pineschi G., & Di Pietro, A. (2013). Anxiety management through psychological techniques: Relaxation and psyching-up in sport. *Journal of Sport Psychology in Action, 4*, 181–190. doi:10.1080/21520704.2013.820247.

Rees, R. J., & Bellon, M. L. (2007). Post concussion syndrome ebb and flow: Longitudinal effects and management. *NeuroRehabilitation, 22*, 229–242. Retrieved from https://content.iospress.com/articles/neurorehabilitation/nre00371.

Ruhe, A., Gansslen, A., & Klein, W. (2013). The incidence of concussion in professional and collegiate ice hockey: Are we making progress? A systematic review of the literature. *British Journal of Sports Medicine, 8*, 102–106. doi:10.1136/bjsports-2012-091609.

Savard, M. (May 2017). *Hell and back*. Players' Tribune. Retrieved from www.theplayerstribune.com/en-us/articles/marc-savard-bruins-hell-and-back.

Sayegh, A. A., Sandford, D., & Carson, A. J. (2010). Psychological approaches to treatment of postconcussion syndrome: A systematic review. *Journal of Neurology, Neurosurgery, & Psychiatry, 81*, 1128–1134. doi:10.1136/jnnp.2008.170092.

Schwab Reese, L. M., Pittsinger, R., & Yang, J. (2012). Effectiveness of psychological intervention following sport injury. *Journal of Sport and Health Science, 1*, 71–79. doi:10.1016/j.jshs.2012.06.003.

Seguin, C. M., & D'Angelo, M. (2016, September). *Stress management and relaxation training: Psychological skills training workshop for adults.* Cornwall, ON.

Snell, D. L., Surgenor, L. J., Hay-Smith, E. J. C., Williman, J., & Siegert, R. J. (2015). The contribution of psychological factors to recovery after mild traumatic brain injury: Is cluster analysis a useful approach? *Brain Injury, 29*, 291–299. doi:10.3109/02699052.2014.976594.

Stoler, D. R., & Hill, B. A. (2013). *Coping with concussion and mild traumatic brain injury: A guide to living with the challenges associated with post concussion syndrome and brain trauma.* New York, NY: Penguin Group.

Terrell, T. R., Nobles, T., Rader, B., Bielak, K., Asif, I., Casmus, R., … Hussein, R. (2014). Sports concussion management: Part I. *Southern Medical Journal, 107*, 115–125. doi:10.1097/SMJ.0000000000000063.

Thomas, R. E., Alves, J., Vaska, M. M., & Magalhaes, R. (2017). Therapy and rehabilitation of mild brain injury/concussion: Systematic review. *Restorative Neurology and Neuroscience, 35*, 643–666. doi:10.3233/RNN-170761.

Venville, A., Sawyer, A. M., Long, M., Edwards, N., & Hair, S. (2015). Supporting people with an intellectual disability and mental health problems: A scoping review of what they say about service provision. *Journal of Mental Health Research in Intellectual Disabilities, 8,* 186–212. doi:10.1080/19315864.2015.1069912.

Waid-Ebbs, J. K., Daly, J., Wu, S. S., Berg, W. K., Bauer, R. M., Perlstein, W. M., & Crosson, B. (2014). Response to goal management training in veterans with blast-related mild traumatic brain injury. *Journal of Rehabilitation Research & Development, 51,* 1555–1566. doi:10.1682/JRRD.2013.12.0266.

Wesch, N., Hall, C., Prapavessis, H., Maddison, R., Bassett, S., Foley, L., ... Forwell, L. (2011). Self-efficacy, imagery use, and adherence during injury rehabilitation. *Scandinavian Journal of Medicine and Science in Sports, 22,* 695–703. doi:10.1111/j.1600-0838.2011.01304.x.

Wilson, G. T. (2011). Behavior therapy. In R. Corsini & D. Wedding (Eds.), *Current psychotherapies* (9th ed., pp. 235–275). Belmont, CA: Brooks/Cole, Cengage Learning.

Yoon, I., & Yoon, Y-J. (2014). Effect of psychological skill training as a psychological intervention for a successful rehabilitation of a professional soccer player: Single case study. *Journal of Exercise Rehabilitation, 10*(5), 295–301. doi:10.12965/jer.140149.

Zimmerman, B. J. (2000). Attaining self-regulation: A social-cognitive perspective. In M. Boekaerts, P. R. Pintrich, & M. Zeidner (Eds.), *Handbook of self-regulation* (pp. 13–42). San Diego, CA: Academic Press.

8 Concussion in athletes with disabilities

Osman Hassan Ahmed, Matthew Slater,
Jamie B. Barker, and Tracy Blake

Introduction

An estimated one billion people around the world are currently living with a disability (World Health Organization, 2011). The term *disability* is defined as "a physical or mental condition that limits a person's movements, senses, or activities" (Oxford Living Dictionaries, 2018). Physical disabilities encompass a range of muscular, orthopedic, and neurological impairments, and can originate from infectious diseases, non-communicable chronic conditions (e.g., cerebral palsy), and injuries sustained (e.g., spinal cord injury; World Health Organization, 2011). Mental disabilities are equally broad in scope and impair an individual's intellectual capacity, with the most common example of this being learning disabilities (Grünke & Cavendish, 2016). There have been increasing numbers of individuals with disabilities participating in both team and independent sports. However, to date there has been little focus or attention on the specific needs and demands of managing concussion within this athlete population.

This chapter explores some of the psychological issues relating to athletes with both physical and mental disabilities—populations that have been omitted from the discourse surrounding concussions to date. It begins with a *precis* of some of the existing literature on concussion in disability sport, including the epidemiological studies that demonstrate why this is an issue of concern. Literature relating to athletes with physical and learning disabilities, as well as attention deficit-hyperactivity disorder, is used to contextualize the clinical implications of concussions among athletes with disabilities. The chapter then discusses the significance of social isolation for athletes with disabilities who have sustained a concussion, before outlining the social identity approach and how this approach (alongside input from a sport psychology consultant) can be of value to these athletes. The chapter closes with practical steps that can be implemented by a multi-disciplinary team, followed by suggestions for future research in the field.

Epidemiology of concussion in disability sport

Despite growing efforts to encourage participation in disability sport (Gibson, 2016), there has not been a similar focus on the care and management of injuries for athletes with disabilities, including sport-related concussions. This section aims to outline some of the existing studies present on concussion in disability sport and includes the example of disability football as one area where preliminary research has taken place.

The gap in knowledge related to concussion in disability sport was highlighted in two recent editorials (Webborn et al., 2018; West et al., 2017). Both of these delivered a call to action to the International Paralympic Committee and research communities for increased evidence-informed safeguards for athletes with disabilities following concussion. Webborn and colleagues (2018) highlighted the duty of care that practitioners have to safeguard the long-term health of athletes with disabilities, especially those who compete in elite disability sports with high rates of head injuries, such as wheelchair basketball, sit-ski alpine athletes, and visually impaired footballers. In a similar vein, West et al. (2017) used the example of cerebral palsy football to discuss the nuances involved in assessing and managing concussion in a disability cohort. Drawing upon discussions with doctors and physiotherapists responsible for the care of cerebral palsy footballers, the authors highlighted that staff working with these disability athletes would welcome a consensus statement on how to best manage concussion within this population. An additional recommendation from West and colleagues was for an increased focus on collecting normative data in disability sport, to make any clinical guidance appropriately evidence-based.

Although injuries in disability sport and Paralympic sport have not historically been subject to rigorous, long-term prospective studies, there have been a few epidemiological studies with respect to sport-related concussion. One of the earliest studies to look at injury in disability sport was from Ferrara et al. (1992), who conducted a retrospective survey that showed 3% of the U.S.-based athletes reported a head injury. This study grouped all injuries to the head together, and therefore determining which head injuries were considered a concussion versus other injuries (e.g., facial lacerations) is not possible. A retrospective, self-report questionnaire approach was also used by Wessels, Broglio, and Sosnoff (2012) to identify the incidence of concussion among wheelchair basketball players in the United States. From the athletes sampled in this study, 6.1% reported sustaining a concussion, and participants included individuals with spinal cord injury, spina bifida, cerebral palsy, and lower limb amputations. The study did not ask the participants about their functional limitations following their concussion, nor about any psychological consequences which may have arisen post-injury.

Building on this preliminary work, subsequent studies adopted more robust methodologies. Willick et al. (2013) used the injury databases from medical professionals at the London 2012 Paralympic Games to generate a high quality and comprehensive prospective cohort study. Using injury data from both medical report forms completed at the time of assessment as well as from daily web-based injury surveys completed by medical staff, the numbers of head/face injuries (2.2% of all injuries reported) were comparable to Ferrara and colleagues' (1992) study, whilst the sport with the highest injury incidence rate of all Paralympic sports was five-a-side football. Another study from Silva et al. (2013) discussed the injuries (including concussions) associated with international-level blind footballers from

Brazil. The sample size for this 4-year study was low ($N = 13$ athletes), and of the 144 injuries reported during this period, 8.6% of injuries were to the head. One factor associated with the greater frequency of reported concussions is the running posture adopted by blind footballers; their anterior trunk posture, leading to the head being positioned ahead of the body, is suggested to leave their heads more susceptible to injury than in mainstream football.

Paralympic football was also the subject of a separate study by Webborn et al. (2016), where injuries to both visually impaired and cerebral palsy footballers competing at the London 2012 Paralympic Games were analyzed. Head/ neck injuries accounted for a large number (25%) of all acute injuries during competition, and the authors suggested that the use of protective headgear may mitigate these injuries specifically in visually impaired football. The history of epidemiology in Paralympic sport was outlined by Webborn and Emery (2014) and reinforced the significant evolution of the level of sports in the Paralympic Games since the first organized disability sport events were held in 1948. Their review cautions against comparing injury rates between older and more contemporary studies, given the significant changes to the style of play in Paralympic sports over the past several decades.

Most recently, Kissick and Webborn (2018) undertook a detailed review outlining concussion in Para sport and summarized much of the existing literature present related to concussion in disability sport. This included data collected by the IPC via their injury and surveillance studies, with these studies commencing in 2002 for the Winter Paralympic Games and in 2012 for the Summer Paralympic Games. The authors noted that there is currently a lack of data-driven research in the area and summarized some of the challenges involved in using existing concussion screening tools in a disability population. Factors such as reduced hearing (e.g., deaf athletes), cognitive impairment (e.g., athletes with a learning disability), and balance/co-ordination impairment (e.g., cerebral palsy athletes) were all mentioned. Their review concluded by emphasizing the need for education to all stakeholders involved in disability sport, enforcement of safety laws to assist those participating in disability sport, and engineering to facilitate the creation of protective equipment. Other important factors that were highlighted by Kissick and Webborn included: The need to develop concussion assessment tools specific to athletes with disabilities; adapting and tailoring principles of rest and return to play (RTP) for these athletes; and gaining a greater understanding of the mechanisms of concussion in disability sport. Implementing the recommendations of these authors would enhance concussion-related care for athletes with disabilities. This could have substantial benefits across disability sport, including in the many formats of disability football, which have been suggested by Ahmed et al. (2015) to be lacking in adequate injury prevention and treatment mechanisms.

Concussion in disability football (soccer)

A recent study from Weiler et al. (2018) compared Sport Concussion Assessment Tool 3 (SCAT3) scores of male and female athletes—both with and without disabilities—who played international football. The disability football cohort consisted of players from the blind, deaf, cerebral palsy, and learning disability squads. Players from the disability squads reported significantly higher symptom scores as compared to players without disability. Female deaf footballers had worse balance error scores than female footballers without disability, and male footballers with learning disabilities had significantly worse performance on immediate memory testing than male football players with no reported learning disabilities.

The knowledge, attitudes, and beliefs of clinicians responsible for the care of disabled footballers towards concussion in sport have also been explored (Griffin et al., 2017). Physiotherapists and medical doctors working with international cerebral palsy football squads were interviewed to gather their perspectives related to cerebral palsy football. Only 29% of the health professionals involved in the study reported using any form of concussion assessment tool following a suspected injury, with 50% reporting difficulty in conducting cognitive assessments in this population. The overwhelming majority (86%), however, agreed that a sport-specific disability consensus statement would be helpful in guiding their practice with these athletes.

The findings from both of these studies (Griffin et al., 2017; Weiler et al., 2018) have several implications for clinicians. The data from Weiler and colleagues' 2018 study confirms what many clinicians would have already been aware of: there are some key differences that should be considered when assessing concussion in a disability cohort. The presence of factors such as visual impairment, gait or co-ordination difficulties, or learning disabilities are all likely to impact upon pre- and post-concussion testing. As such, clinicians need to carefully consider how they interpret information collected using the current battery of concussion screening tools, as the results from these tests may represent the disabled athlete's standard baseline rather than the presence of deficits (i.e. "false positives"). A key element missing from these studies is the disability athlete's perspective towards the management of concussion via quantitative and qualitative methods, which would provide insights that would enrich and enhance their care.

Throughout this section, it has been demonstrated that concussion in disability sport impacts upon athletes across a range of sports. The few data-driven studies in the area also show that the baseline characteristics of athletes with a physical disability vary substantially from those in unimpaired athletes and suggest that there are challenges for clinicians in managing concussion in this population. The following section will summarize some of the existing literature related to athletes with a mental disability, who also require special attention during their assessment and treatment.

Concussion and learning disabilities, attention deficit hyperactivity disorder, and dyslexia

The areas of learning disabilities (LD), attention deficit-hyperactivity disorder (ADHD), and dyslexia are one of the few aspects of mental disability that have been discussed in relation to concussion in sport. Collins et al. (1999) were the first to demonstrate that players with LD and a history of two or more concussions performed significantly worse on neurocognitive testing than players without LD. The authors suggested that the presence of LD might have made the initial diagnosis of concussion challenging, which appears to be a valid conclusion given the intricacies in using concussion screening tools. Much like the challenges present with assessing concussion in athletes with physical disabilities, the presence of mental disability provides challenges for clinicians to consider. At this time, there has been insufficient examination of these issues in the literature. Efforts should be made in future research to examine these issues and provide some guidance to help the clinician with this specialized cohort.

More recently, several studies have explored the influence of LD/ADHD on concussion reporting and concussion history (Iverson et al., 2016; Nelson et al., 2016; Wiseheart & Wellington, 2017). Nelson et al.'s (2016) study included data from over 8,000 athletes in a cross-sectional study. Although this work was limited by the fact that the sample was primarily male football players, it provided insights about the impact of ADHD and LD on concussion reporting. Their results indicated that among athletes without a history of concussion, those with ADHD reported more baseline symptoms, and that athletes with ADHD *and* LD had poorer performances on neurocognitive testing. These outcomes are noteworthy for clinicians working with athletes with LD and ADHD and may help provide context to the neurocognitive data collected at baseline.

Iverson et al. (2016) also explored data from athletes with LD and ADHD to examine their lifetime history of concussion. Using self-reported data from a large sample of adolescent athletes, Iverson and colleagues showed that athletes with LD and/or ADHD had a significantly higher prevalence of prior concussions than athletes without these conditions. The presence of LD is likely to affect an athlete's ability to engage with concussion baseline testing, and this is also applicable to athletes with dyslexia. Wiseheart and Wellington (2017) have outlined a screening protocol for dyslexia into the assessment tools used by athletic trainers involved in the diagnosis of athletes with concussion. Their protocol aims to assist athletic trainers identify dyslexia in the student athletes they assess, which, in turn, enables them to contextualize athletes' concussion baseline testing scores.

In sum, this section has highlighted some of the influences that conditions such as LD, AHDH, and dyslexia have on concussion assessment and recovery. With an increased understanding of the intersection between these conditions and concussion, more nuanced methods of assessing and managing concussion for individuals with these conditions may emerge.

Gaps in current knowledge/understanding of concussion in disability sport

Despite there being a number of consensus/position statements on concussion in sport, there has been no explicit mention of the assessment and management of concussion for athletes with disabilities. Many of the signs/symptoms associated with concussion overlap with signs and symptoms that many athletes with disabilities experience as a result of their disability (e.g., self-reported balance problems, abnormal finger-to-nose coordination). Thus, the first step should be to understand and identify the clinical presentations of a concussion that are appropriate for athletes with disabilities, how they should be measured, and how they should be elevated. It should also be noted that the majority of the understanding of concussion in athletes with disability is derived from formal, organized sport at the elite level. There is very little literature on recreational (i.e., non-elite) athletes with disabilities who would seek care from a general physician/clinician, as opposed to the relatively resource-rich, multidisciplinary healthcare access afforded to many elite, non-disabled athletes. There has also been no research to date on the psychological effects of sports concussion on athletes with disabilities.

In addition to these highlighted gaps in the literature, there is also a need to understand the functional implications of concussion for athletes with disabilities. Epidemiological data suggests that there is a significant burden of concussion in athletes who participate in disability sport (Iverson et al., 2016). It can be argued, therefore, that clinicians have a duty to better appreciate concussion-related consequences within this cohort. Given the well-established benefits of sporting participation to individuals with a disability (Shephard, 1991), future iterations of the Consensus in Sport Group (McCrory et al., 2017) and other consensus/position statements around the world should provide guidance for clinicians about how to better support athletes with disabilities.

Implications of concussion for athletes with disabilities

Given the current gaps in concussion knowledge, it is important to understand the implications that concussion can have on their well-being. This section examines the existing literature related to this, focusing on two key facets for athletes with disabilities: Concussion symptom disclosure and adherence to concussion management recommendations.

Two of the most critical issues in optimizing concussion management lie in concussion evaluation and treatment plan adherence. These issues are made even more difficult when contextualized within the lived experiences of athletes with disabilities. Whilst the last 20 years have seen concerted efforts to standardize the evaluation of concussion within the sport and exercise medicine community, this process is still heavily influenced by the symptoms endorsement of the athlete, and the clinical expertise of the practitioner. There is a paucity of evidence-based concussion assessment tools that specifically cater to athletes with disabilities (e.g., the wheelchair error scoring system from Wessels, 2014). There are also no modifications to existing concussion assessment tools that adequately account for pre-existing disabilities, despite significant differences in pre-injury levels of function (Weiler et al., 2018). This results in concussion evaluation, management, and rehabilitation approaches that are neither patient-centered, nor evidence-based, and which could negatively impact the overall health and performance of the athlete.

The complexities of concussion management are exacerbated for athletes with disabilities. Previous research is rather equivocal regarding the impact of mental health and neurodevelopmental disorders on concussion recovery but suggests that athletes living with depression may have a prolonged recovery (Iverson et al., 2017). Relative rest is considered to be an important part of the concussion management process. Among athletes with physical disabilities (e.g., spinal cord injuries), the physical toll of activities of daily living is higher. Thus, they do not get the same level of relative rest that non-disabled athletes would be able to attain, which may prolong their recovery. Similarly, athletes with intellectual disabilities need more cognitive exertion in the context of daily life, thereby reducing their ability to optimize their recovery through rest.

As previously noted, the impact of concussion on athletes with disabilities has not fully been explored, and there is currently a lack of evidence-based assessment tools and management strategies that are both patient-centered and tailored to this population. The influence of pre-existing depression on recovery from concussion for the athlete with a disability also warrants further research.

Concussion symptom disclosure

Symptom disclosure is an issue in sport injury assessment in general, but it is particularly important with respect to concussion, where accurate diagnosis relies heavily on athletes' self-reported symptom endorsement. Reasons that athletes with disabilities may be reticent to disclose symptoms to health care providers range from coach and parental pressure, to a desire to support the team, to athletic identity (Wessels, Broglio, & Sosnoff, 2012). Athletes with disabilities—particularly ones with "invisible" disabilities, such as attention or learning disorders—may have added reluctance associated with disclosing a concussion (Madaus, 2008; Madaus, Foley, Maguire, & Ruban, 2002). The non-specific nature of concussion symptoms also presents a problem with respect to symptom disclosure.

Many of the symptoms included in post-concussion symptom checklists are not universally applicable to athletes with disabilities. For example, athletes with cerebral palsy may not be able to differentiate balance problems caused by a concussion versus those caused by their condition, and the symptom "sensitivity to light" following a concussion may not be applicable for athletes with visual impairments. In sum, some concussion symptoms could mirror symptoms that an athlete with disability lives with on a daily basis. Chronic desensitization may skew their perception of a symptom's presence, particularly in scenarios where they are not associated with an overt mechanism of injury. This could result in the underestimation or even unawareness of a symptom as being due to concussion, resulting in a lack of timely medical follow-up. Symptom endorsement may also be influenced by the dosage and timing of pharmaceutical management associated with an athlete's pre-existing condition. Medications for conditions such as posttraumatic stress illnesses, ADHD, and chronic migraines, for example, may mask the presence of post-concussion anxiety, trouble focusing, or headaches.

The absence of population and condition-specific tools for athletes with disabilities increases the already significant pressure on the health care providers' clinical decision-making, with respect to concussion evaluation and diagnosis.

Adherence to concussion recommendations

The focus on the uptake, adoption, and sustained adherence to sport and exercise medicine interventions continues to increase as the gap between evidence-based efficacy and real-world effectiveness of interventions persists (Brown, Verhagen, van Mechelen, Lambert, & Draper, 2016; O'Brien & Finch, 2014). The 3rd consensus statement on concussion in sport recommended that athletes be asymptomatic in order to progress through a graduated physical activity protocol and procure medical clearance before unmodified return to sport (McCrory et al., 2009). Wessels, Broglio, and Sosnoff (2012), however, found more than half of the sample of wheelchair basketball players continued to engage in physical activity while symptomatic but could not identify reasons as to why this was the case. Further research is needed in order to better understand determinants of effective concussion management intervention adherence amongst athletes with disabilities (Wessels, Broglio, & Sosnoff, 2012).

The chronic disease sector of health has evaluated the role and impact of treatment burden (i.e. treatment fatigue) on adherence, including amongst individuals with HIV, those with diabetes, as well as with smoking cessation programs (Heckman and Mosso, 2014). Research suggests that treatment fatigue increases when daily withdrawal symptoms increase, and vice versa (Liu, et al., 2013). Athletes with disabilities often have a significant history of medical intervention, which may increase their sensitivity to the additional treatment burdens associated with concussion. This, in turn, may result in an increased susceptibility to treatment fatigue and the risk of non-adherence. As with many issues associated with concussion in athletes with disabilities, this area has not been well researched and warrants further study in order to improve the quality of evidence-based care provided.

In summary, athletes with disabilities who sustain a concussion may have additional complications related to injury disclosure and symptom endorsement, as well as treatment plan adherence. Clinicians treating these athletes need to consider these issues carefully when assessing and managing concussion.

Social isolation and concussion

Social isolation following sports injury has been explored in the literature, but to date there has not been carryover to the area of concussion and athletes with disabilities. This section summarizes current knowledge on social isolation and injury and discusses how this may be especially problematic for athletes with disabilities.

Prolonged concussion recovery may result in isolation from the social networks and support athletes develop through sport (André-Morin, Caron, & Bloom, 2017). Social interaction and improved self-esteem are two of the most commonly listed benefits of engagement in sport and physical activity (Eime et al., 2013). Young athletes, in particular, cite the loss of activities due to concussion as their most pressing concern (Delaney et al., 2015). Post-concussion symptoms in young athletes have also been associated with an increased difficulty with emotions, with influencing their roles in scholastic and social environments, and with being viewed differently by peers (Valovich MacLeod, Wagner, & Bacon, 2017). A study from Shapiro and Martin (2014) indicated that lower self-perceptions of athletic ability were linked to increased isolation amongst young athletes with disabilities. The lack of in-depth qualitative studies related to isolation following concussion in this population warrants further investigation in order to deepen our understanding of the implications of concussion for athletes with disabilities.

Understanding social isolation is particularly important for athletes with disabilities, given the added potential weight of athlete identity. The culture of sport normalizes and valorizes playing through injury. A study of over 300 youth ice hockey players found that, amongst players who sustained an injury, the risk of a second injury was higher in those who scored above the 75th percentile on the Athletic Identity Measurement Scale (McKay et al., 2013). Athletes with a greater connection to their athletic identity may be more inclined to minimize or outright ignore concussion symptoms or not adhere to concussion management and return to play protocol. This may be compounded in athletes with disabilities, for whom the athlete identity may also serve as a means to diminish the impact of marginalization and oppression associated with living with a disability (DePauw, 1997; Huang & Brittain, 2006). Concussions are heterogeneous injuries whose natural history is poorly understood amongst athletes with disabilities. The fear of losing access to the power and privilege of the athlete identity for an indeterminate length of time due to concussion may further motivate athletes with disabilities to push against the boundaries of their health in order to return to play. When considering the safety implications of premature return to play following a concussion, and the increased difficulty to evaluate concussion in athletes with disabilities, ensuring that athletes are active, honest, and adherent participants in their recovery and RTP is critical.

The social identity approach

This section includes two parts. First, we introduce the social identity approach, briefly discuss the research evidence that has demonstrated the positive influence of social identity, and outline the benefits of adopting a social identity approach for concussed athletes with disabilities. Second, we outline the interventions based on the social identity approach to enhance concussion management for athletes with disabilities.

Social identity refers to an "individual's knowledge that he [or she] belongs to certain social groups together with some emotional value and significance to him [or her] of this group membership" (Tajfel, 1972, p. 292). Accordingly, an individual's social identity reflects the part of their self-concept associated with internalized group memberships, which have psychological meaning and value (e.g., "us England players"). As acknowledged by Turner (1982), social identities are distinct to an individual's personal identity, where the self is understood in terms of individual and unique characteristics (e.g., as "I" or "me").

In sport, the social identity approach has emerged over the past few years (Rees, Haslam, Coffee, & Lavallee, 2015). To date, researchers have yet to adopt this approach to concussion in disability sport. There is a plethora of social identity research outside of sport, and it has revealed that high levels of group identification lead to various positive outcomes for individuals and groups (Haslam, 2004). For example, individuals have reported feeling capable and in control (Greenaway et al., 2015), an increased willingness to go above and beyond one's role for the group (Haslam et al., 2004), and greater social support (Reicher & Haslam, 2006), all of which may be of benefit for concussion management in disability sport.

Shifting individuals' focus from "me" to "we" has been found to be crucial for mental health interventions (Greenaway et al., 2015). It may also be crucial in concussion identification and recovery for the athletes with disabilities. Athletes with a shared team identity (i.e., "we") may be more supportive in the context of performance (e.g., poor form) and health (e.g., concussion) issues. Conversely, teams with a lack of shared identity, where athletes are concerned with and operate within their personal identity (i.e., "me"), may be less likely to support one another during a concussion or be committed to the group. The sport psychology consultant (SPC) is well placed to deliver interventions that cultivate a distinct team identity to aid the concussion management of athletes with disabilities.

Using the social identity approach to enhance concussion management

This section will draw on our experiences of practicing in elite sport to highlight strategies that could be adopted to optimize post-concussion RTP for athletes with disabilities. As part of an athlete's rehabilitation team, the SPC has a crucial role in supporting an athlete with disability that may be anxious when preparing for RTP. Beyond this input, the SPC may work to understand and facilitate the disabled athlete's social network within their sport (teammates, coaches, mentors, physiotherapist/the team doctor where applicable) as a crucial part of their concussion rehabilitation. Increasing evidence suggests that multiple social identities (i.e., group memberships) enhance one's perceived health during difficult transitional periods (Steffens et al., 2016). Thus, the role of SPCs in cultivating support networks for athletes with disabilities who have sustained concussions beyond their athletic role (e.g., family member, volunteer, student, etc.) to maintain and enhance well-being should also be explored.

SPCs can develop disability athletes' social networks to aid psychological preparation following concussion. Data indicate that athletes who have a strong athletic identity may experience psychological and/or behavioral disturbances if they are often unable to fulfill their athletic role through injury (Sparkes, 1998). This could be particularly pertinent for athletes with disabilities, whose sporting participation may provide them with a passion and focus. Accordingly, athletes with disabilities could work with SPCs (both proactively and reactively) to optimize their social networks. Specifically, SPCs could raise the awareness of disability athletes' available social networks within which support is harbored and help the athlete develop and implement strategies to enhance the quality of social support within their athletic role and other social roles (e.g., family, friends).

Developing and evolving a shared team and organizational identity may also be beneficial for athletes involved in organized disability sport. Available evidence indicates that informational support is more influential when provided by someone with whom individuals share a group membership (i.e., as part of "us" rather than as part of an out-group; Gallagher, Meaney, & Muldoon, 2014) and thus may be of benefit for recovery following concussion. Messages and support given by key stakeholders (e.g., physiotherapists and team doctors) are more likely to be perceived as intended and have more impact (e.g., increased engagement with a rehabilitation program) if athletes share a common group identity with the provider. Slater and Barker's (2018) study in elite disability football developed and evaluated an intervention that aimed to strengthen disabled footballers' perceived team identification. The social identity intervention was based on the 3R's ("Reflecting," "Representing," and "Realizing") and was implemented twice over the 22-month duration of the study. Compared to baseline data, findings in year one ($d = 0.76$) and year two ($d = 0.82$) indicated large effect size increases in disabled footballers' reported social identification. Creating a shared team identity through the 3Rs may also increase the likelihood that key messages (e.g., concussion procedures) will be perceived as important, meaningful, and well-intended because athletes share the same identity and values as the provider of the information (e.g., support staff).

In sum, research examining social identity interventions in sport is currently in its infancy, and researchers investigating the influence of such interventions involving athletes with disabilities following concussion should be encouraged. The social identity approach emphasizes the importance of developing a shared team identity that in turn provides a unique opportunity to enhance concussion management in disabled athletes. As such, social identity-based interventions could be a way to help develop a strong team identity that could become the foundation for effective support during concussion management.

Future research

Whilst the focus in the past decade has been on a unified approach to concussion evaluation and management, the specific needs of the athlete with a disability would indicate that this population requires a different approach. This chapter has highlighted a number of important avenues for researchers to consider, as there is precious little research on the efficacy of current concussion management strategies in athletes with disabilities. The added value of bespoke interventions that consider or accommodate specific issues that may be faced by athletes with disabilities is desperately needed. But in order for such research to be of use, the paucity of research regarding the burden and concussion, as well as the efficacy of current concussion strategies and effectiveness amongst athletes with disabilities must also be addressed.

Efforts have been made by researchers in Sweden to understand more about the injury experiences of athletes with disabilities (Fagher et al., 2016), and this work highlighted the complexity of athletes with disabilities' perceptions of their injuries. To expand on Fagher and colleagues' study, future research should consider assessing the social status of disabled athletes with a concussion. A fruitful starting point would be to examine athletes' level of social identification and perceived social support (e.g., via the Perceived Available Support in Sport Questionnaire; Freeman, Coffee, & Rees, 2011) at the various stages following concussion and in RTP. The most pertinent for consideration is how an athlete's social support changes (e.g., from when competing compared to following concussion) and the role that an SPC can play. This would provide valuable insight to enable appropriate strategies to put in place for athletes with both physical and mental disabilities following a concussion.

More broadly, the psychological health and well-being of disabled athletes with a concussion has received limited research attention. Previous research has found that athletes with disabilities perceived multiple sources of organizational stressors (Arnold et al., 2017). Suffering a concussion is an additional stressor for disabled athletes, which is likely to have implications for their psychological health and well-being. Therefore, it appears to be important to qualitatively investigate the unique stressors and challenges experienced by these athletes and explore how able they are to cope with these demands. This would provide an opportunity to examine the impact on athletes' understanding of concussion, their capability to manage concussions sustained by them or their teammates, and the social support provided/received following this injury.

Other future research efforts could focus on the use of innovative technologies to facilitate disabled athletes following a concussion. Fagher et al. (2017) described the use of eHealth technologies to facilitate self-reporting of injuries in a Paralympic population, and the promising findings from this feasibility study suggest it may assist the diagnosis of the disabled athlete following concussion. Other innovative approaches to concussion management using eHealth have been attempted with non-disabled athletes (Ahmed et al., 2017), and these could also facilitate the management of athletes with a physical or mental disability following concussion if the technological benefits they provide (e.g. assisting graded RTP, enabling peer support, and reducing social isolation) could be harnessed effectively.

Conclusions

The prevalence of head injuries among athletes with disabilities has been reported as being as high as 25% of all injuries (Webborn et al., 2016), and both physical and mental disabilities have been associated with poorer performance on neuropsychological testing as well as poorer clinical recovery (Nelson et al., 2016;

Weiler et al., 2018). Currently, athletes with disabilities are underrepresented in concussion research; from understanding the burden and patterns of concussion to the development, implementation, and evaluation of concussion management programming. The role of social identity and social support are areas of focus that may constitute valuable approaches to assist the recovery of an athlete with a disability following concussion. In order to make progress with engaging athletes with disabilities in physical activity throughout the lifespan, our ability to provide them with high quality, evidence-informed strategies to optimize their health is essential. An important step in this process will be the inclusion of athletes with disabilities in concussion consensus/agreement statements, alongside the creation of concussion assessment and management guidelines that are tailored towards the athlete with a disability.

References

Ahmed, O. H., Hussain, A. W., Beasley, I., Dvorak, J., & Weiler, R. (2015). Enhancing performance and sport injury prevention in disability sport: moving forwards in the field of football. *British Journal of Sports Medicine, 49*, 566–567.

Ahmed, O. H., Schneiders, A. G., McCrory, P. R., & Sullivan, S. J. (2017). Sport concussion management using Facebook: A feasibility study of an innovative adjunct "iCon." *Journal of Athletic Training, 52*, 339–349.

André-Morin, D., Caron, J. G., & Bloom, G. A. (2017). Exploring the unique challenges faced by female university athletes experiencing prolonged concussion symptoms. *Sport, Exercise, and Performance Psychology, 6*, 289–303.

Arnold, R., Wagstaff, C. R., Steadman, L., & Pratt, Y. (2017). The organisational stressors encountered by athletes with disabilities. *Journal of Sports Sciences, 35*, 1187–1196.

Brown, J. C., Verhagen, E., van Mechelen, W., Lambert, M. I., & Draper, C. E. (2016). Coaches' and referees' perceptions of the BokSmart injury prevention programme. *International Journal of Sports Science & Coaching, 11*, 637–647.

Collins, M. W., Grindel, S. H., Lovell, M. R., Dede, D. E., Moser, D. J., Phalin, B. R., & McKeag, D. B. (1999). Relationship between concussion and neuropsychological performance in college football players. *The Journal of the American Medical Association, 282*, 964–970.

Delaney, J. S., Lamfookon, C., Bloom, G. A., Al-Kashmiri, A., & Correa, A. (2015). Why university athletes choose not to reveal their concussion symptoms during a practice or game. *Clinical Journal of Sport Medicine, 25*, 113–125.

DePauw, K. P. (1997). The (In)Visibility of DisAbility: Cultural contexts and "sporting bodies." *Quest, 49*, 416–430.

Eime, R. M., Young, J. A., Harvey, J. T., Charity M. J., & Payne, W.R. (2013). A systematic review of the psychological and social benefits of participation in sport for children and adolescents: Informing development of a conceptual model of health through sport. *International Journal of Behavioral Nutrition and Physical Activity, 10*, 98.

Fagher, K., Forsberg, A., Jacobsson, J., Timpka, T., Dahlström, Ö., & Lexell J., (2016). Paralympic athletes' perceptions of their experiences of sports-related injuries, risk factors and preventive possibilities. *European Journal of Sport Science, 16*, 1240–1249.

Fagher, K., Jacobsson, J., Dahlström, Ö., Timpka, T., & Lexell, J. (2017). An eHealth application of self-reported sports-related injuries and illnesses in Paralympic sport: Pilot feasibility and usability study. *Journal of Medical Internet Research Human Factors, 29*, 30.

Ferrara, M. S., Buckley, W. E., McCann, B. C., Limbird, T. J., Powell, J. W., & Robl, R. (1992). The injury experience of the competitive athlete with a disability: Prevention implications. *Medicine & Science in Sports & Exercise, 24*, 184–188.

Freeman, P., Coffee, P., & Rees, T. (2011). The PASS-Q: The perceived available support in sport questionnaire. *Journal of Sport and Exercise Psychology, 33*, 54–74.

Gallagher S., Meaney S., & Muldoon O. T. (2014). Social identity influences stress appraisals and cardiovascular reactions to acute stress exposure. *British Journal of Health Psychology, 19*, 566–579.

Greenaway K. H., Haslam S. A., Cruwys T., Branscombe N. R., Ysseldyk R., & Heldreth C. (2015). From "We" to "Me": Group identification enhances perceived personal control with consequences for health and well-being. *Journal of Personality and Social Psychology, 109*, 53–74.

Griffin, S., West, L. R., Ahmed, O. H., & Weiler R. (2017). Concussion knowledge, attitudes and beliefs amongst sports medicine personnel at the 2015 Cerebral Palsy Football World Championships. *British Journal of Sports Medicine, 51*, 325.

Grünke, M., & Cavendish, W. M. (2016). Learning disabilities around the globe: Making sense of the heterogeneity of the different viewpoints. *Learning Disabilities—A Contemporary Journal, 14*, 1–8.

Haslam, S. A. (2004). *Psychology in organizations: The social identity approach* (2nd ed.). Thousand Oaks, CA: Sage Publications.

Haslam, A. S., Jetten, J., O'Brien, A., & Jacobs, E. (2004). Social identity, social influence and reactions to potentially stressful tasks: Support for the self-categorisation model of stress. *Stress and Health, 20*, 3–9.

Heckman, J. J., & Mosso, S. (2014). The economics of human development and social mobility. *Annual Review of Economics, 6*, 689–733.

Huang, C., & Brittain, I. (2006). Negotiating identities through disability sport. *Sociology of Sport Journal, 23*, 352–375.

Iverson, G. L., Wojtowicz, M., Brooks, B. L., Maxwell, B. A., Atkins, J. E., Zafonte, R., & Berkner P. D. (2016). High school athletes with ADHD and learning difficulties have a greater lifetime concussion history. *Journal of Attention Disorders.* DOI: 10.1177/1087054716657410.

Iverson, G. L., Gardner, A. J., Terry, D. P., Ponsford, J. L., Sills, A. K., Broshek, D. K., & Solomon G. S. (2017). Predictors of clinical recovery from concussion: A systematic review. *British Journal of Sports Medicine, 51*, 941–948.

Kissick J., & Webborn N. (2018). Concussion in Para sport. *Physical Medicine and Rehabilitation Clinics of North America, 29*, 299–311.

Liu, X., Li, R., Lanza, S. T., Vasilenko, S., & Piper M. (2013). Understanding the role of cessation fatigue in the smoking cessation process. *Drug and Alcohol Dependency, 133*, 548–555.

Madaus, J. W. (2008). Employment self-disclosure rates and rationales of university graduates with learning disabilities. *Journal of Learning Disabilities, 41*, 291–299.

Madaus, J. W., Foley, T. E., McGuire, J. M., & Ruban, L. M. (2002). Employment self-disclosure of postsecondary graduates with learning disabilities: Rates and rationales. *Journal of Learning Disabilities, 36*, 364–369.

McCrory, P., Meeuwisse, W., Johnston, K., Dvorak, J., Aubry, M., Molloy, M., & Cantu, R. (2009). Consensus statement on Concussion in Sport—The 3rd International Conference on Concussion in Sport held in Zurich, November 2008. *South African Journal of Sports Medicine, 21*, 36–46.

McCrory, P., Meeuwisse, W., Dvorak, J., Aubry, M., Bailes, J., Broglio, S., … Vos, P. E. (2017). Consensus statement on concussion in sport—The 5th international conference on concussion in sport held in Berlin, October 2016. *British Journal of Sport Medicine, 51*, 838–847.

McKay, C., Campbell, T., Meeuwisse, W., & Emery, C. (2013). The role of psychosocial risk factors for injury in elite youth ice hockey. *Clinical Journal of Sport Medicine, 23*, 216–221.

Nelson, L. D., Guskiewicz, K. M., Marshall, S. W., Hammeke, T., Barr W., … McCrea, M.A. (2016). Multiple self-reported concussions are more prevalent in athletes with ADHD and learning disability. *Clinical Journal of Sport Medicine, 26*, 120–127.

O'Brien, J., & Finch, C. F. (2014). The implementation of musculoskeletal injury-prevention exercise programmes in team ball sports: a systematic review employing the RE-AIM framework. *Sports Medicine, 44*, 1305–1318.

Oxford Living Dictionary (2018). Definition of disability in English. Retrieved 20th July 2018 from: https://en.oxforddictionaries.com/definition/disability.

Rees, T., Haslam, S. A., Coffee, P., & Lavallee, D. (2015). A social identity approach to sport psychology: Principles, practice, and prospects. *Sports Medicine, 45*, 1083–1096.

Reicher, S. D., & Haslam, S. A. (2006). Rethinking the psychology of tyranny: The BBC Prison Study. *British Journal of Social Psychology, 45*, 1–40.

Shapiro, D. R., & Martin J. J. (2014). The relationships among sport self-perceptions and social well-being in athletes with physical disabilities. *Disability and Health Journal,7*, 42–48.

Shephard, R. J. (1991). Benefits of sport and physical activity for the disabled: Implications for the individual and for society. *Scandinavian Journal of Rehabilitation Medicine, 23*, 51–59.

Silva, M. P., Morato, M. P., Bilzon, J. L., Duarte, E. (2013). Sports injuries in Brazilian blind footballers. *International Journal of Sports Medicine, 34*, 239–243.

Slater, M. J., & Barker, J. B. (2018). Doing social identity leadership: Exploring the efficacy of an identity leadership intervention on perceived leadership and mobilization in elite disability soccer. *Journal of Applied Sport Psychology*. https://doi.org/10.1080/10413200.2017.1410255.

Sparkes A. C. (1998). Athletic identity: An Achilles' heel to the survival of self. *Qualitative Health Research, 8*, 644–664.

Steffens, N. K., Jetten, J., Haslam, C., Cruwys, T., & Haslam S. A. (2016). Multiple social identities enhance health post-retirement because they are a basis for giving social support. *Frontiers in Psychology, 7*, 1519.

Tajfel, H. (1972). Social categorisation. English manuscript of "La categorisation sociale." In S. Moscovici (Ed.), *Introduction à la psychologie sociale* (Vol. 1, pp. 272–302). Paris: Larousse.

Gibson, O. (2016). Premier League clubs working to help more disabled people get into sport. *The Guardian*. Retrieved 4th January 2018 from: www.theguardian.com/sport/2016/oct/05/premier-league-clubs-disabled-people-sport.

Turner, J. C. (1982). Towards a cognitive redefinition of the social group. In H. Tajfel (Ed.), *Social identity and intergroup relations* (pp. 15–40). Cambridge: Cambridge University Press.

Valovich McLeod, T. C., Wagner, A. J., & Bacon, C. E. W. (2017). Lived experiences of adolescent athletes following sport-related concussion. *Orthopaedic Journal of Sports Medicine, 5*, 1–10.

Webborn, N., Blauwet, C. A., Derman, W., Idrisova, G., Lexell, J., Stomphorst, J., ... Kissick, J. (2018). Heads up on concussion in Para sport. *British Journal of Sports Medicine, 52*(18), 1157–1158.

Webborn, N., & Emery C. (2014). Descriptive epidemiology of Paralympic sports injuries. *PM&R, 6*, S18–S22.

Webborn, N., Cushman, D., Blauwet, C. A., Emery, C., Derman, W., Schwellnus, M., ... Willick, S. E. (2016). The epidemiology of injuries in football at the London 2012 Paralympic Games. *Physical Medicine and Rehabilitation, 8*, 545–552.

Weiler, R., van Mechelen, W., Fuller, C., Ahmed, O. H., & Verhagen, E. (2018). Do neurocognitive SCAT3 baseline test scores differ between footballers (soccer) living with and without disability? A cross-sectional study. *Clinical Journal of Sport Medicine, 28*, 43–50.

Wessels, K. K., Broglio, S. P., & Sosnoff, J. J. (2012). Concussions in wheelchair basketball. *Archives of Physical Medicine and Rehabilitation, 93*, 275–278.

Wessels, K. (2014). *Concussions in wheelchair users: Quantifying seated postural control.* (Doctoral dissertation, University of Illinois at Urbana-Champaign).

West, L. R., Griffin, S., Weiler, R., & Ahmed, O. H. (2017). Management of concussion in disability sport: A different ball game? *British Journal of Sports Medicine, 51*, 1050–1051.

Willick, S. E., Webborn, N., Emery, C., Blauwet, C. A., Pit-Grosheide, P., Stomphorst, J., ... Derman, W. (2013). The epidemiology of injuries at the London 2012 Paralympic Games. *British Journal of Sports Medicine, 47*, 426–432.

Wiseheart, R., & Wellington, R. (2017). Identifying dyslexia risk in student-athletes: A preliminary protocol for concussion management. *Journal of Athletic Training, 52*, 982–986.

World Health Organization. (2011). World report on disability. Retrieved 6th July 2018 from: www.who.int/disabilities/world_report/2011/en/index.html.

9 Sex differences of sport-related concussion

Tracey Covassin, Morgan Anderson, Kyle M. Petit, Jennifer L. Savage, and Abigail C. Bretzin

Introduction

According to the American Psychological Association, sex is operationally defined as the physical and biological traits that distinguish between males and females (American Psychological Association, 2013). Due to the physical and biological differences between males and females, such as neck strength (Mansell et al., 2005) and hormonal differences (Roof & Hall, 2000), "sex difference" is used throughout the chapter when comparing males and females. The injured athlete's sex should be considered when developing management and treatment approaches due to the differences observed in symptom reporting, neurocognitive outcomes, and negative psychological outcomes that could result following a sport-related concussion (SRC). Understanding sex differences in concussion risk and recovery outcomes between males and females will drive management and treatment approaches in order for the athlete to return to play in a safe and efficient time period.

This chapter will address numerous areas related to sex and psychological aspects of SRC. First, a brief overview of the most recent injury rates among male and female athletes at both the high school and collegiate level will be provided. Second, sex differences in concussion symptoms, neurocognitive outcomes, recovery, and treatment will be presented. Third, sex differences in psychological aspects of SRC will be discussed. Specifically, we will examine if there are differences between males and females for depression, anxiety, suicide, and health-related quality of life following an SRC. Lastly, we will discuss if males and females cope differently and use different social support mechanisms following their head injury.

Sex differences in the epidemiology of SRC

Approximately 1.6 to 3.8 million sport and recreational concussions occur each year in the United States (Langlois, Rutland-Brown, & Wald, 2006). In a recent epidemiological study by Zuckerman and colleagues (2015), the highest National Collegiate Athletic Association (NCAA) injury rate per 10,000 athlete exposures were wrestling (10.9), followed by men's ice hockey (7.9), women's ice hockey

(7.5), and American football (6.7). In one of the largest high school studies conducted within the United States, the National Athletic Treatment Injury and Outcomes Network (NATION) study reported the highest injury rates in American football (9.2), followed by boys' lacrosse (6.5), girls' soccer (6.1), and girls' lacrosse (5.5) (see Table 9.1).

Over the past decade, research has been consistent when reporting on sex comparable sports. Specifically, female high school and collegiate athletes participating in soccer, basketball, and softball have been at a greater risk for an SRC compared to males participating in the same sports (Covassin, Moran, & Elbin, 2016; O'Connor et al., 2017; Zuckerman et al., 2015). At the collegiate level, softball players are at a 3.65 times greater risk for an SRC compared to baseball players, with female soccer athletes just under a 2 times greater risk for an SRC compared to male soccer athletes (1.83) (Zuckerman et al., 2015). Female basketball (1.5) and lacrosse (1.64) players are at over 1.5 times greater risk for an SRC compared to their counterparts (Zuckerman et al., 2015). Similar results have been reported at the high school level. Girls who participated in softball were at a four times greater risk for an SRC than baseball players (Zuckerman et al., 2015). Girls were also 1.76 and 1.53 times more likely to incur an SRC in

Table 9.1 Injury rates per 10,000 athlete exposures for high school and collegiate athletes

Sport	High School	College
	NATION Study (2011–2014) (O'Connor et al., 2017)[a]	NCAA (2009–2014) (S. Zuckerman et al., 2015)[b]
American Football	9.21	6.71
Ice Hockey (W)	–	7.50
Ice Hockey (M)	–	7.91
Lacrosse (W)	5.54	5.21
Lacrosse (M)	6.65	3.18
Soccer (W)	6.11	6.31
Soccer (M)	3.98	3.44
Wrestling	5.76	10.92
Field Hockey	4.42	4.02
Basketball (W)	4.44	5.95
Basketball (M)	2.52	3.89
Softball	3.57	3.29
Baseball	0.86	0.90
Volleyball	2.50	3.57

a O'Connor, K. L., Baker, M. M., Dalton, S. L., Dompier, T. P., Broglio, S. P., & Kerr, Z. Y. (2017). Epidemiology of sport-related concussions in high school athletes: National athletic treatment, injury and outcomes network (NATION), 2011–2012 through 2013–2014. *Journal of Athletic Training, 52*, 175–185.
b Zuckerman, S. L., Kerr, Z. Y., Yengo-Kahn, A., Wasserman, E., Covassin, T., & Solomon, G. S. (2015). Epidemiology of sports-related concussion in NCAA athletes from 2009–2010 to 2013–2014: Incidence, recurrence, and mechanisms. *American Journal of Sports Medicine, 43*, 2654–2662.

basketball and soccer compared to boys, respectively. However, when examining Division I and III NCAA ice hockey athletes, Rosene and colleagues (2017) found no differences between male and female collegiate athletes.

Sex differences have also been reported with respect to the mechanism of an SRC. The majority of researchers have reported that males have a higher proportion of SRCs due to player-to-player contact compared to females (O'Connor et al., 2017; Rosene et al., 2017; Zuckerman et al., 2015). Interestingly, in women's ice hockey, almost half (48.1%) of all SRCs occur due to player contact (Rosene et al., 2017), even though checking is not allowed in women's ice hockey. Female collegiate soccer athletes had over a two times greater risk for an SRC due to contact with an apparatus (i.e., ball, goalpost) and playing surface compared to male collegiate soccer athletes (Chandran et al., 2017).

There are several reasons why females incur more SRCs than males in sex comparable sports. First, females are more honest in reporting their SRC to a healthcare professional than males (Kerr et al., 2016). Second, researchers have suggested that female soccer athletes tend to sustain more SRCs due to a larger head to ball ratio (Boden, Kirkendall, & Garrett, 1998). Third, researchers have shown that females have an increased head-neck segment length and decreased neck girth (Mansell et al., 2005), as well as lower neck strength compared to males. This may potentially lead to a greater proportion of SRCs, due to females being subject to higher forces of angular acceleration (Tierney et al., 2008; Tierney et al., 2005). Lastly, females may be more susceptible to SRCs due to having a greater amount of estrogen (Roof & Hall, 2000). However, more research is needed to determine if hormonal variations contribute to sex differences in SRCs.

Sex differences in symptom reporting, neurocognitive function, recovery, and treatment

Symptom reporting

Concussed athletes can present with a wide variety of signs and symptoms that may go unrecognized by sports medicine professionals or unreported by athletes (Wallace, Covassin, & Beidler, 2017). More importantly, the signs and symptoms of an SRC may occur alone or in combination with each other, thus making every concussed athlete a unique case. The most commonly reported SRC symptoms are headache (94.7%), followed by dizziness (74.8%), difficulty concentrating (61%), sensitivity to light (46.6%), and sensitivity to noise (39.3) (O'Connor et al., 2017). The majority of athletes report symptom resolution approximately 14 days post-concussion (McCrory et al., 2017).

Several studies have reported sex differences in SRC symptoms (Covassin et al., 2013; Neidecker et al., 2017; Sandel et al., 2017). The majority of research supports sex differences in total symptom severity (Broshek et al., 2005; Covassin et al., 2013; Sandel et al., 2017; Zuckerman et al., 2014) and symptom recovery following an SRC (Covassin et al., 2013; O'Connor et al., 2017). Female high school and collegiate athletes also reported more symptoms on the migraine-cognitive-fatigue cluster (i.e., headache, dizziness, fatigue, sensitivity to light/noise, difficulty remembering/concentrating) and sleep cluster (i.e., trouble falling asleep, sleeping less than usual) when compared to males (Covassin et al., 2013). When considering individual symptoms, Frommer and colleagues (2011) reported male high school athletes had greater symptoms in amnesia, confusion, and disorientation than female high school athletes; whereas, female high school athletes had greater symptom reports in drowsiness and sensitivity to noise. Researchers have also indicated that males had a higher incidence of anterograde amnesia and loss of consciousness compared to females (Neidecker et al., 2017). However, other researchers found no sex differences in individual symptoms following an SRC (O'Connor et al., 2017; Zuckerman et al., 2014).

Although the majority of research suggests sex differences exist on symptom severity and total symptoms, additional research is needed to determine if females truly have different individual symptoms than males or if they just report more total symptoms compared to males. In addition, future research should concentrate on examining if female athletes have a different symptom trajectory than male athletes following an SRC. Understanding differences in symptom trajectories between male and female athletes may help healthcare professionals target specific symptoms to reduce recovery time.

Neurocognitive function

Current consensus statements recommend the utilization of a multifaceted assessment and treatment approach following an SRC (Broglio et al., 2014; McCrory et al., 2017). This multifaceted approach includes an objective assessment of neurocognitive function at baseline (i.e., pre-injury) and post-injury time points (McCory et al., 2017). Previous research indicates neurocognitive sex differences exist (Sandel et al., 2017), specifically in relation to reaction time (Broshek et al., 2005; Colvin et al., 2009), visual memory (Covassin et al., 2012; Covassin, Schatz, & Swanik, 2007), and visual motor speed (Majerske et al., 2008).

For example, Sandel and colleagues (2017) compared neurocognitive performance between male and female soccer and lacrosse athletes within three days after sustaining an SRC. Concussed female athletes performed significantly worse than male athletes across all neurocognitive domains (Sandel et al., 2017). Additionally, the degree of neurocognitive impairment demonstrated by females post-injury was significantly greater than the degree of impairment demonstrated by males (Sandel et al., 2017). In fact, 74% of female athletes demonstrated at least one reliable change from baseline compared to 59% of male athletes (Sandel et al., 2017). Reliable change indices, established by Iverson, Lovell, & Collins (2003), are objective cutoff scores for neurocognitive domains in order to detect meaningful change between baseline and re-test assessments. Therefore, the majority of concussed female athletes examined by Sandel and colleagues (2017) produced neurocognitive scores above clinically meaningful change on at least one neurocognitive domain when compared to their baseline. Interestingly, these results reflect the findings of Broshek and colleagues (2005), which revealed concussed female athletes' neurocognitive performance declined approximately one reliable change from baseline performance. Specifically, concussed female athletes demonstrated significantly greater declines in simple and complex reaction time compared to males (Broshek et al., 2005). In addition, female athletes were 1.5 times more likely to have neurocognitive impairments after sustaining an SRC compared to male athletes (Broshek et al., 2005). However, these results are limited by the fact that the majority of female athletes in this study played a variety of sports (e.g., soccer and lacrosse), whereas the majority of males participated in American football only (Covassin et al., 2013). In order to address this limitation, several studies have investigated sex differences in neurocognitive function in comparable sports (e.g., soccer) (Colvin et al., 2009; Covassin et al., 2013; Zuckerman et al., 2012).

Research conducted by Colvin and colleagues (2009) examined neurocognitive sex differences in male and female soccer athletes following an SRC. Concussed female athletes demonstrated significantly slower reaction time compared to male athletes (Colvin et al., 2009). In addition, Covassin et al. (2013) reported female soccer athletes demonstrated visual memory impairments at eight days post-concussion compared to male soccer athletes. Similarly, Majerske et al. (2008) observed visual motor speed impairments in high school aged female athletes after an SRC, but no other significant differences were observed in neurocognitive performance. Future research should continue to investigate which neurocognitive domains are most impaired following an SRC in order to implement individualized treatment options.

Contrary to the evidence presented above, other studies have reported no significant sex differences in neurocognitive function after an SRC (Sufrinko et al., 2016; Zuckerman et al., 2012). Zuckerman et al. (2012) compared neurocognitive performance between concussed male and female high school soccer athletes. Results of this study revealed no sex differences on any neurocognitive domain. In addition, Sufrinko and colleagues (2016) compared neurocognitive performance between concussed male and female athletes and found no sex differences on any of the neurocognitive domains. However, these results may be due to the wide age range (i.e., 9–18 years) of athletes sampled (Sufrinko et al., 2016).

Overall, research suggests that there are significant sex differences in neurocognitive function following an SRC. Female athletes are observed to have significantly more neurocognitive impairments compared to male athletes and are more likely to be impaired for longer periods of time. Understanding sex differences in neurocognitive function following an SRC will help healthcare professionals better understand recovery patterns and individualize treatment options between male and female athletes.

Recovery

SRCs affect athletes differently, thus it is difficult to determine an exact trajectory of recovery for every individual. However, it has been identified that for most athletes, a significant clinical recovery is made within the first two weeks following a head injury (McCrory et al., 2017). Despite these findings, some athletes may report protracted symptoms lasting several weeks to months following an SRC. The primary cause of this protracted recovery remains unclear; however, several factors have been attributed to this delay in recovery. Specifically, younger athletes, as well as females, have been identified to be at a greater risk for a protracted recovery compared to their male counterparts.

Earlier studies reported no sex differences in athletes' recovery following an SRC. Cantu, Guskiewicz, and Register-Mihalik (2010) observed no differences between male and female athletes in symptom resolution or return to play time. Additionally, a large study consisting of 812 athletes with SRCs over the span of two years reported that males and females presented with no differences in recovery time (Frommer et al., 2011). Yet, the emergence of new literature suggests that sex differences in recovery from an SRC may exist.

Recent literature suggests that females take longer to recover and have a greater risk of persistent symptoms compared to males (Baker et al., 2016; Covassin et al., 2016; Iverson et al., 2017; Neidecker et al., 2017; Stone et al., 2017). Specifically, utilizing a qualitative interview approach, André-Morin, Caron, and Bloom (2017) reported that collegiate female athletes cited academic difficulties, emotional symptoms, such as frustration and depression, and concerns about their weight throughout their protracted recovery (10 weeks to 14 months). When comparing recovery time between males and females, Baker and colleagues (2016) reported adolescent females took significantly longer to recover following an SRC than their male counterparts (24 days vs. 14 days). Similar results were found in a larger study of 579 middle school, high school, and collegiate athletes, with females taking nearly 29 days to recovery, while males only took 22 days (Stone et al., 2017). More specifically, when evaluating sex comparable sports, female soccer and basketball athletes took longer to return to full participation than males of the same sport (Covassin et al., 2016). However, the same study also reported no differences between males and females for ice hockey, lacrosse, and baseball/softball (Covassin et al., 2016).

Although early research found no sex differences in recovery time, recent research suggests female athletes take significantly longer to recover from SRC compared to male athletes. However, this finding may only be observed in specific sports such as soccer and basketball and may not be generalizable to other sex comparable sports. Further research is needed to confirm the extent of these differences. In addition, future research should determine the most appropriate treatment strategies for males and females as they recover from an SRC.

Treatment

The idea of proactive treatment for athletes with an SRC has progressed tremendously in recent years. Treatments such as rest, academic accommodations, medication, and vestibular therapy have become common when treating an athlete with protracted concussion symptoms (Kostyun & Hafeez, 2015). More specifically, research suggests that females average more of these treatment interventions (2.2 interventions) than males (1.3 interventions) (Kostyun & Hafeez, 2015).

Physical and cognitive rest has been the cornerstone of SRC management and is often recommended initially following injury (McCrory et al., 2017). Precautionary in nature, rest is often utilized to prevent the exacerbation of symptoms one may experience following a head injury. Differences have been reported between males and females and the prescription of rest following an SRC. Females have been found to be prescribed rest 95% of the time compared to 73% for males (Kostyun & Hafeez, 2015). Researchers have speculated that these results may be due to females reporting more post-concussive symptoms than males (Sufrinko et al., 2016). However, emerging research suggests that too much rest may actually extend recovery following an SRC (Grool et al., 2016; Thomas et al., 2015). Further research is warranted to not only determine the effectiveness of rest but also if sex differences exist in the amount of rest athletes are prescribed.

Similar to rest, sex differences have been reported for academic accommodations following an SRC. Females were prescribed academic accommodations 72% of the time, while males were prescribed only 42% of the time (Kostyun & Hafeez, 2015). These accommodations may range from extended deadlines to environmental accommodations for light or noise sensitivity (Kostyun & Hafeez, 2015). Differences seen in accommodations may reflect females becoming more anxious or concerned over missing assignments or examinations, thus easing these symptoms may improve recovery outcomes.

Research indicates that females report dizziness more often than males following a head injury (Broshek et al., 2005). Similarly, females perform worse on a vestibular ocular reflex test when compared to males (Sufrinko et al., 2016). These findings may explain why females are more commonly prescribed vestibular therapy than males. Recent findings have concluded that females were prescribed vestibular therapy eight times more often than males (Kostyun & Hafeez, 2015). It is probable that this treatment is less common than rest and academic accommodations, as a trained professional must conduct the vestibular therapy (Collins et al., 2014).

To date, there has been no clear evidence to support the use of medication in treating an SRC, unless it is related to long-term effects of SRC. Furthermore, the use of medication shortly after a head injury may mask associated symptoms, making return to play decisions more difficult (McCrory et al., 2017). If pharmacotherapy is utilized, the return to play decision must be carefully considered by a medical professional (McCrory et al., 2017). Despite the lack of evidence to support pharmacotherapy, sex differences have been reported, with females receiving this treatment four times more than males (Kostyun & Hafeez, 2015).

Sex differences have been well documented in SRC recovery and intervention strategies. Females not only demonstrate a more protracted recovery but are also prescribed more intervention strategies compared to males. Female athletes may be prescribed more treatment interventions due to increased symptom reporting and increased risk for developing anxiety following SRC. However, little is known as to why females receive interventions following an SRC more often compared to males. Further research is needed to evaluate why females take longer to recover, as well as which intervention strategies are most successful for each sex. Sex-specific interventions would provide a more individualized treatment path, thus potentially reducing recovery time in athletes with an SRC.

Sex differences with respect to psychological aspects of SRC

Depression

Collegiate athletes are no different than the typical college student population who face daily stress in their studies, concerns for their future, and financial issues. Researchers have reported that depressive symptoms range from 5% to 22% in NCAA athletes (Kerr et al., 2014; Yang et al., 2007). Athletes who suffer from depression exhibit signs and symptoms of sadness, emptiness, hopelessness, diminished interest or pleasure in activities of daily living, decrease or increase in appetite or sleep, and fatigue (American Psychological Association, 2013). Additionally, female athletes have reported higher symptoms of depression compared to male athletes (Wolanin et al., 2016).

Depression is considered the most prevalent psychological disturbance in traumatic brain injury (TBI) patients, including those with mild TBI (Kreutzer, Seel, & Gourley, 2001). Mainwaring, Hutchison, Bisschop, Comper, and Richards (2010) found that concussed patients reported 3 times greater depression symptoms compared to their baseline depression scores. Concussed athletes have also been shown to exhibit depression symptoms at 1 week (Roiger, Weidauer, & Kern, 2015) and 14 days post-concussion (Kontos et al., 2012). However, when examining long-term depression symptoms in concussed athletes, researchers reported no differences at one and three months compared to non-concussed athletes (Roiger, Weidauer, Kern, 2015). These findings are similar to the clinical trajectory of SRC recovery where approximately 80% of concussed athletes recover within 14 days (McCrory et al., 2017). As a result, it is difficult to disentangle SRC symptoms from depression symptoms.

With regard to sex, only two studies have examined depression among concussed male and female athletes. Kontos and colleagues (2012) examined depression symptoms in high school and collegiate athletes following an SRC. Results of this study found that there were no sex differences between concussed male and female athletes. However, this study was limited to a small sample size, with only 24 female athletes compared to 51 male athletes included in the study. Recently, Stazyk et al. (2017) examined depression symptomology in a large sample of youth and adolescent athletes following a mild TBI/SRC, with 23% of females and 19% of males reporting depression symptoms. However, the depression inventory utilized in this study was administered three months following their injury, and this study included individuals who had been hospitalized as a result of a severe head injury (Stazyk et al., 2017).

Although previous research suggests concussed athletes experience depression symptoms, limited research exists investigating depression symptoms among male and female athletes following an SRC. Therefore, additional research is warranted to determine if sex differences exist in depression symptoms following an SRC. Early identification of depression symptoms in athletes with an SRC may help healthcare professionals develop intervention strategies to combat these symptoms.

Anxiety

Anxiety symptom prevalence is more common among female athletes compared to males. In college, the percentage of female athletes with anxiety symptoms ranges from 10.2% (Gulliver et al., 2015) to 37.3% (Storch et al., 2005), in comparison to a range of 3.8% (Gulliver et al., 2015) to 22.2% (Storch et al., 2005) among male athletes. Similarly, female high school athletes (38%) demonstrate a higher prevalence of anxiety compared to male high school athletes (26%) (Merikangas et al., 2010). If these symptoms are mismanaged or ignored, using interventions such as prolonged strict rest (i.e., no exercise, no school) and limited social interaction with friends may develop emotional changes into clinical anxiety or even more extreme consequences (DiFazio et al., 2016; Gibson et al., 2013; Kontos, Deitrick, & Reynolds, 2016; Sandel et al., 2017; Thomas et al., 2015).

Specifically related to SRCs, approximately 34% of collegiate athletes reported experiencing anxiety after their injury (Yang et al., 2015). Current research suggests that SRC symptoms and impaired function may lead to emotional changes (e.g., anxiety, depression) approximately one or more weeks after injury (Kontos et al., 2012). Previous literature suggests that sex differences in anxiety exist in general athletic populations (Gulliver et al., 2015; Merikangas et al., 2010; Storch et al., 2005), as well as in symptom reporting and neurocognitive function following an SRC (Covassin et al., 2013; Covassin et al., 2012). Therefore, it can be hypothesized that there may be significant sex differences in anxiety prevalence following an SRC. However, there is a lack of empirical evidence to support this hypothesis. More research is needed to investigate sex differences in anxiety after an SRC and recovery outcomes in athletes that report anxiety.

There are very few studies that compare the emotional response between male and female athletes following an SRC. Previous research suggests that healthy females are better and faster at recognizing emotions than males. Given this finding, it is probable that there may be sex differences in emotion recognition following an SRC (Leveille et al., 2017). In a recent study, male and female athletes with a history of concussion were compared to same-sex controls on their ability to recognize emotions (Leveille et al., 2017). Interestingly, concussed male athletes performed worse at recognizing negative emotions than same-sex controls. In fact, concussed male athletes needed more intensity of the emotion in order to identify the emotion when compared to same-sex controls (Leveille et al., 2017). However, when compared to healthy same-sex controls, concussed female athletes performed similarly at recognizing emotions (Leveille et al., 2017). These results suggest sex may be a factor that influences emotion recognition following an SRC.

Previous research suggests female athletes experience greater anxiety in the general athletic population. Interestingly, there is a lack of research investigating differences between male and female anxiety levels following an SRC, given the recent emphasis on the comprehensive targeted treatment approach, which includes an anxiety/mood trajectory (Collins et al., 2014). Due to little empirical evidence, more research is needed to explore sex differences in emotional responses—specifically anxiety—following an SRC. Understanding sex differences in pre-injury anxiety levels and post-injury emotional changes may help sports medicine professionals to develop targeted treatment options.

Suicide

Suicide is a major public health epidemic across the globe and is among the leading causes of death in the United States. According to the Centers for Disease Control and Prevention (2015), suicide was the tenth leading cause of death overall in the United States, claiming the lives of more than 44,000 people. Suicide is the third leading cause of death among individuals aged 10–14, and the second leading cause of death among individuals aged 15–34 (Centers for Disease Control and Prevention, 2015). Studies evaluating whether athletes are at an increased risk of suicide are inconclusive, and very little research has examined sex differences among this specific population. In the general population, females attempt suicide more often than males, whereas males complete suicide more often than females (Baum, 2005). Researchers suggest that NCAA athletes have a higher risk of committing suicide compared with the general collegiate population (Rao et al., 2015).

Very little is known concerning sex differences in the risk of suicide in athletes. When examining athletes and the risk of suicide, some studies revealed that male athletes had a higher rate of suicide when compared to female athletes. Baum (2005) suggested that males had a greater ratio of a suicide rate compared to females (5:1), which was higher than the general population (3:1). In contrast, Rao and colleagues (2015) reported that male non-athletes were 2.5 times as likely to be suicidal than their male athlete peers, while female non-athletes were 1.67 times as likely to report suicidal behavior than their female athlete peers. Furthermore, the risk of suicide in male athletes was 3.67 times higher compared to female athletes (Rao et al., 2015). Lastly, Kokotailo et al. (1996) surveyed student-athletes at two large Midwestern universities and concluded that male athletes demonstrated greater risk than non-athletes, whereas female athletes showed fewer risk behaviors than non-athletes for suicide.

Despite sex-differences in the risk of suicide reported among athletes, results are even more conflicting when examining concussed athletes and the risk of suicide. Research has found that the long-term risk of suicide among those with a concussion was three times higher than the general population (Fralick et al., 2016). Some researchers suggest that females have a higher rate of suicide compared to males with mTBIs (Cancelliere, Donovan, & Cassidy, 2016; Ilie et al., 2014). Furthermore, Andre-Morin and colleagues (2017) interviewed five female university athletes who experienced protracted recovery (10 weeks to 14 months) following their concussion. One female athlete reported that she had attempted suicide three months following her concussion diagnosis due to academic diffi- culties. In contrast, one study found that males and females had similar levels of depression and risk of suicide, regardless of concussion history (Rabelo, 2017).

Very few studies have explored sex differences in the risk of suicide among the general population and specifically athletes with an SRC. Further research is needed to understand the incidence of suicide in concussed athletes and to determine if sex differences truly exist. Understanding sex differences in suicide risk may help healthcare professionals identify athletes at high risk to implement targeted interventions early in the SRC recovery process.

Health-related quality of life

Health-related quality of life (HRQOL) has become a recent topic of SRC man- agement measuring physical and mental wellbeing (Iadevaia, Roiger, & Zwart, 2015). General HRQOL assessments include physical, social, functional, and emotional domains (Iadevaia et al., 2015). TBI and mTBI, including SRC, have been reported to influence sleep patterns, fatigue, anxiety, depression, and cogni- tive function, while also impacting social and behavioral changes following injury, therefore impacting HRQOL (Siponkoski et al., 2013). Thus, SRCs and post- concussion syndrome can put patients at risk for HRQOL impairments, which has been a topic of interest, especially in pediatric athletes (Moran et al., 2012).

Collegiate and adolescent athletes with a history of SRC were reported to have worse HRQOL scores, specifically reporting deficits in bodily pain, general health, vitality, mental health, and social functioning compared to athletes with no SRC history (Kuehl et al., 2010; Valovich McLeod, Bay, & Snyder, 2010). Additionally, athletes with a history of three or more SRCs perceived adverse effects in bodily pain and social functioning compared to athletes with no his- tory or one to two previous SRCs (Kuehl et al., 2010). These results may aid in explaining why researchers encourage a whole-person clinical examination, including psychological and mental health following an SRC (McLeod, Fraser, & Johnson, 2017).

One of the few studies evaluating sex differences in HRQOL following an SRC found that there may be acute differences after injury (Russell et al., 2017). Males reported better emotional HRQOL scores compared to females within one week of an SRC, however, there were no sex differences in any other domains of the HRQOL over time (Russell et al., 2017). Similarly, a study assessing HRQOL after severe TBI reported no significant differences between sexes one year after injury (Saban et al., 2011).

Current research suggests there may be acute differences in HRQOL among male and female athletes acutely following SRC. Yet, it is important for research- ers to continue to investigate if sex differences in HRQOL exist. In addition, researchers should explore long-term differences in HRQOL among male and female athletes after an SRC.

Sex differences in social support and coping strategies

Social support

As previously mentioned, once an athlete has reported an SRC, it is not uncommon for them to experience some level of psychological disturbance, such as depression or anxiety (van Wilgen, Kaptein, & Brink, 2010; Wiese-Bjornstal, 2010). Research has shown that social support is imperative to combating these psychological conditions following injury (Bianco, 2001). Specifically, emotional, tangible, and informational support may contribute significantly to the recovery of an athletic injury (Clement & Shannon, 2011).

Individuals such as parents, friends, teammates, coaches, and healthcare professionals may serve as viable options for social support (Covassin et al., 2014). When evaluating sex differences and social support for common orthopedic injuries, it was suggested that male athletes sought more sources of support than females (Yang et al., 2010). However, females reported greater satisfaction with their sources of social support compared to males (Yang et al., 2010). Following an SRC, athletes have been shown to seek support from family most often (89%), followed by friends (78%) and teammates (65%) (Covassin et al., 2014).

Despite this knowledge, research has yet to evaluate if sex differences exist when seeking social support and to what extent. Insight into these possible sex differences would allow for more specific strategies when seeking support following injury. Such information may improve supporting strategies and help athletes cope with injuries such as an SRC.

Coping strategies

An emotional reaction to consider with SRCs is an individual's coping resources. Coping is defined as a constantly changing process of cognitive and behavioral approaches designed to manage internal and external demands that exceed one's resources. Coping is organized into cognitive/behavioral, problem/emotion focused, or approach/avoidance groupings (Lazarus & Folkman, 1984). Researchers are beginning to examine coping resources in athletes with SRCs, orthopedic injuries, and non-injured match controls. Recently, researchers suggested high school and collegiate athletes who sustained an SRC reported less adaptive responses than athletes with orthopedic injuries or match controls, while no differences were found between the orthopedic and match control groups (Kontos et al., 2013). Similarly, a study conducted by Wells, Langdon, and Hunt (2017) also suggested coping strategies of behavioral disengagement and social isolation were seen throughout the SRC recovery process. Additionally, emotion-focused strategies were positively related to injury symptoms in both the SRC and orthopedic injury groups; whereas, higher problem-focused disengagement strategies were associated with more postconcussion symptoms (Woodrome et al., 2011). Lastly, concussed athletes who had increased symptoms and lower visual memory on neurocognitive performance reported higher levels of avoidance coping behaviors three and eight days post-injury (Covassin et al., 2013). However, these findings are in contrast to Woodrome and colleagues (2011), who reported that among children with an SRC, problem-focused disengagement resources were positively associated with symptoms. Similarly, Snell et al. (2011) reported that concussed patients used more coping behaviors three months following their injury.

The interaction of sex differences and coping resources in injured and concussed athletes are scarce and suggest that females have increased scores on a few coping resources. Furthermore, findings across studies are difficult to synthesize given the various categorizations of coping (i.e., problem versus emotion focused, approach versus avoidance focused, etc.). However, in one study conducted by Kontos and colleagues (2013), females were reported to have more frequent self-distraction, active coping, instrumental support, humor, and self-blame than males among injured and concussed athletes. Additionally, female concussed athletes demonstrated increased levels of humor coping behaviors compared to female orthopedic injuries and match controls (Kontos et al., 2013). Lastly, female concussed athletes demonstrated higher levels of acceptance compared with match controls (Kontos et al., 2013).

The differences in coping resources across both SRC and orthopedic injury groups between males and females may relate to injured male athletes feeling more pressure to return to sport from teammates and minimizing the effects of injury compared to injured female athletes. Lower levels of reported coping responses have been demonstrated by males and may be characterized by pressure to hide any signs of injury (Granito, 2001). In contrast, females tend to appraise stressors as more threatening than males and may reflect different stress appraisals (Tamres, Janicki, & Helgeson, 2002). In addition, females may be more honest in their reporting of coping, whereas males may be more guarded in their responses (Deroche et al. 2011).

Ultimately, healthcare professionals should consider an athlete's sex when providing positive coping strategies and resources to injured athletes. Clinicians should be aware of the different coping strategies, and future research should focus on teaching SRC athletes to utilize more positive coping strategies instead of maladaptive coping strategies. Positive coping techniques could include deep breathing, relaxation techniques, and seeking assistance. Lastly, healthcare providers could administer coping assessments to identify which male and female athletes might benefit from coping interventions, which may enhance the recovery process and its negative effects.

Conclusions

In conclusion, sex differences have been reported between male and female athletes participating in similar sports. Female athletes are at a higher risk of sustaining a concussion than male athletes in sex comparable sports. However, little is known exactly why female athletes are more susceptible to injury. Several reasons have been proposed for these reported differences such as neck strength (Mansell et al., 2005), hormonal differences (Roof & Hall, 2000), style of play

(Sandel et al., 2017), and equipment rules (Hinton et al., 2005; Sandel et al., 2017). In addition, sex differences have been found in self reported symptoms and neurocognitive performance following an SRC. Female athletes take longer to recover and demonstrate increased symptom scores and neurocognitive deficits following concussion. Therefore, healthcare professionals should develop individualized treatment approaches and appropriate intervention strategies given the differences observed in recovery process between male and female athletes. Although these sex differences have been well documented in the literature, more research is needed to investigate psychological symptoms that may develop after an SRC.

Following an SRC, both male and female athletes have reported psychological symptoms (i.e., depression, anxiety) that could be attributed to their SRC, however there are very few studies that have examined sex differences in these mental health issues. More research is needed to understand mental health issues following an SRC between male and female athletes. Specifically, researchers should determine if these psychological symptoms are directly related to their SRC. Understanding the relationship between psychological symptoms and overall SRC recovery may help healthcare professionals to develop targeted intervention strategies to reduce the likelihood of athletes developing depression or anxiety after an SRC. Finally, more research is needed to understand the long-term effects of SRC between male and female athletes. Much of the literature included in this chapter investigated acute effects of SRC between male and female athletes. However, very few studies have explored sex differences in long-term effects of SRC.

References

American Psychological Association. (2013). *Diagnostic and statistical manual of mental disorders* (6th ed.). Washington, DC: American Psychiatric Association.

André-Morin, D., Caron, J.G., & Bloom, G.A. (2017). Exploring the unique challenges faced by female university athletes experiencing prolonged concussion symptoms. *Sport, Exercise, and Performance Psychology, 6*, 289–303. doi:10.1037/spy0000106.

Baker, J. G., Leddy, J. J., Darling, S. R., Shucard, J., Makdissi, M., & Willer, B. S. (2016). Gender differences in recovery from sports-related concussion in adolescents. *Clinical Pediatrics, 55*, 771–775. doi:10.1177/0009922815606417.

Baum, A. L. (2005). Suicide in athletes: A review and commentary. *Clinics in Sports Medicine, 24*, 853–869. doi:10.1016/j.csm.2005.06.006.

Bianco, T. (2001). Social support and recovery from sport injury: Elite skiers share their experiences. *Research Quarterly for Exercise and Sport, 72*, 376–388. doi:10.1080/02701367.2001.10608974.

Boden, B. P., Kirkendall, D. T., & Garrett, W. E. (1998). Concussion incidence in elite college soccer players. *The American Journal of Sports Medicine, 26*, 238–241.

Broglio, S. P., Cantu, R. C., Gioia, G. A., Guskiewicz, K. M., Kutcher, J., Palm, M., & McLeod, T. C. V. (2014). National athletic trainers' association position statement: Management of sport concussion. *Journal of Athletic Training, 49*, 245–265.

Broshek, D. K., Kaushik, T., Freeman, J. R., Erlanger, D., Webbe, F., & Barth, J. T. (2005). Sex differences in outcome following sports-related concussion. *Journal of Neurosurgery*, 102, 856–863. doi:10.3171/jns.2005.102.5.0856.

Cancelliere, C., Donovan, J., & Cassidy, J. D. (2016). Is sex an indicator of prognosis after mild traumatic brain injury: A systematic analysis of the findings of the World Health Organization collaborating centre task force on mild traumatic brain injury and the international collaboration on mild traumatic brain injury prognosis. *Archives of Physical Medicine and Rehabilitation*, 97, S5–S18. doi:10.1016/j. apmr.2014.11.028.

Cantu, R. C., Guskiewicz, K., & Register-Mihalik, J. K. (2010). A retrospective clinical analysis of moderate to severe athletic concussions. *Physical Medicine and Rehabilitation*, 2, 1088–1093. doi:10.1016/j.pmrj.2010.07.483.

Centers for Disease Control and Prevention. (2015). *Leading cause of death in the United States*. Retrieved from https://webappa.cdc.gov/cgi-bin/broker.exe.

Chandran, A., Barron, M. J., Westerman, B. J., & DiPietro, L. (2017). Multifactorial examination of sex-differences in head injuries and concussions among collegiate soccer players: NCAA ISS, 2004–2009. *Injury Epidemiology*, 4, 28–35.

Clement, D., & Shannon, V. R. (2011). Injured athletes' perceptions about social support. *Journal of Sport Rehabilitation*, 20, 457–470. doi:10.1123/jsr.20.4.457.

Collins, M. W., Kontos, A. P., Reynolds, E., Murawski, C. D., & Fu, F. H. (2014). A comprehensive, targeted approach to the clinical care of athletes following sport-related concussion. *Knee Surgery Sports Traumatology Arthroscopy*, 22, 235–246. doi:10.1007/s00167-013-2791-6.

Colvin, A. C., Mullen, J., Lovell, M. R., West, R. V., Collins, M. W., & Groh, M. (2009). The role of concussion history and gender in recovery from soccer-related concussion. *The American Journal of Sports Medicine*, 37, 1699–1704. doi:10.1177/0363546509332497.

Covassin, T., Crutcher, B., Bleecker, A., Heiden, E. O., Dailey, A., & Yang, J. Z. (2014). Postinjury anxiety and social support among collegiate athletes: A comparison between orthopaedic injuries and concussions. *Journal of Athletic Training*, 49, 462–468. doi:10.4085/1062-6059-49.2.03.

Covassin, T., Elbin, R. J., Bleecker, A., Lipchik, A., & Kontos, A. P. (2013). Are there differences in neurocognitive function and symptoms between male and female soccer players after concussions? *The American Journal of Sports Medicine*, 41, 2890–2895. doi:10.1177/0363546513509962.

Covassin, T., Elbin, R. J., Crutcher, B., Burkhart, S., & Kontos, A. (2013). The relationship between coping, neurocognitive performance, and concussion symptoms in high school and collegiate athletes. *The Sport Psychologist*, 27, 372–379. doi:10.1123/tsp.27.4.372.

Covassin, T., Elbin, R. J., Harris, W., Parker, T., & Kontos, A. (2012). The role of age and sex in symptoms, neurocognitive performance, and postural stability in athletes after concussion. *The American Journal of Sports Medicine*, 40, 1303–1312. doi:10.1177/0363546512444554.

Covassin, T., Moran, R., & Elbin, R. J. (2016). Sex differences in reported concussion injury rates and time loss from participation: An update of the national collegiate athletic association injury surveillance program from 2004–2005 through 2008–2009. *Journal of Athletic Training*, 51, 189–194. doi:10.4085/1062-6050-51.3.05.

Covassin, T., Schatz, P., & Swanik, C. B. (2007). Sex differences in neuropsychological function and post-concussion symptoms of concussed collegiate athletes. *Neurosurgery, 61,* 345–351. doi:10.1227/01.neu.0000279972.95060.cb.

Deroche, T., Woodman, T., Stephan, Y., Brewer, B. W., & Le Scanff, C. (2011). Athletes' inclination to play through pain: A coping perspective. *Anxiety Stress and Coping, 24,* 579–587. doi:10.1080/10615806.2011.552717.

DiFazio, M., Silverberg, N. D., Kirkwood, M. W., Bernier, R., & Iverson, G. L. (2016). Prolonged activity restriction after concussion: Are we worsening outcomes? *Clinical Pediatrics (Phila), 55,* 443–451. doi:10.1177/0009922815589914.

Fralick, M., Thiruchelvam, D., Tien, H. C., & Redelmeier, D. A. (2016). Risk of suicide after a concussion. *Canadian Medical Association Journal, 188,* 497–504. doi:10.1503/cmaj.150790.

Frommer, L. J., Gurka, K. K., Cross, K. M., Ingersoll, C. D., Comstock, R. D., & Saliba, S. A. (2011). Sex differences in concussion symptoms of high school athletes. *Journal of Athletic Training, 46,* 76–84. doi:10.4085/1062-6050-46.1.76.

Gibson, S., Nigrovic, L. E., O'Brien, M., & Meehan, W. P., 3rd. (2013). The effect of recommending cognitive rest on recovery from sport-related concussion. *Brain Injury, 27,* 839–842. doi:10.3109/02699052.2013.775494.

Granito V. J., Jr. (2001). Athletic injury experience: A qualitative focus group approach. *Journal of Sport Behavior, 24,* 63–82.

Grool, A. M., Aglipay, M., Momoli, F., Meehan, W. P., Freedman, S. B., Yeates, K. O., … Zemek, R. (2016). Association between early participation in physical activity following acute concussion and persistent postconcussive symptoms in children and adolescents. *Journal of the American Medical Association, 316,* 2504–2514. doi:10.1001/jama.2016.17396.

Gulliver, A., Griffiths, K. M., Mackinnon, A., Batterham, P. J., & Stanimirovic, R. (2015). The mental health of Australian elite athletes. *Journal of Science and Medicine in Sport, 18,* 255–261. doi:10.1016/j.jsams.2014.04.006.

Hinton, R. Y., Lincoln, A. E., Almquist, J. L., Douoguih, W. A., & Sharma, K. M. (2005). Epidemiology of lacrosse injuries in high school-aged girls and boys: A 3-year prospective study. *The American Journal of Sports Medicine, 33,* 1305–1314. doi:10.1177/0363546504274148.

Iadevaia, C., Roiger, T., & Zwart, M. B. (2015). Qualitative examination of adolescent health-related quality of life at 1 year postconcussion. *Journal of Athletic Training, 50,* 1182–1189. doi:10.4085/1062-6050-50.11.02.

Ilie, G., Adlaf, E. M., Mann, R. E., Boak, A., Hamilton, H., Asbridge, M., … Cusimano, M. D. (2014). The moderating effects of sex and age on the association between traumatic brain injury and harmful psychological correlates among adolescents. *Plos One, 9.* doi:10.1371/journal.pone.0108167.

Iverson, G. L., Gardner, A. J., Terry, D. P., Ponsford, J. L., Sills, A. K., Broshek, D. K., & Solomon, G. S. (2017). Predictors of clinical recovery from concussion: A systematic review. *British Journal of Sports Medicine, 51,* 941–948. doi:10.1136/bjsports-2017-097729.

Iverson, G. L., Lovell, M. R., & Collins, M. W. (2003). Interpreting change on ImPACT following sport concussion. *Clinical Neuropsychology, 17*(4), 460–467. doi:10.1076/clin.17.4.460.27934.

Kerr, Z. Y., Evenson, K. R., Rosamond, W. D., Mihalik, J. P., Guskiewicz, K. M., & Marshall, S. W. (2014). Association between concussion and mental health in former collegiate athletes. *Injury Epidemiology, 1,* 28–38.

Kerr, Z. Y., Register-Mihalik, J. K., Kroshus, E., Baugh, C. M., & Marshall, S. W. (2016). Motivations associated with nondisclosure of self-reported concussions in former collegiate athletes. *The American Journal of Sports Medicine*, *44*, 220–225.

Kokotailo, P. K., Henry, B. C., Koscik, R. E., Fleming, M. F., & Landry, G. L. (1996). Substance use and other health risk behaviors in collegiate athletes. *Clinical Journal of Sport Medicine*, *6*, 183–189. doi:10.1097/00042752-199607000-00008.

Kontos, A. P., Covassin, T., Elbin, R. J., & Parker, T. (2012). Depression and neurocognitive performance after concussion among male and female high school and collegiate athletes. *Archives of Physical Medicine and Rehabilitation*, *93*, 1751–1756. doi:10.1016/j.apmr.2012.03.032.

Kontos, A. P., Deitrick, J. M., & Reynolds, E. (2016). Mental health implications and consequences following sport-related concussion. *British Journal of Sports Medicine*, *50*, 139–140. doi:10.1136/bjsports-2015-095564.

Kontos, A. P., Elbin, R. J., Newcomer Appaneal, R., Covassin, T., & Collins, M. W. (2013). A comparison of coping responses among high school and college athletes with concussion, orthopedic injuries, and healthy controls. *Research in Sports Medicine*, *21*, 367–379. doi:10.1080/15438627.2013.825801.

Kostyun, R. O., & Hafeez, I. (2015). Protracted recovery from a concussion: A focus on gender and treatment interventions in an adolescent population. *Sports Health—A Multidisciplinary Approach*, *7*, 52–57. doi:10.1177/1941738114555075.

Kreutzer, J. S., Seel, R. T., & Gourley, E. (2001). The prevalence and symptom rates of depression after traumatic brain injury: A comprehensive examination. *Brain Injury*, *15*, 563–576.

Kuehl, M. D., Snyder, A. R., Erickson, S. E., & McLeod, T. C. V. (2010). Impact of prior concussions on health-related quality of life in collegiate athletes. *Clinical Journal of Sport Medicine*, *20*, 86–91. doi:10.1097/JSM.0b013e3181cf4534.

Langlois, J. A., Rutland-Brown, W., & Wald, M. M. (2006). The epidemiology and impact of traumatic brain injury: A brief overview. *The Journal of Head Trauma Rehabilitation*, *21*, 375–378.

Lazarus, R. S., & Folkman, S. (1984). *Stress, appraisal, and coping*. New York, NY: Springer.

Leveille, E., Guay, S., Blais, C., Scherzer, P., & De Beaumont, L. (2017). Sex-related differences in emotion recognition in multi-concussed athletes. *Journal of International Neuropsychology Society*, *23*, 65–77. doi:10.1017/s1355617716001004.

Majerske, C. W., Mihalik, J. P., Ren, D., Collins, M. W., Reddy, C. C., Lovell, M. R., & Wagner, A. K. (2008). Concussion in sports: Postconcussive activity levels, symptoms, and neurocognitive performance. *Journal of Athletic Training*, *43*, 265–274. doi:10.4085/1062-6050-43.3.265.

Mansell, J., Tierney R., Sitler M., Swanik K., & Stearne, D. (2005). Resistance training and head-neck segment dynamic stabilization in male and female collegiate soccer players. *Journal of Athletic Training*, *40*, 310–319.

Mainwaring, L., Hutchison, M., Bisschop, S., Comper, P., & Richards, D. (2010). Emotional response to sport concussion compared to ACL injury. *Brain Injury*, *24*, 589–597

McCrory, P.,Meeuwisse, W. H., Dvořák, J., Echemendia, R. J., EngebretsenL., Feddermann-Demont, N., … Vos, P.E. (2017). 5th International conference on concussion in sport (Berlin): *British Journal of Sports Medicine*, 51, 837–847.

McLeod, T. C. V., Fraser, M. A., & Johnson, R. S. (2017). Mental health outcomes following sport-related concussion. *Athletic Training and Sports Health Care, 9,* 271–282.

Merikangas, K. R., He, J. P., Burstein, M., Swanson, S. A., Avenevoli, S., Cui, L., ... Swendsen, J. (2010). Lifetime prevalence of mental disorders in U.S. adolescents: Results from the National Comorbidity Survey Replication—Adolescent supplement (NCS-A). *Journal of American Academy of Child Adolescent Psychiatry, 49,* 980–989. doi:10.1016/j.jaac.2010.05.017.

Moran, L. M., Taylor, H. G., Rusin, J., Bangert, B., Dietrich, A., Nuss, K. E., ... Yeates, K. O. (2012). Quality of life in pediatric mild traumatic brain injury and its relationship to postconcussive symptoms. *Journal of Pediatric Psychology, 37,* 736–744. doi:10.1093/jpepsy/jsr087.

Neidecker, J. M., Gealt, D. B., Luksch, J. R., & Weaver, M. D. (2017). First-time sports-related concussion recovery: The role of sex, age, and sport. *Journal of the American Osteopathic Association, 117,* 635–642.

O'Connor, K. L., Baker, M. M., Dalton, S. L., Dompier, T. P., Broglio, S. P., & Kerr, Z. Y. (2017). Epidemiology of sport-related concussions in high school athletes: National athletic treatment, injury and outcomes network (NATION), 2011–2012 through 2013–2014. *Journal of Athletic Training, 52,* 175–185.

Rabelo, J. L. (2017). *Sports-related concussions and depression.* (Doctor of Psychology), Alliant International Unviersity, San Diego, CA.

Rao, A. L., Asif, I. M., Drezner, J. A., Toresdahl, B. G., & Harmon, K. G. (2015). Suicide in national collegiate athletic association (NCAA) athletes: A 9-year analysis of the NCAA resolutions database. *Sports Health—A Multidisciplinary Approach, 7,* 452–457. doi:10.1177/1941738115587675.

Roiger, T., Weidauer, L., & Kern, B. (2015). A longitudinal pilot study of depressive symptoms in concussed and injured/nonconcussed National Collegiate Athletic Association division I student-athletes. *Journal of Athletic Training, 50,* 256–261.

Roof, R., & Hall, E. (2000). Gender differences in acute CNS trauma and stroke: Neuroprotective effects of estrogen and progesterone. *Journal of Neurotrauma, 17,* 367–388.

Rosene, J. M., Raksnis, B., Silva, B., Woefel, T., Visich, P. S., Dompier, T. P., & Kerr, Z. Y. (2017). Comparison of concussion rates between NCAA division I and division III Men's and Women's ice hockey players. *The American Journal of Sports Medicine, 45,* 2622–2629.

Russell, K., Selci, E., Chu, S., Fineblit, S., Ritchie, L., & Ellis, M. J. (2017). Longitudinal assessment of health-related quality of life following adolescent sports-related concussion. *Journal of Neurotrauma, 34,* 2147–2153. doi:10.1089/neu.2016.4704.

Saban, K. L., Smith, B. M., Collins, E. G., & Pape, T. L. B. (2011). Sex differences in perceived life satisfaction and functional status one year after severe traumatic brain injury. *Journal of Women's Health, 20,* 179–186. doi:10.1089/jwh.2010.2334.

Sandel, N., Reynolds, E., Cohen, P. E., Gillie, B. L., & Kontos, A. P. (2017). Anxiety and mood clinical profile following sport-related concussion: From risk factors to treatment. *Sport Exercise, Performance, and Psychology, 6,* 304–323. doi:10.1037/spy0000098.

Sandel, N. K., Schatz, P., Goldberg, K. B., & Lazar, M. (2017). Sex-based differences in cognitive deficits and symptom reporting among acutely concussed adolescent lacrosse and soccer players. *The American Journal of Sports Medicine, 45,* 937–944. doi:10.1177/0363546516677246.

Siponkoski, S. T., Wilson, L., von Steinbuchel, N., Sarajuuri, J., & Koskinen, S. (2013). Quality of life after traumatic brain injury: Finnish experience of the qolibri in residential rehabilitation. *Journal of Rehabilitation Medicine, 45,* 835–842. doi:10.2340/16501977-1189.

Snell, D. L., Siegert, R. J., Hay-Smith, E. J. C., & Surgenor, L. J. (2011). Factor structure of the brief COPE in people with mild traumatic brain injury. *Journal of Head Trauma Rehabilitation, 26,* 468–477. doi:10.1097/HTR.0b013e3181fc5e1e.

Stazyk, K., DeMatteo, C., Moll, S., & Missiuna, C. (2017). Depression in youth recovering from concussion: Correlates and predictors. *Brain Injury, 31,* 631–638.

Stone, S., Lee, B., Garrison, J. C., Blueitt, D., & Creed, K. (2017). Sex differences in time to return-to-play progression after sport-related concussion. *Sports Health—A Multidisciplinary Approach, 9,* 41–44. doi:10.1177/1941738116672184.

Storch, E. A., Storch, J. B., Killiany, E. M., & Roberti, J. W. (2005). Self-reported psychopathology in athletes: A comparison of intercollegiate student-athletes and non-athletes. *Journal of Sport Behavior, 28,* 86–98.

Sufrinko, A. M., Mucha, A., Covassin, T., Marchetti, G., Elbin, R. J., Collins, M. W., & Kontos, A. P. (2016). Sex differences in vestibular/ocular and neurocognitive outcomes after sport-related concussion. *Clinical Journal of Sport Medicine, 27,* 133–138. doi:10.1097/jsm.0000000000000324.

Tamres, L. K., Janicki, D., & Helgeson, V. S. (2002). Sex differences in coping behavior: A meta-analytic review and an examination of relative coping. *Personality and Social Psychology Review, 6,* 2–30. doi:10.1207/S15327957PSPR0601_1.

Thomas, D. G., Apps, J. N., Hoffmann, R. G., McCrea, M., & Hammeke, T. (2015). Benefits of strict rest after acute concussion: A randomized controlled trial. *Pediatrics, 135,* 213–223. doi:10.1542/peds.2014-0966.

Tierney, R., Higgins, M., Caswell, S., Brady, J., McHardy, K., Driban, J., & Darvish, K. (2008). Sex differences in head acceleration during heading while wearing soccer headgear. *Journal of Athletic Training, 43,* 578–584.

Tierney, R., Sitler, M., Swanik, B., Swanik, K., Higgins, M., & Torg, J. (2005). Gender differences in head-neck segment dynamic stabilization during head acceleration. *Medicine and Science in Sports and Exercise, 37,* 272–279.

Valovich McLeod, T. C., Bay, R. C., & Snyder, A. R. (2010). Self-reported history of concussion affects health-related quality of life in adolescent athletes. *Athletic Training & Sports Health Care, 2,* 219–226.

van Wilgen, C. P., Kaptein, A. A., & Brink, M. S. (2010). Illness perceptions and mood states are associated with injury-related outcomes in athletes. *Disability and Rehabilitation, 32,* 1576–1585. doi:10.3109/09638281003596857.

Wallace, J., Covassin, T., & Beidler, E. (2017). Sex differences in high school athletes' knowledge of sport-related concussion symptoms and reporting behaviors. *Journal of Athletic Training, 52,* 682–688.

Wells, P., Langdon, J. L., & Hunt, T. N. (2017). The emotions, coping and social support perceived by NCAA division I athletes during concussion recovery. *Journal of Athletic Training, 52,* S198.

Wiese-Bjornstal, D. M. (2010). Psychology and socioculture affect injury risk, response, and recovery in high-intensity athletes: A consensus statement. *Scandinavian Journal of Medicine and Science in Sports, 20,* 103–111. doi:10.1111/j.1600-0838.2010.01195.x.

Wolanin, A., Hong, E., Marks, D., Panchoo, K., & Gross, M. (2016). Prevalence of clinically elevated depressive symptoms in college athletes and differences by gender and sport. *British Journal of Sports Medicine, 50,* 167–171.

Woodrome, S. E., Yeates, K. O., Taylor, H. G., Rusin, J., Bangert, B., Dietrich, A., ... Wright, M. (2011). Coping strategies as a predictor of post-concussive symptoms in children with mild traumatic brain injury versus mild orthopedic injury. *Journal of the International Neuropsychological Society, 17,* 317–326. doi:10.1017/S1355617710001700.

Yang, J., Peek-Asa, C., Corlette, J., Cheng, G., Foster, D., & Albright, J. (2007). Prevalence of and risk factors associated with symptoms of depression in competitive collegiate student athletes. *Clinical Journal of Sport Medicine, 17,* 481–487.

Yang, J. Z., Peek-Asa, C., Lowe, J. B., Heiden, E., & Foster, D. T. (2010). Social support patterns of collegiate athletes before and after injury. *Journal of Athletic Training, 45,* 372–379. doi:10.4085/1062-6050-45.4.372.

Yang, J., Peek-Asa, C., Covassin, T., Torner, J. C. (2015). Post-concussion symptoms of depression and anxiety in division I collegiate athletes. *Developmental Neuropsychology, 40,* 18–23.

Zuckerman, S. L, Apple, R. P., Odom, M. J., Lee, Y. M., Solomon, G. S., & Sills, A. K. (2014). Effect of sex on symptoms and return to baseline in sport-related concussion. *Journal of Neurosurgery: Pediatrics, 13,* 72–81.

Zuckerman, S. L., Kerr, Z. Y., Yengo-Kahn, A., Wasserman, E., Covassin, T., & Solomon, G. S. (2015). Epidemiology of sports-related concussion in NCAA athletes from 2009–2010 to 2013–2014: Incidence, recurrence, and mechanisms. *The American Journal of Sports Medicine, 43,* 2654–2662.

Zuckerman, S. L., Solomon, G. S., Forbes, J. A., Haase, R. F., Sills, A. K., & Lovell, M. R. (2012). Response to acute concussive injury in soccer players: Is gender a modifying factor? *Journal of Neurosurgery Pediatrics, 10* (6), 504–510. doi:10.3171/2012.8.peds12139.

10 Child and adolescent athletes

Laura Purcell

Introduction

Concussions are common injuries in sports and recreational activities, particularly in the pediatric population. About 70% of sport-related concussions (SRC) occur in persons under 20 years of age and the majority (about 70%) occur in males (Browne & Lam, 2006; Harris et al., 2012; Meehan & Mannix, 2010). In Canada, the highest incidence of SRC occur among 10–14-year-olds. More than 50% of concussions in males occur in hockey, whereas most concussions (36%) in girls occur during soccer (see Figure 10.1; Government of Canada, 2017).

Not only is the high incidence of concussions in children and adolescents concerning, but the differences between children and adults impact concussion diagnosis and management, which presents unique challenges for practitioners. These differences include continuous growth, development, and maturation during childhood and adolescence; differences in injury presentation, assessment, and recovery; and different management priorities, including return to school (RTS; Davis et al., 2017; Davis & Purcell, 2014; McCrory et al., 2004; Patel & Pratt, 2009). In addition, return to activity and sport/play (RTP) is managed differently in children and adolescents compared to adults. Although RTP strategies are based on adult guidelines, they should be more conservative in pediatric athletes (Davis et al., 2017; McCrory et al., 2017; Purcell, 2009; Purcell, 2014).

Another area of concern during concussion recovery is emotional issues that athletes may encounter. Psychological aspects of concussion, including depression and anxiety, may negatively impact concussion recovery and lead to persistent symptoms (Chertok & Martin, 2013; Covassin et al., 2017; Putukian & Echemendia, 2003; Sandel et al., 2017; Vargas et al., 2015). Adolescents appear to be at particular risk for prolonged recovery and development of affective symptoms post-concussion (Zemek et al., 2016). Recently, there has been increasing focus on the psychological aspects of concussion in research and management.

This chapter addresses concussion in children and adolescents, highlighting the differences between them and adults with respect to concussion management. More specifically, the importance of return to school and differences in return to sport management will be emphasized. Finally, psychological aspects of concussion in youth athletes will be discussed.

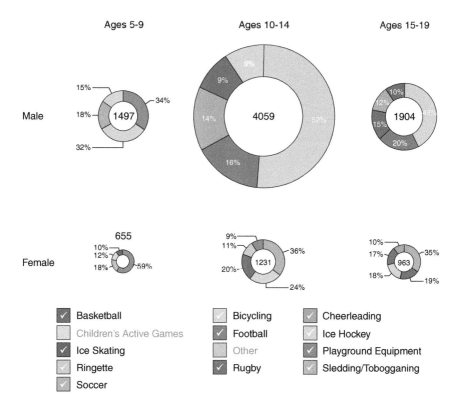

Figure 10.1 Injury statistics from the database of the Canadian Hospitals Injury Reporting and Prevention Program (CHIRPP), Public Health Agency of Canada.

Uniqueness of children and adolescents

Children are unique to adults in many ways. They are in a constant state of change as they grow and develop, and this may make them more vulnerable to injury, prolong recovery, and complicate concussion diagnosis and management.

Maturation, growth, and development

Children and adolescents are undergoing three simultaneous and continuous processes of growth (i.e., increase in body size over time), maturation (i.e., progress towards a biologically mature state), and development (i.e., acquisition of behavioral competence, or learning the appropriate behavior expected by one's society and culture). They are growing and maturing cognitively, physically, emotionally, and socially throughout childhood and adolescence. These three processes occur in concert and interact, but there is wide variation in the tempo and achievement of these processes within individuals and between sexes. Growth, maturation, and development are largely controlled by genetic and neuroendocrine factors; however, environmental factors, such as nutrition, opportunity, and social context, can influence these processes (Baxter-Jones & Malina, 2001; Patel & Pratt, 2009).

Neuropsychological tests have shown that children undergo rapid cognitive development up to age 18 years, with substantial improvements in reaction time, working memory, and learning, with the greatest changes occurring between 9–15 years of age (McCrory et al., 2004). Cognitive and psychosocial development throughout childhood and adolescence impacts injury management. In middle childhood (ages 6–10 years), children cannot think futuristically. Thinking at this age is very concrete (i.e., in the here and now), and they cannot appreciate the consequences of their actions. Attention spans are limited, and children can be easily distracted. So, children may not fully appreciate what can happen if they go back to play before they have fully recovered from a concussion (Patel & Pratt, 2009).

During early adolescence (ages 11–13 years), thinking remains concrete, with failure to fully comprehend long-term consequences of actions and injuries. Peer acceptance is very important, so injured adolescents may not seek medical attention for head injuries or adhere to management recommendations, so as not to risk peer disapproval. Middle adolescence (age 14–16 years) is marked by development of abstract thinking and an improving ability to comprehend behavior consequences. There is increasing independence and separation from parents, with greater influence from peers and media. Sport participation can be very important to gain social acceptance. Adolescents may not be willing to risk their social position by adhering to treatment recommendations. Older adolescents (17 years and older) are capable of more abstract thinking, are more mature in their understanding of personal and social relationships and are better able to appreciate the potential consequences of injuries. Therefore, they will likely be more compliant with recommended management (Greydanus & Pratt, 2009).

Vulnerability to injury

Neuropsychological tests in concussed athletes have shown impairments in reaction time, concentration/attention, processing speed, and memory. Younger athletes appear to have more significant neurological deficits following concussion and take longer to recover from sport-related concussion than older athletes. Memory dysfunction, in particular, appears to be more affected in high school athletes compared with college athletes, lasting up to 10–14 days post-concussion in high school athletes, whereas college athletes had symptom resolution by day 3 (Fazio et al., 2007; Field et al., 2003; McClincy et al, 2006; Sim, Terryberry-Spohr, & Wilson, 2008). Although adults typically recover within ten days following concussion, children and adolescents typically take up to four weeks to recover, with a substantial percentage (16–33%) taking more than four weeks to recover (Grubenhoff et al., 2016; Grubenhoff et al., 2015; Purcell, Harvey, & Seabrook, 2016; Zemek et al., 2016). There are very few studies in younger children aged 5–12 years, hence many unknowns remain regarding how this population is affected by concussion and how they recover.

Symptom self-report

Diagnosis of concussion is largely based on self-report of symptoms following injury—there is no definitive diagnostic test that accurately diagnoses or excludes concussion. As a result, clinicians must rely on athletes to honestly and accurately report their symptoms at the time of injury to make a diagnosis, as well as throughout the recovery phase to monitor progress and resolution of symptoms. For younger athletes, the ability to verbalize how they are feeling can be challenging because they have not yet attained the cognitive and emotional maturity to recognize and report symptoms (Lovell & Fazio, 2008; Patel & Pratt, 2009; Purcell, 2014). Getting input from parents can be very valuable to ascertain types and severity of symptoms and monitor progress (Davis et al., 2017).

There is also evidence that neurocognitive deficits may persist beyond report of resolution of physical symptoms. Prospective case-control studies have demonstrated persistent decreases in memory, processing speed, and reaction time post-concussion despite athletes reporting symptom resolution (Fazio et al., 2007; Lovell et al., 2003; Van Campen et al., 2006). These studies indicate that self-report of symptoms may be inadequate to diagnose concussion injury and monitor recovery and resolution of symptoms (Fazio et al., 2007).

Medical supervision

Unlike college/university and professional sports, there is typically no medical team present during youth sporting events. There are no team physicians, there may be no trainers, and coaches may be less experienced and knowledgeable. A large number of children and adolescents also participate in recreational activities with little to no adult supervision. The absence of trained supervision may result in under-recognition and underreporting of concussions (Lovell & Fazio, 2008; Purcell, 2009). Subsequently, appropriate management of injury may not be instituted at the time of injury, and guidance for return to activity may be lacking, leading to potential complications and prolonged recovery (Purcell, 2009). It is therefore vitally important that all participants in youth sport (athletes, parents, coaches, teachers, officials/referees) are educated in recognizing possible concussions, so that athletes with potential concussive injuries are safely removed from play. The Concussion Recognition Tool 5 (see Figure 10.2) has been developed to help non-medically trained individuals to recognize the signs and symptoms of possible concussion (2017). It also provides guidance for removing an injured athlete from play/sport and seeking medical assessment.

Figure 10.2 The Concussion Recognition Tool-5©.
© Concussion in Sport Group 2017

The use of this tool will hopefully increase the identification of potential concussions in youth athletes and lead to better management.

Assessment tools

The Sport Concussion Assessment Tool (SCAT) was developed for assessment of athletes on the field of play following the 2nd International Conference on Concussion in Sport in 2004. The SCAT has gone through several revisions, the most current version being the SCAT5, recommended for use in athletes 13 years and older (Sport Concussion Assessment Tool-5, 2017).

Given the developmental differences in younger children, it has been recognized that concussion assessment tools for this group need to be developmentally appropriate. This recognition led to the creation of the ChildSCAT3 assessment tool for children aged 5–12 years following the 4th International Consensus Conference on Concussion in Sport in 2012 (Davis et al., 2017; McCrory et al., 2013). This was updated to the Child SCAT5 following the 5th International Consensus Conference on Concussion in Sport in 2016 (Child Sport Concussion Assessment Tool-5, 2017).

The ChildSCAT5 uses the Health and Behavior Inventory, a validated symptom list that includes a child-friendly symptom report and a parent symptom report (see Figure 10.3). In addition, more developmentally appropriate assessments of cognition and balance are incorporated into the ChildSCAT5. In contrast to the SCAT5, the Digits Backwards starts with a string of two digits, because many children cannot do three, and the Months in Reverse Order was changed to days of the week because many children are unable to recite the months of the year in reverse order. The Balance assessment for children less than ten years includes only double leg stance and tandem stance, because many young children are unable to balance on one leg (Davis et al., 2017; McCrory et al., 2013; McCrory et al., 2017). The ChildSCAT5 also includes information regarding return to school for child athletes.

Return to school

In the past, the emphasis for concussion management has been on RTP. However, recently RTS has become a priority of concussion management for pediatric patients. For student-athletes, RTS following a concussive injury is of particular concern because school is their primary "work" (Master et al., 2012). Post-concussion symptoms such as headaches, dizziness, and fatigue, as well as memory, attention, and concentration deficits, may have a negative impact on a student's ability to RTS (Fazio et al., 2007; Field et al., 2003; McClincy et al., 2006; Sim, Terryberry-Spohr, & Wilson, 2008). Students who have numerous symptoms and more severe symptoms may experience exacerbation of symptoms upon RTS (Silverberg et al., 2016).

Many position/consensus statements and guidelines have addressed RTS following a concussion, but these resources are not evidence-based because there

STEP 2: SYMPTOM EVALUATION

The athlete should be given the symptom form and asked to read this instruction paragraph out loud then complete the symptom scale. For the baseline assessment, the athlete should rate his/her symptoms based on how he/she typically feels and for the post injury assessment the athlete should rate their symptoms at this point in time.

To be done in a resting state

Please Check: ☐ Baseline ☐ Post-Injury

Name: _____

DOB: _____

Address: _____

ID number: _____

Examiner: _____

2

Child Report[3]

	Not at all/ Never	A little/ Rarely	Somewhat/ Sometimes	A lot/ Often
I have headaches	0	1	2	3
I feel dizzy	0	1	2	3
I feel like the room is spinning	0	1	2	3
I feel like I'm going to faint	0	1	2	3
Things are blurry when I look at them	0	1	2	3
I see double	0	1	2	3
I feel sick to my stomach	0	1	2	3
My neck hurts	0	1	2	3
I get tired a lot	0	1	2	3
I get tired easily	0	1	2	3
I have trouble paying attention	0	1	2	3
I get distracted easily	0	1	2	3
I have a hard time concentrating	0	1	2	3
I have problems remembering what people tell me	0	1	2	3
I have problems following directions	0	1	2	3
I daydream too much	0	1	2	3
I get confused	0	1	2	3
I forget things	0	1	2	3
I have problems finishing things	0	1	2	3
I have trouble figuring things out	0	1	2	3
It's hard for me to learn new things	0	1	2	3
Total number of symptoms:				of 21
Symptom severity score:				of 63
Do the symptoms get worse with physical activity?			Y	N
Do the symptoms get worse with trying to think?			Y	N

Overall rating for child to answer:

	Very bad										Very good
On a scale of 0 to 10 (where 10 is normal), how do you feel now?	0	1	2	3	4	5	6	7	8	9	10

If not 10, in what way do you feel different?:

Parent Report

The child:

	Not at all/ Never	A little/ Rarely	Somewhat/ Sometimes	A lot/ Often
has headaches	0	1	2	3
feels dizzy	0	1	2	3
has a feeling that the room is spinning	0	1	2	3
feels faint	0	1	2	3
has blurred vision	0	1	2	3
has double vision	0	1	2	3
experiences nausea	0	1	2	3
has a sore neck	0	1	2	3
gets tired a lot	0	1	2	3
gets tired easily	0	1	2	3
has trouble sustaining attention	0	1	2	3
is easily distracted	0	1	2	3
has difficulty concentrating	0	1	2	3
has problems remembering what he/she is told	0	1	2	3
has difficulty following directions	0	1	2	3
tends to daydream	0	1	2	3
gets confused	0	1	2	3
is forgetful	0	1	2	3
has difficulty completing tasks	0	1	2	3
has poor problem solving skills	0	1	2	3
has problems learning	0	1	2	3
Total number of symptoms:				of 21
Symptom severity score:				of 63
Do the symptoms get worse with physical activity?			Y	N
Do the symptoms get worse with mental activity?			Y	N

Overall rating for parent/teacher/coach/carer to answer

On a scale of 0 to 100% (where 100% is normal), how would you rate the child now?

If not 100%, in what way does the child seem different?

Figure 10.3 The Child Sport Concussion Assessment Tool-5©.

Child SCAT5 © Concussion in Sport Group 2017

is currently little available research in this area (Halstead et al., 2013; McCrory, Davis, & Makdissi, 2012; Purcell, 2014; Zemek et al., 2014). A recent systematic review looking at the differences in concussion management between children and adults addressed RTS (Davis et al., 2017), and a subsequent systematic review of RTS following concussion identified the current state of evidence in the literature (Purcell, Davis, & Gioia, 2018). The systematic reviews identified a number of factors that should be considered in the RTS process, including:

- Symptomatology: Students who experienced more symptoms, more severe symptoms, more persistent symptoms, and specific symptoms, such as executive dysfunction, difficulty concentrating, visual abnormalities, and vestibular deficits, had more prolonged recoveries and had more difficulty with RTS (Baker et al., 2015; Corwin et al., 2015; Corwin et al., 2014; Purcell et al., 2016; Ransom et al., 2015)
- Age/school level: Adolescents/high school students typically have more symptoms, more severe symptoms, and more difficulty with RTS than younger students, and tended to have more prolonged recoveries (Carson et al., 2014; Purcell et al., 2016; Ransom et al., 2015; Zuckerbraun et al., 2014). Age 13 years old and greater was a predictor of persistent concussion symptoms in a recent prospective, multi-center ED cohort study (Zemek et al., 2016)
- Course load: Particular subjects, including math and reading/language, may be more difficult for students returning to school after a concussion and may require targeted interventions (Ransom et al., 2015)
- Rest after injury: Lack of cognitive and physical rest immediately after a concussive injury has been associated with persistent post-concussive symptoms. High levels of cognitive activity, such as school attendance, may exacerbate post-concussion symptoms and prolong recovery, as well as prolong RTS (Brown et al., 2014; Makki et al., 2016; Silverberg et al., 2016; Taubman et al., 2016). In addition, student athletes who continued to play after injury took twice as long to recover and were almost nine times as likely to have prolonged recovery (>21 days) compared with those who stopped play immediately (Elbin et al., 2016). Cognitive performance was lower and symptoms higher in adolescents not removed from play immediately after concussion (Elbin et al., 2016)

Practitioners should screen for the presence of risk factors/predictors of persistent symptoms to identify athletes who may have difficulty with RTS and may need more supports (Davis & Purcell, 2014; Purcell et al., 2018).

The systematic review on RTS following concussion also identified a number of strategies to aid RTS. The strategies identified include the provision of symptom-specific accommodations, such as temporary school absence (see Table 10.1); the development of school concussion policies; regular medical follow-up after injury; and the provision of a RTS letter (Davis & Purcell, 2014; Purcell et al., 2018).

Table 10.1 Symptom-specific academic accommodations

Post-concussion symptom	Effect on school learning	Accommodation
Physical symptoms		
Headache	Difficulty concentrating	Frequent breaks, quiet area, hydration
Fatigue	Decreased attention, concentration, low energy	Frequent breaks, shortened day, attendance in fewer classes
Light/noise sensitivity	Worsening symptoms (headache)	Sunglasses, ear plugs/headphones, avoid noisy areas (cafeterias, assemblies, sport events, music class), limit computer work
Dizziness/balance	Unsteadiness when walking, room feels like it is spinning	Elevator/lift pass (if available) Class transition before bell
Cognitive symptoms		
Difficulty concentrating	Limited focus on schoolwork	Shorter assignments, decreased workload, frequent breaks, having someone read out loud, more time to complete assignments/tests, quiet area to complete work
Working/short-term memory	Forgetting instructions, oral lecture, reading material, thoughts during tasks	Repetition; written instructions Provide student with teacher-generated class notes
Difficulty remembering	Difficulty retaining new information, remembering instructions, accessing learned information	Written instructions, smaller amounts to learn, repetition
Slow speed of performance/process	Unable to keep pace with work load, slower reading/writing/calculation Difficulty processing verbal information effectively	Extended time to complete coursework, assignments, tests Reduce/slow down verbal information and check for comprehension
Emotional symptoms		
Anxiety	Decreased attention or concentration, overexertion to avoid falling behind	Reassurance and support from teachers about accommodations, reduced workload
Irritability	Poor tolerance for stress (social, academic load)	Reduce stimulation and stressors (e.g., overwhelmed with missing work)

Note: Reproduced with permission of Taylor & Francis from Gioia, G. A. (2017). Return to school: When and how should return to school be organized after a concussion? In I. Gagnon & A. Ptito (Eds.), *Sports concussions: A complete guide to recovery and management* (pp. 241–262), Boca Raton, FL: CRC Press; permission conveyed through Copyright Clearance Center, Inc.

Initially following a concussion, students may need to stay home from school with relative restriction of physical and cognitive activity to allow acute symptoms to subside. Worsening of post-concussion symptoms upon RTS has been shown to occur in up to 45% of students (Carson et al., 2014), and may be caused by students pushing through symptoms or by suboptimal accommodations/support (Davis & Purcell, 2014; Purcell et al., 2018). However, symptom exacerbation may be unrelated to physical or mental activity but rather other factors, such as stress or poor sleep (Silverberg et al., 2016). On the other hand, there is evidence that longer restriction of activity, including school absence, may delay recovery and worsen symptoms (Thomas, Apps, Hoffman, McCrea, & Hammeke, 2015). Therefore, school absence should be minimized to reduce the occurrence of secondary problems, such as anxiety about missed school, social isolation, and depression (Davis & Purcell, 2014; Halstead et al., 2013; Master et al., 2012; Purcell et al., 2018). Typically, students should be able to RTS with or without accommodations within two to five days post-injury (Grubenhoff et al., 2015; Purcell et al., 2016; Thomas et al., 2015).

Current clinical and consensus-based recommendations state that as post-concussion symptoms improve, students can increase cognitive activity at home. Once students can tolerate about 30 minutes of cognitive activity at home without significant worsening of their symptoms, they can try RTS with accommodations as needed (Davis & Purcell, 2014; Halstead et al., 2013; Master et al., 2012; McGrath, 2010; Sady, Vaughan, & Gioia, 2011). Students do not need to be symptom-free to RTS. RTS may be facilitated by following a stepwise, symptom-limited program of gradually increasing cognitive activity (see Table 10.2; Gioia, 2016; Master et al., 2012; McCrory et al., 2017; Purcell, 2014).

School concussion policies have been shown to be effective in supporting students returning to school after concussion and have improved provision of academic accommodations (Davies, Sandlund, & Lopez, 2016; Glang et al., 2015). A key factor for successfully implementing an RTS protocol is concussion education, particularly of school staff and parents (Davies et al., 2016; Halstead et al., 2013; Master et al., 2012; McGrath, 2010). Online educational tools and evidence-based education programs can be effective to increase knowledge of concussion and current management recommendations (Glang et al., 2015; Graff & Caperell, 2016; Hunt et al., 2016). Government legislation can be instrumental in the development of school concussion policies (Gioia, Glang, Hooper, & Brown, 2016; Hachem et al., 2016; Ontario Ministry of Education, 2014).

Regular medical follow-up for students after concussion is essential to guide the RTS process and monitor recovery (Grubenhoff et al., 2015). Effective communication between the student/parents, medical team, and school personnel (including a RTS letter) is necessary to ensure successful RTS (Gioia, 2016; Hachem et al., 2016). This support network can decrease a student's anxiety about missing school, allowing the student to focus on recovery and help facilitate symptom improvement (Davies et al., 2016; Halstead et al., 2013; Master et al., 2012; McGrath, 2010; Sady et al., 2011).

Table 10.2 Graduated return to school strategy

Mental activity	Activity at each step	Goal of each step
1. Daily activities that do not give the child symptoms	Typical activities that the child does during the day as long as they do not increase symptoms (e.g. reading, texting, screen time). Start with 5–15 minutes at a time and gradually build up	Gradual return to typical activities
2. School activities at home	Homework, reading or other cognitive activities outside of the classroom	Increase tolerance to cognitive work
3. Return to school part-time	Gradual introduction of school work; may need to start with a partial school day or with increased breaks during the day	Increase academic activities
4. Return to school full-time	Gradually progress school activities until a full day can be tolerated	Return to full academic activities and catch up on missed work

Note: Reproduced with permission from "Consensus Statement on Concussion in Sport—The 5th International Conference on Concussion in Sport Held in Berlin, October 2016," by P. McCrory, W. Meeuwisse, J. Dvorak, M. Aubry, J. Bailes, S. Broglio, … G. A. Davis, 2017, *British Journal of Sports Medicine, 51,* 838–847. doi: 10.1136/bjsports-2017-097699.

Return to play/sport

Limited research has been conducted looking at RTP following an SRC in youth. RTP recommendations in children and adolescents have been extrapolated from adult consensus guidelines (e.g., McCrory et al., 2013; McCrory et al., 2017). This is the area of concussion management with the highest risk of complications and potentially catastrophic injury (i.e., second impact syndrome) if athletes RTP before full recovery. As such, caution is warranted given that repeated concussions can result in cumulative effects negatively affecting concentration and attention (Moser, Schatz, & Jordan, 2005), as well as increased vulnerability to recurrent concussive injury (Collins et al., 2002; Guskiewicz et al., 2000). Second impact syndrome rarely occurs in young athletes less than 20 years of age when an athlete sustains a second head injury while still symptomatic from a previous injury, resulting in brain edema and death (Cantu, 1998; McCrory et al., 2012).

In Canada, a 17-year-old girl died from second impact syndrome in 2014 following recurrent head injuries sustained while playing rugby. After her death, a coroner's inquest was conducted, followed by the formation of an advisory committee to examine the recommendations of the inquest. This led to the passing of Rowan's Law in Ontario in 2018—the first concussion safety legislation in Canada. The law establishes removal from sport and return to sport protocols following concussion, education for teachers and coaches, and a concussion code of conduct to reduce the incidence of concussions in sports (Legislative Assembly of Ontario, 2018).

Given that younger athletes take longer to recover from concussion compared with adults, RTP recommendations are more conservative (Davis et al., 2017;

Davis & Purcell, 2014; Halstead & Walter, 2010; McCrory et al., 2017; Purcell, 2009; Purcell, 2014). However, specific criteria are lacking. If a youth athlete is suspected to have sustained a concussion, they should be immediately removed from play and not allowed to return the same day and not RTP until medically cleared. Current recommendations include initial cognitive and physical rest in the first couple of days after injury, followed by gradual increase in activity, guided by symptoms (see Table 10.3; McCrory et al., 2017). As symptoms subside, athletes can begin a stepwise exertion strategy of increasing physical activity. This exertion protocol should be supervised by a qualified medical practitioner with expertise in managing SRC. Children and adolescents should not RTP (contact training or game play) until they have successfully RTS and all concussion symptoms have resolved at rest and with exertion (Davis et al., 2017; Halstead & Walter, 2010; McCrory et al., 2017; Purcell, 2014). Because of individual differences in presentation and recovery from concussion and longer recovery times, RTP decisions should be made cautiously in children and adolescents. Guidelines can be used as a reference point, but each athlete should be assessed individually, using clinical signs and symptoms and regular follow-up (Collins et al., 2014; Purcell, 2009).

Table 10.3 Graduated return to sport strategy

Stage	Aim	Activity	Goal of each step
1	Symptom-limited activity	Daily activities that do not provoke symptoms	Gradual reintroduction of work/school activities
2	Light aerobic exercise	Walking or stationary cycling at slow to medium pace. No resistance training	Increase heart rate
3	Sport-specific exercise	Running or skating drills. No head impact activities	Add movement
4	Non-contact training drills	Harder training drills, e.g., passing drills. May start progressive resistance training	Exercise, coordination, and increased thinking
5	Full-contact practice	Following medical clearance, participate in normal training activities	Restore confidence and assess functional skills by coaching staff
6	Return to sport	Normal game play	

Note: An initial period of 24–48 hours of both relative physical rest and cognitive rest is recommended before beginning the return to sport progression. There should be at least 24 hours (or longer) for each step of the progression. If any symptoms worsen during exercise, the athlete should go back to the previous step. Resistance training should be added only in the later stages (Stage 3 or 4 at the earliest).

Note: Reproduced with permission from "Consensus Statement on Concussion in Sport— The 5th International Conference on Concussion in Sport Held in Berlin, October 2016," by P. McCrory, W. Meeuwisse, J. Dvorak, M. Aubry, J. Bailes, S. Broglio, ... G. A. Davis, 2017, *British Journal of Sports Medicine, 51*, 838–847. doi: 10.1136/bjsports-2017-097699.

Psychological aspects

The psychological aspects of SRC recovery are not well studied, particularly in the pediatric age group, but emerging evidence indicates that athletes with prolonged recoveries and persistent post-concussion symptoms are often associated with predominantly mental health and emotional disturbances after concussive injury (Corwin et al., 2014).

Emotional symptoms

SRC is associated with a constellation of symptoms that include cognitive symptoms, physical symptoms, sleep disturbances, and emotional changes. Cognitive symptoms (e.g., difficulty concentrating) and physical symptoms (e.g., headache) typically occur immediately following injury; sleep disturbances and emotional symptoms tend to develop later in recovery (usually beyond the first week). Following concussion, up to 20% of college athletes may experience significant emotional symptoms, including mood disturbances, anxiety, depression, irritability, sadness, anger, fear, loss of self-esteem, feelings of helplessness, and social isolation (Chertok & Martin, 2013; Putukian & Echemendia, 2003; Sandel et al., 2017; Vargas et al., 2015). Younger athletes may develop similar symptoms after injury (Covassin et al., 2017; Patel, Greydanus, & Pratt, 2009). There is marked overlap of post-concussion symptoms, particularly vestibular and cervical deficits, with psychological responses to injury, so it can be difficult to determine what is directly caused by concussion and how much is a secondary response to the injury (Bloom et al., 2004; Putukian & Echemendia, 2003).

Athletes may experience a sense of loss following concussion, secondary to a lack of team involvement, decreased physical activity, and lack of a structured routine schedule (MacPherson, Kerr, & Stirling, 2016; Patel et al., 2009; Putukian & Echemendia, 2003; Turner et al., 2017). Emotional symptoms may develop in response to poor SRC management with overly strict restrictions on activity and social interactions (Gibson et al., 2013; Leddy et al., 2012; Thomas et al., 2015; Turner et al., 2017). Limiting social interactions for adolescents can be detrimental to recovery, causing emotional distress and a sense of isolation because of the significance of social activity in personal development during adolescence (Gibson et al., 2013; Greydanus & Pratt, 2009; MacPherson et al., 2016; Sandel et al., 2017). In addition, concurrent psychosocial stressors (i.e., family dysfunction, death in family, sick family member, moving, financial concerns, etc.) can impact on recovery and lead to persistent symptoms (Sandel et al., 2017). One particularly detrimental stressor is negative reaction from coaches, teammates, friends, and family members who may question the validity of the injury, leading to pressure to RTP or even bullying from peers (Chertok & Martin, 2013).

Risk factors

Risk factors associated with the development of post-concussion mental health, emotional symptoms, as well as persistent symptoms, include pre-existing mental health/emotional history, female gender, and age (adolescents 13 years and older) (Heyer et al., 2016; Sandel et al., 2017; Zemek et al., 2016). A number of psychosocial factors have also been identified as risk factors for prolonged recovery in youth athletes including:

- Somatization: Children who have a preinjury tendency to somaticize have been shown to have delayed recovery from concussion (Grubenhoff et al., 2016)
- Higher athletic identity: Because of the significant degree of psychological investment in sport, concussion injury threatens their self-identity and overall sense of competence, straining their ability to cope, leading to symptom hypervigilance and symptom exacerbation from emotional distress (O'Rourke et al., 2017; Putukian & Echemendia, 2003)
- Amotivation: Athletes who were less motivated to RTP recovered more slowly; the injury provides a good excuse to not participate in sport, with no incentive to minimize symptoms (O'Rourke et al., 2017)
- Performance anxiety: Greater anxiety associated with longer recoveries; may become hypervigilant about symptoms and interpret anxiety symptoms as indicators of incomplete concussion recovery (O'Rourke et al., 2017)

Additionally, coping style may affect injury recovery. Athletes with poor coping skills who adopt maladaptive behaviors may prolong their recovery. For instance, fear of exacerbating symptoms may cause an athlete to develop avoidance behaviors and elect not to RTS, which may prolong recovery and result in development or worsening of emotional symptoms (Sandel et al., 2017; Thomas et al., 2015). Furthermore, capacity for emotional regulation can influence the development of postinjury emotional symptoms. Athletes who are more resilient in the face of adversity tend to recover better than those who have difficulty with adverse events (Sandel et al., 2017). Children and adolescents in particular lack life experience and familiarity with the psychological consequences of injury, as well as coping skills and resources to deal with injury (Covassin et al., 2017).

Management of emotional symptoms

Throughout concussion recovery, emotional and mental health symptoms should be assessed, and treatment should be instituted in athletes whose symptoms become significant, to facilitate recovery (Collins et al., 2014; Patel et al., 2009; Putukian & Echemendia, 2003; Sandel et al., 2017). Social support, both informational and emotional, from family, friends, teammates, coaches, trainers, and doctors is very important to help with recovery and to decrease social isolation and anxiety. Therefore, children and adolescents should be encouraged to maintain their social networks during injury recovery (Bloom et al., 2004; Chertok & Martin, 2013; Covassin et al., 2017; Putukian & Echemendia, 2003; Zemek et al., 2014).

Treatment options for significant affective symptoms include:

- Psychoeducation: Information about the injury and expected recovery (Sandel et al., 2017)
- Behavioral regulation strategies: Maintenance of healthy lifestyle factors such as nutrition and hydration, sleep hygiene, physical activity, stress management (Collins et al., 2014; Purcell, 2014; Sandel et al., 2017; Thomas et al., 2015; Zemek et al., 2014)
- Cervical and vestibular rehabilitation (Purcell, 2014; Schneider et al., 2013; Schneider et al., 2017; Zemek et al., 2014)
- Desensitization to environmental stimuli (Sandel et al., 2017)
- Support groups: May help injured athletes realize they are not alone and can reduce anxiety, depression, and isolation (Bloom et al., 2004)
- Psychotherapy, such as cognitive behavioral therapy and coping strategies (Collins et al., 2014; Patel et al., 2009; Sandel et al., 2017; Zemek et al., 2014)

Specific psychological techniques that may be helpful during recovery include goal-setting, which has been shown to enhance healing following injury; relaxation training, which increases body awareness, enhances muscular relaxation at rest, and increases muscular efficiency during performance; biofeedback; imagery; and cognitive restructuring (Bloom et al., 2004; Chertok & Martin, 2013; Putukian & Echemendia, 2003). In severe cases, patients may require referral to psychology/psychiatry as well as pharmacological treatment in addition to the aforementioned solutions (Collins et al., 2014; Patel et al., 2009; Purcell, 2014; Zemek et al., 2014).

Conclusions

Although the majority of SRC occur in children and adolescents, there has been a relative lack of research in this age group, particularly in children aged 5–12 years. Because children are developing, diagnosis of concussion can be more challenging, and different assessment tools are necessary. Children and adolescents take longer to recover from concussion than adults and have different management priorities. RTS is a priority for children and adolescents following concussion, and RTP should be more conservative, with return to contact training and game play occurring only once full RTS has occurred. Persistent post-concussion symptoms are often associated with mental health and emotional disturbances following concussion. Significant psychological issues, such as anxiety and depression, if unrecognized and unaddressed, may prolong recovery. Therefore, mental health issues and emotional disturbances should be monitored throughout concussion recovery and specific interventions instituted when necessary, to facilitate recovery.

There remain many unanswered questions with respect to how children and adolescents are affected by concussion and what the best management should be in this age group. Rigorous, high-quality research is urgently needed to inform management guidelines, particularly regarding RTS and RTP, and develop evidence-based best practices.

References

Baker, J. G., Leddy, J. J., Darling, S. R., Rieger, B. P., Mashtare, T. L., Sharma, T., & Willer, B. S. (2015). Factors associated with problems for adolescents returning to the classroom after sport-related concussion. *Clinical Pediatrics, 54,* 961–968. doi: 10.1177/0009922815588820.

Baxter-Jones, A. D. G., & Malina, R. M. (2001). Growth and maturation issues in elite young athletes: Normal variation and training. In N. Maffulli, K. Chan, R. Malina, & T. Parker (Eds.), *Sport medicine for specific ages and abilities* (pp. 95–108). London: Churchill Livingstone.

Bloom, G. A., Horton, A. S., McCrory, P., & Johnston, K. M. (2004). Sport psychology and concussion: New impacts to explore. *British Journal of Sports Medicine, 38,* 519–521. doi: 10.1136/bjsm.2004.011999.

Brown, N. J., Mannix, R. C., O'Brien, M. J., Gostine, D., Collins, M. W., & Meehan, W. P. (2014). Effect of cognitive activity level on duration of post-concussion symptoms. *Pediatrics, 133,* e299–e304. doi: 10.1542/peds.2013-2125.

Browne, G. J., & Lam, L. T. (2006). Concussive head injury in children and adolescents related to sports and other leisure physical activities. *British Journal of Sports Medicine, 40,* 163–168. doi: 10.1136/bjsm.2005.021220.

Cantu, R. C. (1998). Second-impact syndrome. *Clinics in Sports Medicine, 17,* 37–44. doi: 1016/S0278-5919(05)70059-4.

Carson, J. D., Lawrence, D. W., Kraft, S. A., Garel, A., Snow, C. L., Chatterjee, A., ... Frémont, P. (2014). Premature return to play and return to learn after a sport-related concussion: Physician's chart review. *Canadian Family Physician, 60,* e310–e315.

Chertok, G. J., & Martin, I. H. (2013). Psychological aspects of concussion recovery. *International Journal of Athletic Therapy and Training, 18,* 7–9. doi: 10.1123/ijatt.18.3.7.

Child Sport Concussion Assessment Tool-5. (2018, May). Retrieved from: http://bjsm. bmj.com/content/51/11/862.

Collins, M. W., Kontos, A. P., Reynolds, E., Murawski, C. D., & Fu, F.H. (2014). A comprehensive, targeted approach to the clinical care of athletes following sport-related concussion. *Knee Surgery, Sports Traumatology, Arthroscopy, 22,* 235–246. doi: 10.1007/s00167-013-2791-6.

Collins, M. W., Lovell, M. R., Iverson, G. L., Cantu, R. C., Maroon, J. C., & Field, M. (2002). Cumulative effects of concussion in high school athletes. *Neurosurgery, 51,* 1175–1181. doi: 10.1097/00006123-200211000-00011.

Concussion Recognition Tool-5. (2017). Retrieved from: http://bjsm.bmj.com/content/51/11/872.

Corwin, D. J., Wiebe, D. J., Zonfrillo, M. R., Grady, M. F., Robinson, R. L., Goodman, A. M., & Master, C. L. (2015). Vestibular deficits following youth concussion. *The Journal of Pediatrics, 166,* 1221–1225. doi: 10.1016/j.jpeds.2015.01.039.

Corwin, D. J., Zonfrillo, M. R., Master, C. L., Arbogast, K. B., Grady, M. F., Robinson, R. L., ... Wiebe, D. J. (2014). Characteristics of prolonged concussion recovery in a pediatric subspecialty referral population. *The Journal of Pediatrics, 165,* 1207–1215. doi: 10.1016/j.jpeds.2014.08.034.

Covassin, T., Elbin, R. J., Beidler, E., LaFevor, M., & Kontos, A. P. (2017). A review of psychological issues that may be associated with a sport-related concussion in youth and collegiate athletes. *Sport, Exercise, and Performance Psychology, 6,* 220. doi: 10.1037/spy0000105.

Davies, S. C., Sandlund, J. M., & Lopez, L. B. (2016). School-based consultation to improve concussion recognition and response. *Journal of Educational and Psychological Consultation, 26*, 49–62. doi: 10.1080/10474412.2014.963225.

Davis, G. A., Anderson, V., Babl, F. E., Gioia, G. A., Giza, C. C., Meehan, W., ... Takagi, M. (2017). What is the difference in concussion management in children as compared with adults? A systematic review. *British Journal of Sports Medicine, 51*, 949–957. doi: 10.1136/bjsports-2016-097415.

Davis, G. A., & Purcell, L. K. (2014). The evaluation and management of acute concussion differs in young children. *British Journal of Sports Medicine, 48*, 98–101. doi: 10.1136/bjsports-2012-092132.

Elbin, R. J., Sufrinko, A., Schatz, P., French, J., Henry, L., Burkhart, S., ... Kontos, A. P. (2016). Removal from play after concussion and recovery time. *Pediatrics,* e20160910. doi: 10.1542/peds.2016-0910.

Fazio, V. C., Lovell, M. R., Pardini, J. E., & Collins, M. W. (2007). The relation between postconcussion symptoms and neurocognitive performance in concussed athletes. *Neurorehabilitation, 22*, 207–216.

Field, M., Collins, M. W., Lovell, M. R., & Maroon, J. (2003). Does age play a role in recovery from sports-related concussion? A comparison of high school and collegiate athletes. *The Journal of Pediatrics, 142*, 546–553. doi: 10.1067/mpd.2003.190.

Gibson, S., Nigrovic, L. E., O'Brien, M., & Meehan, W. P. III (2013). The effect of recommending cognitive rest on recovery from sport-related concussion. *Brain Injury, 27*, 839–842. doi: 10.3109/02699052.2013.775494.

Gioia, G. A. (2016). Medical-school partnership in guiding return to school following mild traumatic brain injury in youth. *Journal of Child Neurology, 31*, 93–108. doi: 10.1177/0883073814555604.

Gioia, G. A., Glang, A. E., Hooper, S. R., & Brown, B. E. (2016). Building statewide infrastructure for the academic support of students with mild traumatic brain injury. *The Journal of Head Trauma Rehabilitation, 31*, 397–406.doi: 10.1097/HTR.0000000000000205.

Gioia, G. A. (2017). Return to school: When and how should return to school be organized after a concussion? In I. Gagnon & A. Ptito (Eds.), *Sports concussions: A complete guide to recovery and management* (pp. 241–262). Boca Raton, FL: CRC Press.

Glang, A. E., Koester, M. C., Chesnutt, J. C., Gioia, G. A., McAvoy, K., Marshall, S., & Gau, J. M. (2015). The effectiveness of a web-based resource in improving postconcussion management in high schools. *Journal of Adolescent Health, 56*, 91–97. doi: 10.1016/j.jadohealth.2014.08.011.

Government of Canada. (2017). *Concussion & Brain Injuries in Canadian Children and Youth.* Retrieved from https://infobase.phac-aspc.gc.ca/datalab/head-injury-interactive-en.html.

Graff, D. M., & Caperell, K. S. (2016). Concussion management in the classroom. *Journal of Child Neurology, 31*, 1569–1574. doi: 10.1177/0883073816666205.

Greydanus, D. E., & Pratt, H. D. (2009). Adolescent Growth and Development, and Sport Participation. In D. R. Patel, D. E. Greydanus, & R. J. Baker (Eds.), *Pediatric practice: Sports medicine* (pp. 15–25). New York, NY: McGraw-Hill.

Grubenhoff, J. A., Currie, D., Comstock, R. D., Juarez-Colunga, E., Bajaj, L., & Kirkwood, M. W. (2016). Psychological factors associated with delayed symptom resolution in children with concussion. *The Journal of Pediatrics, 174*, 27–32. doi: 10.1016/j.jpeds.2016.03.027.

Grubenhoff, J. A., Deakyne, S. J., Comstock, R. D., Kirkwood, M. W., & Bajaj, L. (2015).Outpatient follow-up and return to school after emergency department evaluation among children with persistent post-concussion symptoms. *Brain Injury*, *29*, 1186–1191. doi: 10.3109/02699052.2015.1035325.

Guskiewicz, K. M., Weaver, N. L., Padua, D. A., & Garrett, W. E. (2000). Epidemiology of concussion in collegiate and high school football players. *The American Journal of Sports Medicine*, *28*, 643–650. doi: 10.1177/03635465000 280050401.

Hachem, L. D., Kourtis, G., Mylabathula, S., & Tator, C. H. (2016). Experience with Canada's first policy on concussion education and management in schools. *Canadian Journal of Neurological Sciences*, *43*, 554–560. doi: 10.1017/cjn.2016.41.

Halstead, M. E., McAvoy, K., Devore, C. D., Carl, R., Lee, M., & Logan, K. (2013). Returning to learning following a concussion. *Pediatrics*, *132*, 948–957. doi: 10.1542/peds.2013-2867.

Halstead, M. E., & Walter, K. D. (2010). Sport-related concussion in children and adolescents. *Pediatrics*, *126*, 597–615. doi: 10.1542/peds.2010-2005.

Harris, A. W., Jones, C. A., Rowe, B. H., & Voaklander, D. C. (2012). A population-based study of sport and recreation-related head injuries treated in a Canadian health region. *Journal of Science and Medicine in Sport*, *15*, 298–304. doi: 10.1016/j.jsams.2011.12.005.

Heyer, G. L., Schaffer, C. E., Rose, S. C., Young, J. A., McNally, K. A., & Fischer, A. N. (2016). Specific factors influence postconcussion symptom duration among youth referred to a sports concussion clinic. *The Journal of Pediatrics*, *174*, 33–38. doi: 10.1016/j.jpeds.2016.03.014.

Hunt, A. W., De Feo, L., Macintyre, J., Greenspoon, D., Dick, T., Mah, K., … Reed, N. (2016). Development and feasibility of an evidence-informed self-management education program in pediatric concussion rehabilitation. *BMC Health Services Research*, *16*, 400. doi: 10.1186/s12913-016-1664-3.

Leddy, J. J., Sandhu, H., Sodhi, V., Baker, J. G., & Willer, B. (2012). Rehabilitation of concussion and post-concussion syndrome. *Sports Health*, *4*, 147–154. doi: 10.1177/1941738111433673.

Legislative Assembly of Ontario. (2018). Bill 193: An act to enact Rowan's law (concussion safety), 2018 and to amend the Education Act. Retrieved from: www.ontla.on.ca/bills/bills-files/41_Parliament/Session2/b193ra_e.pdf.

Lovell, M. R., Collins, M. W., Iverson, G. L., Field, M., Maroon, J. C., Cantu, R., … Fu, F. H. (2003). Recovery from mild concussion in high school athletes. *Journal of Neurosurgery*, *98*, 296–301.

Lovell, M. R., & Fazio, V. (2008). Concussion management in the child and adolescent athlete. *Current Sports Medicine Reports*, *7*, 12–15. doi: 10.1097/01. CSMR.0000308671.45558.e2.

MacPherson, E., Kerr, G., & Stirling, A. (2016). The influence of peer groups in organized sport on female adolescents' identity development. *Psychology of Sport and Exercise*, *23*, 73–81. doi: 10.1016/j.psychsport.2015.10.002.

Makki, A. Y., Leddy, J., Hinds, A., Baker, J., Paluch, R., Shucard, J., & Willer, B. (2016). School attendance and symptoms in adolescents after sport-related concussion. *Global Pediatric Health*, *3*, 2333794X16630493. doi: 10.1177/2333794X16630493.

Master, C. L., Gioia, G. A., Leddy, J. J., & Grady, M. F. (2012). Importance of "return-to-learn" in pediatric and adolescent concussion. *Pediatric Annals*, *41*, 180–185. doi: 10.3928/00904481-20120827-09.

McClincy, M. P., Lovell, M. R., Pardini, J., Collins, M. W., & Spore, M. K. (2006). Recovery from sports concussion in high school and collegiate athletes. *Brain Injury*, *20*, 33–39. doi: 10.1080/02699050500309817.

McCrory, P., Collie, A., Anderson, V., & Davis, G. (2004). Can we manage sport related concussion in children the same as in adults?. *British Journal of Sports Medicine*, *38*, 516–519. doi: 10.1136/bjsm.2004.014811.

McCrory, P., Davis, G., & Makdissi, M. (2012). Second impact syndrome or cerebral swelling after sporting head injury. *Current Sports Medicine Reports*, *11*, 21–23. doi: 10.1249/JSR.0b013e3182423bfd.

McCrory, P., Meeuwisse, W. H., Aubry, M., Cantu, R. C., Dvorak, J., Echemendia, R. J., ... Sills, A. (2013). Consensus statement on concussion in sport—The 4th International Conference on Concussion in Sport held in Zurich, November 2012. *PM&R*, *5*, 255–279. doi: 10.1016/j.pmrj.2013.02.012.

McCrory, P., Meeuwisse, W., Dvorak, J., Aubry, M., Bailes, J., Broglio, S., ... Davis, G. A. (2017). Consensus statement on concussion in sport—The 5th International Conference on Concussion in Sport held in Berlin, October 2016. *British Journal of Sports Medicine*, *51*, 838–847. doi: 10.1136/bjsports-2017-097699.

McGrath, N. (2010). Supporting the student-athlete's return to the classroom after a sport-related concussion. *Journal of Athletic Training*, *45*, 492–498.

Meehan, W. P., & Mannix, R. (2010). Pediatric concussions in United States emergency departments in the years 2002 to 2006. *The Journal of Pediatrics*, *157*, 889–893. doi: 10.1016/j.jpeds.2010.06.040.

Moser, R. S., Schatz, P., & Jordan, B. D. (2005). Prolonged effects of concussion in high school athletes. *Neurosurgery*, *57*, 300–306. doi: 10.1227/01. NEU.0000166663.98616.E4.

Ontario Ministry of Education. (2014). *School board policies on concussion* (Policy/ Program Memorandum No. 158). Retrieved from: www.edu.gov.on.ca/extra/ eng/ppm/158.pdf.

O'Rourke, D. J., Smith, R. E., Punt, S., Coppel, D. B., & Breiger, D. (2017). Psychosocial correlates of young athletes' self-reported concussion symptoms during the course of recovery. *Sport, Exercise, and Performance Psychology*, *6*, 262. doi: 10.1037/spy0000097.

Patel, D. R., Greydanus, D. E., & Pratt, H. D. (2009). Psychosocial aspects of youth sports. In D.R. Patel, D. E. Greydanus, & R. J. Baker (Eds.), *Pediatric practice: Sports medicine* (pp. 26–37). New York, NY: McGraw-Hill.

Patel, D. R., & Pratt, H. D. (2009). Child neurodevelopment and sport participation. In D. R. Patel, D. E. Greydanus, & R. J. Baker (Eds.), *Pediatric practice: Sports medicine* (pp. 1–14). New York, NY: McGraw-Hill.

Purcell, L. (2009). What are the most appropriate return-to-play guidelines for concussed child athletes? *British Journal of Sports Medicine*, *43*, i51–i55. doi: 10.1136/bjsm.2009.058214.

Purcell, L., Harvey, J., & Seabrook, J. A. (2016). Patterns of recovery following sport-related concussion in children and adolescents. *Clinical Pediatrics*, *55*, 452–458. doi: 10.1177/0009922815589915.

Purcell, L. K. (2014). Sport-related concussion: Evaluation and management. *Paediatrics & Child Health, 19*, 153–158. doi: 10.1093/pch/19.3.153.

Purcell, L. K., Davis, G. A., & Gioia, G. A. (2018). What factors must be considered in "return to school" following concussion and what strategies or accommodations should be followed? A systematic review. *British Journal of Sports Medicine*. Advance online publication. doi: 10.1136/bjsports-2017-097853.

Putukian, M., & Echemendia, R. J. (2003). Psychological aspects of serious head injury in the competitive athlete. *Clinics in Sports Medicine, 22*, 617–630.

Ransom, D. M., Vaughan, C. G., Pratson, L., Sady, M. D., McGill, C. A., & Gioia, G. A. (2015). Academic effects of concussion in children and adolescents. *Pediatrics, 135*, 1043–1050. doi: 10.1542/peds.2014-3434.

Sady, M. D., Vaughan, C. G., & Gioia, G. A. (2011). School and the concussed youth: Recommendations for concussion education and management. *Physical Medicine and Rehabilitation Clinics, 22*, 701–719. doi: 10.1016/j.pmr.2011.08.008.

Sandel, N., Reynolds, E., Cohen, P. E., Gillie, B. L., & Kontos, A. P. (2017). Anxiety and mood clinical profile following sport-related concussion: From risk factors to treatment. *Sport, Exercise, and Performance Psychology, 6*, 304. doi: 10.1037/spy0000098.

Schneider, K. J., Iverson, G. L., Emery, C. A., McCrory, P., Herring, S. A., & Meeuwisse, W. H. (2013). The effects of rest and treatment following sport-related concussion: A systematic review of the literature. *British Journal of Sports Medicine, 47*, 304–307. doi: 10.1136/bjsports-2013-092190.

Schneider, K. J., Leddy, J. J., Guskiewicz, K. M., Seifert, T., McCrea, M., Silverberg, N. D., … Makdissi, M. (2017). Rest and treatment/rehabilitation following sport-related concussion: A systematic review. *British Journal of Sports Medicine, 51*, 930–934. doi: 10.1136/bjsports-2016-097475.

Silverberg, N. D., Iverson, G. L., McCrea, M., Apps, J. N., Hammeke, T. A., & Thomas, D. G. (2016). Activity-related symptom exacerbations after pediatric concussion. *JAMA Pediatrics, 170*, 946–953. doi: 10.1001/jamapediatrics.2016.1187.

Sim, A., Terryberry-Spohr, L., & Wilson, K. R. (2008). Prolonged recovery of memory functioning after mild traumatic brain injury in adolescent athletes. *Journal of Neurosurgery, 108*, 511–516. doi: 10.3171/JNS/2008/108/3/0511.

Sport Concussion Assessment Tool-5. (2018, May). Retrieved from: http://bjsm.bmj.com/content/51/11/851.

Taubman, B., Rosen, F., McHugh, J., Grady, M. F., & Elci, O. U. (2016). The timing of cognitive and physical rest and recovery in concussion. *Journal of Child Neurology, 31* , 1555–1560. doi: 10.1177/0883073816664835.

Thomas, D. G., Apps, J. N., Hoffmann, R. G., McCrea, M., & Hammeke, T. (2015). Benefits of strict rest after acute concussion: A randomized controlled trial. *Pediatrics, 135*, 213–223. doi: 10.1542/peds.2014-0966.

Turner, S., Langdon, J., Shaver, G., Graham, V., Naugle, K., & Buckley, T. (2017). Comparison of psychological response between concussion and musculoskeletal injury in collegiate athletes. *Sport, Exercise, and Performance Psychology, 6*, 277–288. doi: 10.1037/spy0000099.

Vargas, G., Rabinowitz, A., Meyer, J., & Arnett, P. A. (2015). Predictors and prevalence of postconcussion depression symptoms in collegiate athletes. *Journal of Athletic Training, 50*, 250–255. doi: 10.4085/1062-6050-50.3.02.

Zemek, R., Barrowman, N., Freedman, S. B., Gravel, J., Gagnon, I., McGahern, C., … Craig, W. (2016). Clinical risk score for persistent postconcussion symptoms among children with acute concussion in the ED. *JAMA, 315*, 1014–1025. doi: 10.1001/jama.2016.1203.

Zemek, R., Duval, S., Dematteo, C., Solomon, B., Keightley, M., & Osmond, M. (2014). *Guidelines for diagnosing and managing pediatric concussion.* Toronto, ON: Ontario Neurotrauma Foundation.

Zuckerbraun, N. S., Atabaki, S., Collins, M. W., Thomas, D., & Gioia, G. A. (2014). Use of modified acute concussion evaluation tools in the emergency department. *Pediatrics, 133*, 635–642. doi: 10.1542/peds.2013-2600.

11 Psychological aspects of concussion in university athletes

Emily Kroshus

Introduction

Across the life course and at all levels of competition, concussions are a prevalent injury in sports that involve routine contact and collision (Pfister et al., 2016; Rosenthal et al., 2014; Zuckerman et al., 2015). University sport, which is comprised of post-secondary students and sponsored by a post-secondary institution, is an important sub-population among which concussion should be explored for several reasons. First, the incidence of diagnosed concussion is higher in university sport as compared to sports in younger age ranges. Among athletes competing in the National Collegiate Athletic Association (NCAA), recent estimates suggest that 3.74 concussions are diagnosed per 1,000 athlete game exposures, as compared to 1.86 per 1,000 athlete game exposures in United States high schools (Dompier et al., 2015). That being said, elevated incidence must be interpreted with caution since medical capabilities are often stronger in university sport as compared to high school or youth, meaning it is possible that the difference reflects differences in diagnoses rather than differences in true incidence (Kroshus et al., 2017). Second, it is a population among which there are unique structural and competitive considerations. For example, university athletes are often living away from home for the first time and dealing with heightened athletic demands and financial considerations like athletic scholarships. Third, relative to professional athletes, there are a large number of participants. In the United States, around 500,000 athletes compete in the NCAA (National Collegiate Athletic Association, 2018b), 65,000 compete in the National Association of Intercollegiate Athletics (National Athletic Intercollegiate Association, 2018), and 60,000 compete in the National Junior College Athletic Association (National Junior Collegiate Athletic Association, 2017). In Canada, around 12,000 athletes compete in U Sports (U Sports, 2018) and 8,000 participate in the Canadian Collegiate Athletic Association (Canadian Collegiate Athletic Association, 2018). University sport is also contested outside of North America, with global sporting championships for university students hosted by the Federation Internationale du Sport Universitaire. Recent championships have been inclusive of participants from 174 countries (International University Sports Federation, 2018). This chapter will focus on university athletes in the United States and Canada, where high-level sport for the young adult age group is often under the organizational umbrella of post-secondary institutions, as compared to European or Australian sport that is often organized in community, regional, or national organizations.

Prevention, identification, and management of concussion

Consistent with broader frameworks of injury and disease prevention, including Gordon's (1983) disease prevention classification system and Haddon's Matrix (Haddon, 1968), this chapter will focus on key concussion-related risk reducing behaviors in the pre-injury period (primary prevention), at the time of injury (secondary prevention), and post-injury (tertiary prevention). The focal strategy for discussion in each of these time periods was informed by recent reviews of concussion prevention strategies (Benson et al., 2013; Emery et al., 2017). In the pre-injury time period, efforts to limit contact from occurring within sports are discussed. For individuals, the most effective primary preventive strategy would be to participate in a sport with a low risk of concussion. However, the assumption put forth in this chapter is that, at least for athletes who have not sustained multiple concussions, this risk-reducing decision is more likely to occur near the outset of sport participation (e.g., prior to high school) rather than in university when athletes have already invested substantially in their sport. In the time of injury period, early identification and removal from play of athletes who are suspected to have sustained a concussion is discussed. In the post-injury period, medically indicated return to play is discussed, which is inclusive of athletes who have recovered from the acute injury but who are reconsidering their sport participation decisions.

Theoretic framework

This chapter on psychosocial aspects of concussion-related behavior among university athletes is framed using a social ecologic model (Bronfenbrenner, 1977; Centers for Disease Control and Prevention, 2019) in which individual athletes are embedded in a broader intrapersonal, institutional, community, and societal context (Kerr et al., 2014; Register-Mihalik et al., 2017). Factors at each of these levels influence the behavior of athletes or of other key stakeholders in the sports environment (e.g., coaches, medical staff) who themselves directly or indirectly impact athlete behavior and concussion-related outcomes. This framework is used to guide the conceptualization of this chapter but does not function as a testable theory. For each of the key strategies discussed, and at each level of influence, relevant psychosocial theories proposed or tested in the extant literature about concussion will be reviewed.

Pre-injury: Limit contact

Fewer head impacts should mean fewer opportunities for concussive or subconcussive brain trauma to occur. A recent meta-analysis of the impact of policy and rule changes related to contact suggests that they help decrease concussion incidence (Emery et al., 2017). Most evidence related to such rule changes has come from Canadian youth ice hockey (e.g., Black et al., 2016; Black et al., 2017; Emery et al., 2010), with some related to youth football (Broglio et al., 2016; Cobb et al., 2013) and some in professional sport (Bjørneboe et al., 2013; Donaldson, Asbridge, & Cusimano, 2013; Ruestow et al., 2015). In university football, a recent rule change among Ivy League institutions related to kickoff returns has been associated with reduced concussion incidence (Wiebe et al., 2018).

At the university level to date, only the NCAA has taken steps to limit head impacts by restricting contact in practices, limiting football program two-a-day contact practices in pre-season football (NCAA, contact restrictions). Other efforts by university governing bodies in the United States and Canada to restrict contact in practices are not known at this time. Even at the youth level there is variability in the extent to which policies limiting contact have been passed and ongoing debate about who should be responsible for limiting contact (Bachynski, 2016; Emery, Hagel, & Morrongiello, 2006). For example, restrictions on contact in youth ice hockey are more extensive than restrictions on contact in youth football (Bachynski, 2016). Such differences have, in part, been explained by differences in perceptions about the cultural embeddedness of the sport by decision makers (Bachynski, 2016).

Despite efforts by the NCAA and the Ivy League, rule changes have not been as consistently implemented at the university level as compared to at the youth level. From a public health perspective, evidence-based policy is considered the gold standard (Brownson, Fielding, & Maylahn, 2009). In reality, policies related to concussion are often the result of shifting public opinion fueled by critical events (Harvey, Koller, & Lowrey, 2015), amplified by media attention (Bandura, 2001; Dorfman, Wallack, & Woodruff, 2005; Hartmann, 2009). Such media communications tend to be most compelling when featuring emotional narratives about individuals as opposed to scientific data. Stories about vulnerable youth have an emotive appeal and public opinion tends to be more in favor of limiting risk to minors through precautionary paternalism. Change at all ages may also arise as a result of lawsuits, support of which can be fueled by media and public opinion. The ban on youth heading by U.S. Soccer stemmed directly from a lawsuit filed against a number of soccer governing bodies (*Mehr v. Fédération Internationale de Football Association*). Lawsuits may also indirectly lead to policy and rule change by increasing the potential threat of maintaining the status quo. The NCAA, leading the way in terms of concussion safety-related rule changes at the university sport level, has been subject to numerous lawsuits. Although the causality of this association cannot be determined definitively, external pressure is undoubtedly part of the bigger picture of how and why policy change occurs in sport settings.

However, even if policies are passed, they still need to be adopted by universities and implemented by coaches. At both levels, adoption may be a function of expectations of the consequences of compliance or non-compliance. In addition to outcomes related to student-athlete health, this could include enforcement by the governing body and the potential exposure to litigation if policies are not enforced. Enforcement by university sport governing bodies is challenging for a number of reasons, including the non-profit status of the organizations limiting resources available to be devoted to enforcement. Even when complying with guidelines related to contact, coaches can still engage in coaching practices that encourage safer or less safe forms of contact. For example, encouraging drills that involve high velocity and repeated player-to-player contact.

Decisions about contact restriction tend to exclude the individual athlete once they've selected a given sport. However, if and when there starts to be substantial variability between different university sport governing bodies, or between athletic conferences or institutions in the rules related to contact restriction and concussion safety, it is possible that this may begin to drive the university selection decisions of high school students and their families. On one hand, families who are concerned about concussion safety may elect to participate in an organization that provides what they view as an acceptable level of contact restriction so as to limit concussion risk. On the other hand, to the extent to which families prioritize athletic achievement and view contact restriction as limiting their child's potential for athletic achievement, they may seek to participate in organizations with fewer restrictions.

Time of injury: Early identification and removal from play

A major concern about continued play while symptomatic post-concussion is that the injured athlete may have a more severe brain injury (e.g., subdural hematoma) that requires immediate medical evaluation, or that because of the brain's metabolic vulnerability in the acute symptomatic period after the initial injury, an additional injury could lead to magnified neurologic consequences (Cantu, 1998). During this symptomatic period, reaction time is impaired (Eckner, Kutcher, Broglio, & Richardson, 2014), and athletes are more likely to sustain all types of injury, including orthopedic injury (Brooks et al., 2016; Cross et al., 2016; Lynall et al., 2015). Finally, athletes who continue participating in their sport while symptomatic may take longer to fully recover (Asken et al., 2016). In sum, continued play while symptomatic is an important risk behavior to address in all sports that involve a high risk of concussion. Despite these risks, concussion under-reporting is endemic at the university level; estimates suggest that care is not sought for around half of all suspected concussions (Kroshus et al., 2015; Llewellyn et al., 2014; Torres et al., 2013).

University sport organizations vary in their policies related to athletes' early identification and removal from play of post-concussion. The NCAA mandates that "all student-athletes who are experiencing signs, symptoms of behaviors consistent with a sports-related concussion, at rest or with exertion, must be removed from practice or competition and referred to an athletic trainer or team physician with experience in concussion management" (National Collegiate Athletic Association, 2017). The NCAA also requires that before the start of the season, institutions provide athletes with education about concussion and that athletes sign a form saying that they accept responsibility for reporting possible injury including concussion (National Collegiate Athletic Association, 2017). Institutions are free to provide educational materials of their choosing to athletes, however the NCAA makes available an informational handout for athletes and coaches. The NAIA and NJCAA similarly mandate that "any athlete suspected of sustaining a concussion should be immediately removed from participation and evaluated by a physician or designate" (National Athletic Intercollegiate Association, 2018), and "any athlete suspected of having a concussion should be removed from play immediately and evaluated by a licensed healthcare provider trained in the evaluation and management of concussions" (National Junior College Athletic Association, 2017). In Canadian university sport, there are fewer mandates related to concussion identification and removal from play. U Sport has not publicly disclosed their guidelines, whereas the CCAA focuses only on the evaluation of suspected concussions occurring during national championship competitions (Canadian Collegiate Athletic Association, 2018).

Even in the presence of these policies, many athletes continue to play through suspected concussions (Kroshus, Garnett, et al., 2015; Llewellyn et al., 2014; Torres et al., 2013). Because many concussion symptoms are not immediately evident to external observers, early identification often requires honest report by the injured athlete themselves, meaning that policy mandates about the role of external stakeholders (e.g., coaches and medical staff) have proscribed potential for impact. A growing body of research has sought to understand why athletes who are experiencing symptoms of a possible concussion don't seek immediate medical attention. Initial models proposed that it was driven by inadequate awareness (e.g., athletes not realizing that the symptoms they are experiencing may be from a concussion or knowing that care should be sought for a suspected concussion) (Fedor & Gunstad, 2015; Kaut, DePompei, Kerr, & Congeni, 2003; Miyashita et al., 2013). This knowledge is a necessary precondition for concussion care-seeking. However, subsequent research has suggested that concussion knowledge alone does not explain low rates of care-seeking. Much recent focus has been on individual athlete level psychological theories of behavior, primarily the Theory of Planned Behavior (Ajzen, 1991), as explanatory for concussion under-reporting (Chrisman, Quitiquit, & Rivara, 2013; Kroshus et al., 2014; Register-Mihalik et al., 2017). Consistent with this theory, expectancies about the consequences of concussion reporting, perceived norms related to reporting, and perceived behavioral control are all important determinants of concussion reporting intentions and behavior. Among university athletes, important expectancies relate to the athletic consequences of reporting (e.g., I'll lose my spot on the team) and what they believe are relational consequences of reporting (e.g., my teammates will think less of me) (Kroshus et al., 2014). While long-term health consequences are undoubtedly important behavioral motivators for some athletes, they are far in the future and may not feel immediately relevant enough to many athletes in this age group. Adolescents and young adults tend to find social approval particularly reinforcing (Steinberg, 2008, 2010), meaning that social expectancies will be particularly strong drivers of behavior.

At an interpersonal level, group norms are among the strongest drivers of concussion reporting behaviors (Kroshus et al., 2015). There is evidence to suggest that perceived and actual group norms about concussion reporting are misperceived among university athletes (Kroshus et al., 2014; Kroshus et al., 2015), consistent with evidence about misperceived norms among university students about other risk behaviors such as binge drinking (Borsari & Carey, 2003). Athletes tend to overestimate teammate unlikelihood of reporting a suspected concussion, thinking that they themselves would be more likely to behave in a safe way than their teammates (Kroshus et al., 2014, 2015). This finding is consistent with spiral of silence theory (Noelle-Neumann, 1974), in which individuals who believe that their attitudes are consistent with the group's norm are most likely to speak up (e.g., express support for the norms), whereas those who believe their beliefs are not normative tend to stay quiet. This helps unsafe perceived norms persist because, independent of the actual beliefs, the only voices heard tend to be those that reflect the "unsafe" behavior. The importance of norms in motivating behavior, and the need for them to be corrected, speaks to the importance of multilevel education that engages team members in speaking up about concussion safety to disrupt perceptions of unsafe norms. To date, athlete-focused educational efforts have tended to focus on the cognitions of the injured athlete themselves. However, there is a need for approaches to education that get team members talking about concussion safety, disrupting the spiral of silence and creating new norms related to concussion safety.

Even though university athletes are typically living away from home, parents can still play an important role in shaping attitudes about concussion reporting. Among male and female athletes competing in the NCAA, around 10% indicated that they had experienced pressure from a parent to continue playing their sport with concussion symptoms (Kroshus et al., 2015). It is possible that this pressure is not communicated directly by parents. Rather, athletes may make inferences about parental preferences based on parent investment in their sport (monetary and time). It is also possible that some parents do truly want their child to engage in this unsafe behavior, either because they themselves are not adequately informed about concussion consequences or because what they see as the potential rewards for sport success outweigh the potential risks. Among parents of youth athletes, the Health Belief Model (Rosenstock, 1974) has been used to understand parent communication with their child about concussion care-seeking behavior (Kroshus, Chrisman, & Rivara, 2017). Parents who viewed concussions as more of a threat were more likely to encourage care-seeking. However, perhaps most concerning is that those parents who most strongly valued their child's sport achievement were less likely to encourage care-seeking at any given level of perceived threat. To date, there have been no efforts to engage parents of university athletes in supporting concussion care seeking. Although athletes are no longer living at home, parents are an important influence on their behavior and a potentially important stakeholder group to engage in future educational initiatives by organizations governing university sport.

Coaches have the potential to play a critical role in the early identification and removal from play of athletes with concussion through both direct and indirect processes. In many university sports settings there is a medical professional (e.g., athletic trainer) on the sidelines of games and practices. However, even if this person is present, their attention may be directed elsewhere, and they may not be able to notice all potentially injurious instances of contact and collision. Coaches can function as an extra set of eyes and help notice when an athlete may be symptomatic and requiring of further evaluation. Perhaps most critically, coaches influence concussion identification indirectly by shaping their team's culture related to health and safety (Baugh et al., 2014; Kroshus et al., 2015; Kroshus et al., 2017). When athletes believe that their coach values concussion safety, they are more likely to speak up about their own injury or a teammate's injury (Kroshus et al., 2015; Kroshus et al., 2016). Coaches are themselves influenced in their communication with athletes by their own knowledge about concussion and expectancies about the consequences of encouraging care-seeking (Kroshus et al., 2015). Among wrestling coaches in the NCAA, there was more support for removing a hypothetical athlete with a suspected concussion from an early season match as compared to a championship match (Kroshus et al., 2017). This speaks to the influence of competitive pressures and the way in which these pressures interact with individual sport structures. For example, in the sport of wrestling no substitution is allowed in the middle of a match, meaning that removal from play of an injured athlete results in a forfeit of points. Comparatively, in a sport like ice hockey or football, athletes can be replaced with relatively limited competitive cost. While policies related to concussion identification and removal from play tend to be implemented at the governing body level (e.g., NCAA), there is also a need for sport-specific analysis of potential structural barriers to removing injured athletes from play that could be addressed through sport-level rule changes.

At a societal level, cultural narratives related to gender and athletic identities influence athlete reporting behaviors. The strength of an athlete's identification with the athlete role has been found to moderate the association between perceived athlete norms and reporting intentions (Kroshus et al., 2015). Individuals who see themselves more strongly as athletes are more likely to behave in ways that they think are normative for this role, which almost always means being less likely to report a concussion (Kroshus et al., 2015). At present, cultural narratives about what it means to be an athlete are often rooted in traditional masculinity, with toughness and playing through pain viewed as desirable and socialized within sports contexts from the outset of youth sport participation (Anderson, 2009; Howe, 2004; Stafford, Alexander, & Fry, 2013). Among both male and female university athletes, those who conform more strongly to traditionally masculine norms are less likely to report a suspected concussion (Kroshus et al., 2017). While this association was similarly observed in both male and female athletes, there was a mean difference between males and females in their conformity to these norms, explaining differences in reporting behavior (Kroshus et al., 2017). Kuhn and colleagues (2017) similarly found that male athletes, and in particular football players, were less likely to report a suspected concussion than female athletes. Thus, particular attention may need to be paid to the cultural messages being shared to young boys about masculinity and sport participation, with additional scrutiny of certain sports contexts where emphasis of traditional masculinity may be heightened. However, all athletes, including female athletes, are consuming messages about what it means to be a tough athlete, so there is a need for a broader conversation about what it means to be an athlete and how concussion safety can coexist with contemporary conceptualizations of the sport ethos.

Post-injury: Medically-indicated return to play

As with the immediate post-injury period, full recovery before return to play is critical to minimize the prolonged nature of symptoms and to ensure the brain isn't additionally vulnerable to a subsequent injury (Harmon et al., 2013). Additionally, even if an individual has fully recovered from the acute concussive injury, there is another important decision about return to play, particularly among athletes who have sustained multiple concussions: Whether they cease participation in their sport altogether. This decision is important in light of a growing body of evidence that athletes who have sustained multiple concussions are at elevated risk of long-term neurologic and behavioral consequences (Manley et al., 2017; McAllister & McCrea, 2017).

Different university sport governing bodies have different guidelines about returning to play after recovery from the concussive acute injury. The NCAA provides detailed information about best practices during the return-to-play process, including the utilization of a stepwise protocol where activity is gradually introduced over a series of days (National Collegiate Athletic Association, 2017). The NAIA and NJCAA similarly recommend a graded progression with oversight by a healthcare provider trained in concussion management (National Junior College Athletic Association 2017; National Athletic Intercollegiate Association, 2018). Guidance about the return-to-play process is not provided by Canadian university sport governing bodies. No university sport governing bodies provide guidance about sport cessation after full recovery from multiple concussions. This is understandable because presently there is no medical consensus about when this should occur (Broglio et al., 2014; Harmon et al., 2013; McCrory et al., 2017), and numerous clinical risk modifiers need to be considered in the decision (e.g., injury magnitude, interval between injuries, age, premorbid health conditions).

Although one would hope that a policy related to athlete health and well-being would be followed be all sport stakeholders, some coaches try to rush the process. More than half of sports medicine personnel working in NCAA sport have experienced pressure from a coach to prematurely clear an athlete to return them to play (Kroshus et al., 2015). This doesn't mean that the medical staff did in fact clear them prematurely, however sport stakeholders are not immune to social pressure when it comes to following concussion-related rules (Kroshus, Parsons, & Hainline, 2017). Institutional structure makes a difference in the experience of clinicians related to clearing an athlete to return to play post-concussion. Pressure experienced by clinicians was observed to be greater at universities where medical staff were under the umbrella of the athletic department, as compared to when they were under the umbrella of an external medical body (e.g., campus health services) (Kroshus et al., 2015). One interpretation of this finding is that coaches take more license in their communication with medical staff when they believe that they have more agency in the medical management of concussion (e.g., the medical staff could theoretically be hired or fired based on coach preferences). Another interpretation is that when medical personnel are in an administrative structure where their employment is under the control of athletic administrators, they may perceive coach communication about returning an athlete to play as carrying more weight or being more pressuring.

At the athlete level, there is some evidence of efforts by athletes to rush their return to play. For example, some athletes try to "sandbag" the initial preseason (baseline) neurocognitive test to allow for greater leeway in deficits during the season (Erdal, 2012; Schatz et al., 2017; Schatz et al., 2012; Schatz & Glatts, 2013). It is not evident the extent to which this impacts return to play decisions. To the extent there is scope for athlete subjectivity in the medical evaluation of concussion recovery (e.g., symptom self-report), similar expectancies as have been found to be important in the concussion reporting period (e.g., social and athletic contingencies) will likely also influence athlete behavior during the return-to-play period. It is possible that because the recovering athlete has some distance from the emotional and physiologically arousing field of play, they may be making decisions using a more deliberative and rational process (Schwarz, 2000). Thus, it is possible that they may be more likely to consider longer-term health consequences in their appraisal of the costs and benefits trying to rush back to play. However, as cognitively immature young adults, there is still a limit to their focus on long-term outcomes (Steinberg, 2008, 2010).

There has been little research to date about individual, interpersonal, and contextual determinants of decision-making related to sport retirement after multiple concussions. In the absence of definitive medical guidelines, this decision is preference-sensitive, meaning that individual goals, values, and preferences can reasonably influence the decision. The risk-return framework of behavioral decision theory (Weber, Blais, & Betz, 2002) has been used in recent research related to athletic trainer communication about sport cessation post-concussion (Kroshus, Baugh, & Viswanath, 2018). Consistent with this framework, perceptions about the riskiness of a given decision as well as the individual's willingness to accept that level of risk (risk attitude or risk tolerance) are important, with these risks are balanced against the perceived benefits of the decision and the individual's subjective willingness to accept benefits (Weber et al., 2002). Among clinicians, their own risk tolerance is an important determinant of when they would initiate a conversation about possible sport retirement, as are their perceptions about the athlete's potential for achievement on and off the field of play. A similar framework could be applied to the athlete's own conceptualization of the costs and benefits of sport cessation after multiple concussions, however more research is needed in this area. There is also a need for further research to understand how factors at different levels of the socioecological framework (e.g., institutional pressures, family pressures, scholarship status) influence communication and decision-making about possible sport cessation following multiple concussions.

Gaps, limitations, and future directions

A primary limitation of the present discussion about university sport is that most of the research published to date focuses on NCAA sport in the United States. Information related to concussion in university sport outside of North America is limited. For example, the governing body for Australian university sport has issued guidance about concussion management (UniSport, 2018), however similar guidance has not been provided by the governing body for British university sport (British Universities & College Sport, 2018). Even when present, the implementation of such policies has not been studied, nor have the individual or interpersonal determinants of concussion safety-related behavior been studied in university settings outside of North America. That most research in this area in the United States is not surprising given the large number of institutions that sponsor NCAA sports teams and the revenues available to fund research related to university sport in these settings (National Collegiate Athletic Association, 2018a). Critically, research focused solely on NCAA has found variability in institutional resources available for implementation of health and safety-related guidelines (Kroshus, 2016). This finding underscores the importance of understanding how different university sports contexts—with different resources and pressures—vary in their approach to concussion safety. On one hand, NCAA athletes may have more pressures on them as compared to other university athletes, and this could lead to greater pressure to play through injury or attempt to return to play in time for a big game. On the other hand, they may have access to more medical personnel and may have more medical oversight of their injury. When thinking about concussion safety behaviors within a social ecological model, where individual cognitions and decisions are nested in the contexts within which they live, learn, and play, it is critical to learn more about the range of contexts to which university athletes are exposed.

Another limitation of existing research related to psychological dimensions of concussion safety among university athletes is the largely single-level rather than multilevel nature of studies. Whereas this chapter has proposed that individual behaviors related to concussion-related outcomes need to be understood within a multilevel framework that views the individual as nested within broader interpersonal, institutional, and cultural contexts, extant research tends to focus on individual behaviors. Research is needed that models individuals as nested within teams and schools. Such information can provide critical guidance about the levels at which intervention may be most effective. Conducting such research requires large sample sizes, with multiple institutions. At present, much research among university athletes tends to be in single institutions or small groups of institutions. University sport governing bodies can help promote research of this nature, supporting or encouraging large-scale studies or the collection of common data elements across studies conducted at different institutions so as to be able to aggregate data for subsequent multilevel analyses. Even in the absence of multilevel studies, qualitative research would be useful to explore institutional factors that facilitate or constrain the ability and motivation of individual stakeholders to put concussion safety-related behaviors into practice.

References

Ajzen, I. (1991). The theory of planned behavior. *Organizational Behavior and Human Decision Processes, 50,* 179–211. doi: 10.1016/0749-5978(91)90020-T.

Anderson, E. (2009). The maintenance of masculinity among the stakeholders of sport. *Sport Management Review, 12,* 3–14.

Asken, B. M., McCrea, M. A., Clugston, J. R., Snyder, A. R., Houck, Z. M., & Bauer, R. M. (2016). "Playing through it": Delayed reporting and removal from athletic activity after concussion predicts prolonged recovery. *Journal of Athletic Training, 51,* 329–335. doi: 10.4085/1062-6050-51.5.02.

Bachynski, K. E. (2016). Tolerable risks? Physicians and youth tackle football. *The New England Journal of Medicine, 374,* 405–407. doi: 10.1056/NEJMp1513993.

Bandura, A. (2001). Social cognitive theory of mass communication. *Media Psychology, 3,* 265–299. doi: 10.1207/S1532785XMEP0303_03.

Baugh, C. M., Kroshus, E., Daneshvar, D. H., & Stern, R. A. (2014). Perceived coach support and concussion symptom-reporting: Differences between freshmen and non-freshmen college football players. *The Journal of Law, Medicine & Ethics, 42*(3), 314–322. doi: 10.1111/jlme.12148.

Benson, B. W., McIntosh, A. S., Maddocks, D., Herring, S. A., Raftery, M., & Dvorák, J. (2013). What are the most effective risk-reduction strategies in sport concussion? *British Journal of Sports Medicine, 47,* 321–326. doi: 10.1136/bjsports-2013-092216.

Bjørneboe, J., Bahr, R., Dvorak, J., & Andersen, T. E. (2013). Lower incidence of arm-to-head contact incidents with stricter interpretation of the Laws of the Game in Norwegian male professional football. *British Journal of Sports Medicine, 47*(8), 508–514. doi: 10.1136/bjsports-2012-091522.

Black, A. M., Macpherson, A. K., Hagel, B. E., Romiti, M. A., Palacios-Derflingher, L., Kang, J., ... Emery, C. A. (2016). Policy change eliminating body checking in non-elite ice hockey leads to a threefold reduction in injury and concussion risk in 11- and 12-year-old players. *British Journal of Sports Medicine, 50*(1), 55–61. doi: 10.1136/bjsports-2015-095103.

Black, A., Palacios-Derflingher, L., Schneider, K. J., Hagel, B. E., & Emery, C. A. (2017). The effect of a national body checking policy change on concussion risk in youth ice hockey players. *British Journal of Sports Medicine, 51*(11), A70–A71. doi: 10.1136/bjsports-2016-097270.183.

Borsari, B., & Carey, K. B. (2003). Descriptive and injunctive norms in college drinking: A meta-analytic integration. *Journal of Studies on Alcohol, 64*(3), 331–341.

British Universities and College Sports. (2018). *Rules and Regulations.* Retrieved June 2018 from: www.bucs.org.uk/athlete.asp?section=19287&sectionTitle=Rules+and+Regulations.

Broglio, S. P., Cantu, R. C., Gioia, G. A., Guskiewicz, K. M., Kutcher, J., Palm, M., & McLeod, T. C. V. (2014). National Athletic Trainers' Association position statement: Management of sport concussion. *Journal of Athletic Training*, *49*(2), 245–265.

Broglio, S. P., Williams, R. M., O'Connor, K. L., & Goldstick, J. (2016). Football players' head-impact exposure after limiting of full-contact practices. *Journal of Athletic Training*, *51*(7), 511–518. doi: 10.4085/1062-6050-51.7.04.

Bronfenbrenner, U. (1977). Toward an experimental ecology of human development. *American Psychologist*, *32*(7), 513–531. doi: 10.1037/0003-066X.32.7.513.

Brooks, M. A., Peterson, K., Biese, K., Sanfilippo, J., Heiderscheit, B. C., & Bell, D. R. (2016). Concussion increases odds of sustaining a lower extremity musculoskeletal injury after return to play among collegiate athletes. *The American Journal of Sports Medicine*, *44*(3), 742–747. doi: 10.1177/0363546515622387.

Brownson, R. C., Fielding, J. E., & Maylahn, C. M. (2009). Evidence-based public health: A fundamental concept for public health practice. *Annual Review of Public Health*, *30*, 175–201. doi: 10.1146/annurev.pu.30.031709.100001.

Canadian Collegiate Athletic Association. (2018). *Index*. Retrieved from www.ccaa.ca/splash/index.

Cantu, R. C. (1998). Second-impact syndrome. *Clinics in Sports Medicine*, *17*(1), 37–44.

Center's for Disease Control and Prevention. (2019). *The Social-Ecological Model: A framework for prevention*. Retrieved from www.cdc.gov/violenceprevention/overview/social-ecologicalmodel.html.

Chrisman, S. P., Quitiquit, C., & Rivara, F. P. (2013). Qualitative study of barriers to concussive symptom reporting in high school athletics. *Journal of Adolescent Health*, *52*(3), 330–335.e3. doi: 10.1016/j.jadohealth.2012.10.271.

Cobb, B. R., Urban, J. E., Davenport, E. M., Rowson, S., Duma, S. M., Maldjian, J. A., ... Stitzel, J. D. (2013). Head impact exposure in youth football: Elementary school ages 9–12 years and the effect of practice structure. *Annals of Biomedical Engineering*, *41*(12), 2463–2473. doi: 10.1007/s10439-013-0867-6.

Cross, M., Kemp, S., Smith, A., Trewartha, G., & Stokes, K. (2016). Professional Rugby Union players have a 60% greater risk of time loss injury after concussion: A 2-season prospective study of clinical outcomes. *British Journal of Sports Medicine*, *50*(15), 926–931. doi: 10.1136/bjsports-2015-094982.

Dompier, T. P., Kerr, Z. Y., Marshall, S. W., Hainline, B., Snook, E. M., Hayden, R., & Simon, J. E. (2015). Incidence of concussion during practice and games in youth, high school, and collegiate American football players. *JAMA Pediatrics*, *169*(7), 659–665. doi: 10.1001/jamapediatrics.2015.0210.

Donaldson, L., Asbridge, M., & Cusimano, M. D. (2013). Bodychecking rules and concussion in elite hockey. *PLOS ONE*, *8*(7), e69122. doi: 10.1371/journal.pone.0069122.

Dorfman, L., Wallack, L., & Woodruff, K. (2005). More than a message: Framing public health advocacy to change corporate practices. *Health Education & Behavior*, *32*(3), 320–336. doi: 10.1177/1090198105275046.

Eckner, J. T., Kutcher, J. S., Broglio, S. P., & Richardson, J. K. (2014). Effect of sport-related concussion on clinically measured simple reaction time. *British Journal of Sports Medicine*, *48*(2), 112–118. doi: 10.1136/bjsports-2012-091579.

Emery, C. A., Black, A. M., Kolstad, A., Martinez, G., Nettel-Aguirre, A., Engebretsen, L., ... Schneider, K. (2017). What strategies can be used to effectively reduce the risk of concussion in sport? A systematic review. *British Journal of Sports Medicine*, *51*(12), 978–984. doi: 10.1136/bjsports-2016-097452.

Emery, C. A., Hagel, B., & Morrongiello, B. A. (2006). Injury prevention in child and adolescent sport: Whose responsibility is it? *Clinical Journal of Sport Medicine, 16*(6), 514–521. doi: 10.1097/01.jsm.0000251179.90840.58.

Emery, C. A., Kang, J., Shrier, I., Goulet, C., Hagel, B. E., Benson, B. W., … Meeuwisse, W. H. (2010). Risk of injury associated with body checking among youth ice hockey players. *JAMA, 303*(22), 2265–2272. doi: 10.1001/jama.2010.755.

Erdal, K. (2012). Neuropsychological testing for sports-related concussion: How athletes can sandbag their baseline testing without detection. *Archives of Clinical Neuropsychology, 27*(5), 473–479. doi: 10.1093/arclin/acs050.

Fedor, A., & Gunstad, J. (2015). Limited knowledge of concussion symptoms in college athletes. *Applied Neuropsychology: Adult, 22*(2), 108–113. doi: 10.1080/23279095.2013.860604.

Gordon, R. S. (1983). An operational classification of disease prevention. *Public Health Reports, 98*(2), 107–109.

Haddon, W. (1968). The changing approach to the epidemiology, prevention, and amelioration of trauma: The transition to approaches etiologically rather than descriptively based. *American Journal of Public Health and the Nation's Health, 58*(8), 1431–1438.

Harmon, K. G., Drezner, J. A., Gammons, M., Guskiewicz, K. M., Halstead, M., Herring, S. A., … Roberts, W. O. (2013). American Medical Society for Sports Medicine position statement: Concussion in sport. *British Journal of Sports Medicine, 47*(1), 15–26. doi: 10.1136/bjsports-2012-091941.

Hartmann, T. (2009). *Media Choice: A Theoretical and Empirical Overview.* Hoboken, NJ: Taylor & Francis. Retrieved from https://trove.nla.gov.au/work/25122874.

Harvey, H. H., Koller, D. L., & Lowrey, K. M. (2015). The four stages of youth sports TBI policymaking: Engagement, enactment, research, and reform. *The Journal of Law, Medicine & Ethics, 43*, 87–90. doi: 10.1111/jlme.12225.

Howe, P. D. (2004). *Sport, professionalism, and pain: Ethnographies of injury and risk.* London: Routledge.

International University Sports Federation. (2018). *FISU today.* Retrieved from www.fisu.net/about-fisu/today.

Kaut, K. P., DePompei, R., Kerr, J., & Congeni, J. (2003). Reports of head injury and symptom knowledge among college athletes: Implications for assessment and educational intervention. *Clinical Journal of Sport Medicine, 13*(4), 213–221. doi: 10.1097/00042752-200307000-00004.

Kerr, Z. Y., Register-Mihalik, J. K., Marshall, S. W., Evenson, K. R., Mihalik, J. P., & Guskiewicz, K. M. (2014). Disclosure and non-disclosure of concussion and concussion symptoms in athletes: Review and application of the socio-ecological framework. *Brain Injury, 28*(8), 1009–1021. doi: 10.3109/02699052.2014.904049.

Kroshus, E. (2016). Variability in institutional screening practices related to collegiate student-athlete mental health. *Journal of Athletic Training, 51*(5), 389–397. doi: 10.4085/1062-6050-51.5.07.

Kroshus, E., Baugh, C. M., Daneshvar, D. H., Stamm, J. M., Laursen, R. M., & Austin, S. B. (2015). Pressure on sports medicine clinicians to prematurely return collegiate athletes to play after concussion. *Journal of Athletic Training, 50*(9), 944–951. doi: 10.4085/1062-6050-50.6.03.

Kroshus, E., Baugh, C. M., Daneshvar, D. H., & Viswanath, K. (2014). Understanding concussion reporting using a model based on the theory of planned behavior. *Journal of Adolescent Health*, 54(3), 269–274. doi: 10.1016/j.jadohealth.2013.11.011.

Kroshus, E., Baugh, C. M., Hawrilenko, M. J., & Daneshvar, D. H. (2015). Determinants of coach communication about concussion safety in US collegiate sport. *Annals of Behavioral Medicine*, 49(4), 532–541. doi: 10.1007/s12160-014-9683-y.

Kroshus, E., Baugh, C. M., Stein, C. J., Austin, S. B., & Calzo, J. P. (2017). Concussion reporting, sex, and conformity to traditional gender norms in young adults. *Journal of Adolescence*, 54, 110–119. doi: 10.1016/j.adolescence.2016.11.002.

Kroshus, E., Baugh, C. M., & Viswanath, K. V. (2018). Psychosocial subjectivity by sports medicine clinicians in post-concussion recommendations. *Annals of Behavioral Medicine*, 52, S275–S275.

Kroshus, E., Chrisman, S. P. D., & Rivara, F. P. (2017). Parent beliefs about chronic traumatic encephalopathy: Implications for ethical communication by healthcare providers. *The Journal of Law, Medicine & Ethics*, 45(3), 421–430. doi: 10.1177/1073110517737542.

Kroshus, E., Garnett, B., Hawrilenko, M., Baugh, C. M., & Calzo, J. P. (2015). Concussion under-reporting and pressure from coaches, teammates, fans, and parents. *Social Science & Medicine*, 134, 66–75. doi: 10.1016/j.socscimed.2015.04.011.

Kroshus, E., Garnett, B. R., Baugh, C. M., & Calzo, J. P. (2016). Engaging teammates in the promotion of concussion help seeking. *Health Education & Behavior*, 43(4), 442–451.

Kroshus, E., Kerr, Z. Y., DeFreese, J. D., & Parsons, J. T. (2017). Concussion knowledge and communication behaviors of collegiate wrestling coaches. *Health Communication*, 32(8), 963–969. doi: 10.1080/10410236.2016.1196417.

Kroshus, E., Kubzansky, L. D., Goldman, R. E., & Austin, S. B. (2015). Norms, athletic identity, and concussion symptom under-reporting among male collegiate ice hockey players: A prospective cohort study. *Annals of Behavioral Medicine*, 49(1), 95–103. doi: 10.1007/s12160-014-9636-5.

Kroshus, E., Parsons, J., & Hainline, B. (2017). Calling injury timeouts for the medical evaluation of concussion: Determinants of collegiate football officials' behavior. *Journal of Athletic Training*, 52, 1041–1047. doi: 10.4085/1062-6050-52.11.XX.

Kroshus, E., Rivara, F. P., Whitlock, K. B., Herring, S. A., & Chrisman, S. P. D. (2017). Disparities in athletic trainer staffing in secondary school sport: Implications for concussion identification. *Clinical Journal of Sport Medicine*, 27(6), 542–547. doi: 10.1097/JSM.0000000000000409.

Kuhn, A. W., Zuckerman, S. L., Yengo-Kahn, A. M., Kerr, Z. Y., Totten, D. J., Rubel, K. E., … Solomon, G. S. (2017). Factors associated with playing through a sport-related concussion. *Neurosurgery*, 64, 211–216. doi: 10.1093/neuros/nyx294.

Llewellyn, T., Burdette, G. T., Joyner, A. B., & Buckley, T. A. (2014). Concussion reporting rates at the conclusion of an intercollegiate athletic career. *Clinical Journal of Sport Medicine*, 24(1), 76–79. doi: 10.1097/01.jsm.0000432853.77520.3d.

Lynall, R. C., Mauntel, T. C., Padua, D. A., & Mihalik, J. P. (2015). Acute lower extremity injury rates increase after concussion in college athletes. *Medicine and Science in Sports and Exercise*, 47(12), 2487–2492. doi: 10.1249/MSS.0000000000000716.

Manley, G., Gardner, A. J., Schneider, K. J., Guskiewicz, K. M., Bailes, J., Cantu, R. C., ... Iverson, G. L. (2017). A systematic review of potential long-term effects of sport-related concussion. *British Journal of Sports Medicine, 51*(12), 969–977. doi: 10.1136/bjsports-2017-097791.

McAllister, T., & McCrea, M. (2017). Long-term cognitive and neuropsychiatric consequences of repetitive concussion and head-impact exposure. *Journal of Athletic Training, 52*(3), 309–317. doi: 10.4085/1062-6050-52.1.14.

McCrory, P., Meeuwisse, W., Dvořák, J., Aubry, M., Bailes, J., Broglio, S., ... Vos, P. E. (2017). Consensus statement on concussion in sport—The 5th international conference on concussion in sport held in Berlin, October 2016. *British Journal of Sports Medicine, 51*(11), 838–847. doi: 10.1136/bjsports-2017-097699.

Miyashita, T. L., Timpson, W. M., Frye, M. A., & Gloeckner, G. W. (2013). The impact of an educational intervention on college athletes' knowledge of concussions. *Clinical Journal of Sport Medicine, 23*(5), 349–353. doi: 10.1097/JSM.0b013e318289c321.

National Association of Intercollegiate Athletics. (2018). *About the NAIA.* Retrieved from: www.naia.org/ViewArticle.dbml?ATCLID=205323019&DB_OEM_ID=27900.

National Collegiate Athletic Association. (2018a). *About the NCAA.* Retrieved from: www.ncaa.org/about.

National Collegiate Athletic Association. (2018b). *Student-Athlete Participation 1981–82–2016–17.* Retrieved from: www.ncaa.org/sites/default/files/2016-17NCAA-0472_ParticRatesReport-FINAL_20171120.pdf.

National Collegiate Athletic Association. (2017). *Concussion Safety Best Practices for Campuses.* Retrieved from: www.ncaa.org/sport-science-institute/concussion-safety-best-practices-campuses.

National Junior College Athletic Association. (2017) *Handbook & Casebook.* Retrieved from: https://d2o2figo6ddd0g.cloudfront.net/a/1/o4bxsuaw8aflcy/2017-18_NJCAA_Handbook_Jan_4_2018.pdf.

Noelle-Neumann, E. (1974). The spiral of silence: A theory of public opinion. *Journal of Communication, 24*(2), 43–51. doi: 10.1111/j.1460-2466.1974.tb00367.x.

Pfister, T., Pfister, K., Hagel, B., Ghali, W. A., & Ronksley, P. E. (2016). The incidence of concussion in youth sports: A systematic review and meta-analysis. *British Journal of Sports Medicine, 50*(5), 292–297. doi: 10.1136/bjsports-2015-094978.

Register-Mihalik, J., Baugh, C., Kroshus, E., Kerr, Z. Y., & Valovich McLeod, T. C. (2017). A multifactorial approach to sport-related concussion prevention and education: Application of the socioecological framework. *Journal of Athletic Training, 52*(3), 195–205. doi: 10.4085/1062-6050-51.12.02.

Rosenstock, I. M. (1974). Historical origins of the health belief model, historical origins of the health belief model. *Health Education Monographs, 2*(4), 328–335. doi: 10.1177/109019817400200403.

Rosenthal, J. A., Foraker, R. E., Collins, C. L., & Comstock, R. D. (2014). National high school athlete concussion rates from 2005–2006 to 2011–2012. *The American Journal of Sports Medicine, 42*(7), 1710–1715. doi: 10.1177/0363546514530091.

Ruestow, P. S., Duke, T. J., Finley, B. L., & Pierce, J. S. (2015). Effects of the NFL's amendments to the free kick rule on injuries during the 2010 and 2011 seasons. *Journal of Occupational and Environmental Hygiene, 12*(12), 875–882. https://doi.org/10.1080/15459624.2015.1072632.

Schatz, P., Elbin, R. J., Anderson, M. N., Savage, J., & Covassin, T. (2017). Exploring sandbagging behaviors, effort, and perceived utility of the ImPACT Baseline

Assessment in college athletes. *Sport, Exercise, and Performance Psychology, 6*(3), 243–251. doi: 10.1037/spy0000100.

Schatz, P., & Glatts, C. (2013). "Sandbagging" baseline test performance on ImPACT, without detection, is more difficult than it appears. *Archives of Clinical Neuropsychology, 28*(3), 236–244. doi: 10.1093/arclin/act009.

Schatz, P., Moser, R. S., Solomon, G. S., Ott, S. D., & Karpf, R. (2012). Prevalence of invalid computerized baseline neurocognitive test results in high school and collegiate athletes. *Journal of Athletic Training, 47*(3), 289–296.

Schwarz, N. (2000). Emotion, cognition, and decision making. *Cognition and Emotion, 14*(4), 433–440. doi: 10.1080/026999300402745.

Stafford, A., Alexander, K., & Fry, D. (2013). Playing through pain: Children and young people's experiences of physical aggression and violence in sport. *Child Abuse Review, 22*(4), 287–299. doi: 10.1002/car.2289.

Steinberg, L. (2008). A social neuroscience perspective on adolescent risk-taking. *Developmental Review, 28*(1), 78–106.

Steinberg, L. (2010). A dual systems model of adolescent risk-taking. *Developmental Psychobiology, 52*(3), 216–224.

Torres, D. M., Galetta, K. M., Phillips, H. W., Dziemianowicz, E. M. S., Wilson, J. A., Dorman, E. S., ... Balcer, L. J. (2013). Sports-related concussion: Anonymous survey of a collegiate cohort. *Neurology. Clinical Practice, 3*(4), 279–287. doi: 10.1212/CPJ.0b013e3182a1ba22.

UniSport. (2018). *UniSport Australia Guideline Concussion 2018.* Retrieved from https://docs.wixstatic.com/ugd/8e3023_750c978b3e35433dbe257e7f89344 a9b.pdf.

U Sports. (2018). *History.* Retrieved from https://usports.ca/en/about/history.

Weber, E. U., Blais, A.-R., & Betz, N. E. (2002). A domain-specific risk-attitude scale: Measuring risk perceptions and risk behaviors. *Journal of Behavioral Decision Making, 15*(4), 263–290.

Wiebe, D. J., D'alonzo, B. A., Harris, R., Putukian, M., & Campbell-McGovern, C. (2018). Association between the experimental kickoff rule and concussion rates in Ivy League football. *Jama, 320*(19), 2035–2036.

Zuckerman, S. L., Kerr, Z. Y., Yengo-Kahn, A., Wasserman, E., Covassin, T., & Solomon, G. S. (2015). Epidemiology of sports-related concussion in NCAA athletes from 2009–2010 to 2013–2014: Incidence, recurrence, and mechanisms. *American Journal of Sports Medicine, 43*(11), 2654–2662. doi: 10.1177/0363546515599634.

12 Concussions in professional sports

J. Scott Delaney, Michael Orenstein,
and Rebecca Steins

Introduction

A professional athlete who suffers a concussion garners a great deal of media attention, which can prompt discussion and debate about concussive injury and management. This can be very beneficial, as it often involves reviewing the signs, symptoms, and dangers of a concussion. Treatment algorithms are often discussed, and the possibility of prolonged healing has also been highlighted in several high-profile cases. Many researchers believe the increase in diagnoses of concussion over the past few decades have been due in large part from a greater public awareness of concussions stemming from media coverage of professional athletes who have suffered concussions (Hainline & Ellenbogen, 2017; Wennberg & Tator, 2008). Unfortunately, the public has also witnessed professional athletes returning to sport too soon after injury. Cases of athletes returning to competition after a traumatically induced loss of consciousness or before a thorough concussion evaluation has taken place can serve to confuse and misinform the media and viewing audience (Delaney et al., 2000; McLellan & McKinlay, 2011). This chapter will examine the media coverage of concussions in professional sports as well as the concussion rates amongst different professional sports (including the "big four" North American sports), the different protocols and league policies governing concussion diagnosis and management, the reality of concussion underreporting in professional athletes, and the unique aspects of managing professional athletes with concussions.

Rates of concussion in professional sports

Concussions have seemingly been on the rise in professional sports, a fact which is likely in large part due to increased awareness of the signs and symptoms of the injury (Gouttebarge et al., 2017). Despite research on the diagnosis and incidence of concussions increasing in the past several years, it is still difficult to provide an accurate global estimate of concussion incidence and prevalence (Hainline & Ellenbogen, 2017; Putukian, Aubry, & McCrory, 2009). This may be attributable to the fact that concussion rates in many sports and recreational activities have not been studied, and that the concussion rates in different sports which have been examined are often expressed in different numerical formats. These formats may include concussion injuries as a percentage of total injuries, a percentage of all athletes who have suffered a concussion, concussions per 1,000 player match hours, or the number of concussions per 1,000 athlete exposures.

Despite the inherent challenges in providing global accounts of concussions in professional sports, researchers have been able to estimate concussion rates for different professional sports in specific countries. Concussion incidence in English professional rugby has been reported as 13.4 concussions per 1,000 player hours (England Professional Rugby Injury Surveillance Project Steering Group, 2016), 0.03–0.07 concussions per 1,000 player hours for men's European professional soccer (Waldén et al., 2013), and 17.6 per 1,000 player hours for Australian Rules Football (Gibbs & Watford, 2017). These statistics provide a glimpse into the rates of concussions in professional sports worldwide.

When interpreting concussion rates, it is important to understand that much of this data is collected prospectively and is usually dependent on an athlete volunteering his or her symptoms to medical staff. There is no loss of consciousness nor obvious external signs in the vast majority of sport related concussions (McCrory et al., 2013; McCrory et al., 2017). Many of the initial signs indicative of a concussion exhibited by an athlete may be transient and not observed by medical personnel. As such, medical staff often rely on athletes coming forward to volunteer their symptoms in order to make the diagnosis of a concussion. Athletes may not come forward to be assessed by medical staff if they do not understand they may have suffered a concussion. Furthermore, they may deliberately choose not to reveal their symptoms despite understanding the possibility that they may have sustained a concussion (Caron et al., 2013; Delaney et al., 2002; McCrea et al., 2004). Because of these reasons and others, some researchers have estimated that the vast majority of sport related concussions go unreported and undiagnosed (Ragnarsson et al., 1999).

North American "big four" professional sports

The "big four" professional sports organizations in North America are the National Football League (NFL), National Hockey League (NHL), Major League Baseball (MLB), and National Basketball Association (NBA). These four leagues receive the highest media attention, have the most extensive fan bases, and garner greater economic profits than other professional sports leagues in North America such as the Women's National Basketball Association, the Canadian Football League (CFL), and Major League Soccer (Brown, 2017; Makhni et al., 2014). Not surprisingly, most of the empirical research on professional sports in North America has focused on these four leagues. Makhini et al. (2014) conducted a review of the medical literature investigating the extent of injury reporting of the "big four" sport leagues in North America from 1975 to 2013. Of the publications evaluated, they found that the NFL and NHL had the highest percentages of articles related to concussions and/or neurology within the non-orthopedic and/or medical issues category, coming in at 30% (33 of 109) and 15% (6 of 41) respectively.

Researchers have noted that data on the rate of concussions in the NFL are difficult to obtain (Yengo-Kahn et al., 2016). One study found a rate of 0.61 concussions per game (Nathanson et al., 2016), however, issues such as under-reporting and league policy changes continue to plague epidemiological data on concussions in the NFL (Kerr et al., 2017; Yengo-Kahn et al., 2016). There is a need for more research in this area to better understand the true occurrence of concussions in the NFL.

With regards to the NHL, concussion incidence per regular season ranged from 1.04/1,000 athlete exposures to 1.81/1,000 athlete exposures over a 10-year period (Wennberg & Tator, 2008). Over the time period studied, there was an increase in the time lost per injury.

A study on NBA players found that from 2006 to 2014, an average of 14.9 concussions per season occurred in the approximately 450 players who play each year in the league (Padaki, Cole, & Ahmad, 2016). Although the incidence of NBA player concussions per season did not change significantly during that time period, similar to the NHL data on time lost from concussions, the average number of games missed following a concussion increased from 1.6 (2006 to 2010) to 5 games (2011 to 2014). This finding coincides with the start of the NBA's concussion protocol in 2011 (Padaki, Cole, & Ahmed, 2016).

Finally, the MLB has received the least empirical attention on the topic of concussions among the four major professional sports leagues in North America (Makhni et al., 2014). In reviewing data from 2 MLB seasons (30 teams playing 162 games each), Green and colleagues (2015) found that concussions represented approximately 1% of injuries, with an average of 9 days lost to injury. They found that MLB players incurred an estimated 0.26 concussions per 1,000 athlete exposures (game or practice played), with catchers experiencing the most concussions (Green et al., 2015). The statistics from the "big four" North American professional sports are further complicated by the differences in concussion policies and protocols in each league.

Policy surrounding concussions in professional sports

Despite a general consensus that return to play guidelines should be the same for all concussed athletes regardless of the level of competition, there is a tendency for high-performance athletes to return to play faster due in part to better access to specialized medical care, neuropsychological evaluation, and multidisciplinary resources compared to their non-elite counterparts (Putukian, Aubry, & McCrory, 2009). Cochrane et al. (2017) summarized the different concussion policies within the "big four" sports leagues in North America. Each league has a specified educational intervention that is typically implemented during preseason training. The NFL's concussion education consists of distributing printed materials to players and staff about the potential symptoms and signs of a concussion, and it emphasizes that athletes should disclose possible symptoms to trained medical personnel. Similarly, the NBA educates players and staff on the mechanisms of concussion, common symptoms, how to properly manage the injury, and possible long-term implications. The MLB has a specific preseason concussion education program, although the details of the program are not explicitly stated. Finally, the NHL has an informational video that all players, coaches, medical personnel, and club administrators must watch before being able to participate in preseason training camps. Additionally, players' family and friends are given a brochure to help them recognize a possible concussion (Cochrane et al., 2017).

It can be difficult for a medical staff to closely observe all athletes on the field of play. This is especially true in a professional environment where the sidelines are often filled with media, team officials, advertisements, and stadium or event staff, all of which can obstruct the view of the medical staff. In team sports, there may be many athletes involved in the competition, a large field may be involved, and athletes may be many meters away from the medical staff. To help provide another set of eyes and very often utilize television feed and coverage of the event, several professional leagues now employ "spotters," who are responsible for observing competitions for any visible signs of concussion or any concussion-like behavior among the participants (Seravalli, 2015; Wagner-McGough, 2015). Visible signs after contact may include loss of consciousness, motor incoordination, blank facial expression, difficulty or slowness to stand, or rubbing the head or helmet (Bruce et al., 2017; Echemendia et al., 2017a; Echemendia et al., 2017b). The spotters watch the television feed or from the stands for visible signs or behaviors related to a concussion and can notify the medical staff of the affected athlete. The medical staff can then observe and/or remove the athlete for further evaluation. Expedient sideline access to video of the injury is becoming more common where available and can allow the sport medicine team to visualize and review the mechanism of injury and the athlete's subsequent signs and behaviors (McCrory et al., 2017).

One tactic employed by the NFL and the NHL in diagnosing concussion at the point of injury is the use of a "quiet room," which is an off-field space where an initial concussion evaluation is performed on athletes. In the NHL, athletes are removed from the bench and examined in a separate room by a team physician (e.g., the team's dressing room or in-arena medical room). The NFL has designated tents on the sidelines where medical professionals can initially evaluate an athlete's injury with some degree of privacy. If the preliminary evaluation indicates a possible concussion, further testing is conducted, usually inside the locker room, and a management plan is put in place upon the formal medical diagnosis of a concussion (Dixon, 2011; NFL.com, 2017). Although no empirical-based evidence currently exists for the effectiveness of these protocols, the league-mandated procedures are still an indication of the growing concern for the proper diagnosis and management of concussions in high-contact professional sports.

All four leagues have graduated return to play strategies, with the NFL, NHL, and NBA not allowing athletes to return to play on the same day of a suspected concussion. The MLB is the only organization of the "big four" that requires minimum time off (seven days) before returning to play (Cochrane et al., 2017). The Sport Concussion Assessment Tool 5 (SCAT-5), developed by the Concussion in Sport Group (CISG), accounts for mood-related symptoms such as "More emotional, Irritability, Sadness, Nervous, or Anxious" (Echemendia et al., 2017b). Given the profound types of psychological symptoms an athlete can experience following a concussion (e.g., depression and anxiety), it is important that athletes are evaluated for psychological symptoms as part of making return to play decisions (McCrory et al., 2017).

Media coverage of concussions in professional sports

While league-mandated policies and procedures on concussions in professional sports largely dictate the timeline for an athlete's return from a concussion, the media plays an important role in narrating athletes' return to sport. Traditionally, media outlets have generated heroic narratives of an athlete's commitment to winning by praising the athlete who triumphs despite injury or illness (McGannon, Cunningham, & Schinke, 2013). Such narratives may help perpetuate a "culture of risk," wherein playing through pain or illness reflects desired athlete qualities such as commitment and durability. Athletes who prioritized their health over continuing to play with an injury have risked embarrassment and having their fortitude publicly questioned (Anderson & Kian, 2012; Donnelly, 2004).

Fortunately, this narrative has started to change. In analyzing the media coverage surrounding NHL superstar player Sydney Crosby's 2011 concussion, researchers found a central theme concerning "the culture of risk and its impact on athletes" (McGannon et al., 2013). The story of this high-profile athlete's concussion, which sidelined him for ten months, was used as a cautionary tale and a platform to stimulate concussion management reform (McGannon et al., 2013). Anderson and Kian (2012) further studied the media's attitudes towards concussions and addressed the evolving themes surrounding concussions. Their study focused on analyzing media reports surrounding NFL star quarterback Aaron Rodgers' decision to remove himself from a game following a hit to his head. They found that the media praised Rodgers and his teammate, Donald Driver, who encouraged Rodgers that his health was more important than "just a game." Despite these case studies of media narratives of high-profile professional athletes, much of the media coverage of concussions focuses solely on the physical signs and symptoms and less attention is afforded to the psychological issues associated with concussions (Bloom et al., 2004; Caron et al., 2013; McGannon et al., 2013).

Chronic traumatic encephalopathy in the media

Chronic traumatic encephalopathy (CTE) was first reported in the 1920s and was known as "punch drunk" (Martland, 1928) or "dementia pugilistica" (Millspaugh, 1937). The first contemporary study was led by Dr. Bennett Omalu in the early 2000s. He published a single-participant case study of a retired NFL player whose brain showed distinct areas of amyloid plaques, neurofibrillary tangles, and tau-positive threads on autopsy, which he determined was CTE (Omalu et al., 2005). Prior to his death, the player had dealt with issues of cognitive impairment, mood disorder, and parkinsonian symptoms (Omalu et al., 2005). The 2015 movie "Concussion," which portrayed Dr. Omalu's discovery of CTE in the deceased former NFL athlete, has fueled conversations about the short- and long-term health implications involved in sport participation.

As of 2013, there was a mixed cohort of 110 former professional athletes who had been diagnosed with CTE (Solomon & Zuckerman 2015). The majority of these came from football (57 cases) and boxing (48 cases), with the remaining coming from professional wrestlers and one soccer player (McKee et al., 2009; McKee et al., 2013). A more recent 2017 review from the same group of researchers found that the number of diagnosed CTE cases amongst former professional football players had increased up to 117 cases (Mez et al., 2017). It should be noted that the findings from the aforementioned papers are from case studies or pathological case series and thus do not allow definite causality to be determined as to whether concussions and subconcussive hits are a proven risk factor for CTE (e.g., Asken et al., 2016; Manley et al., 2017; McCrory et al., 2013). There have yet to be any epidemiological, prospective, or cross-sectional studies evaluating concussions as a risk factor for CTE. In the most recent CISG consensus statement, the group stated that "a cause-and-effect relationship has not yet been demonstrated between CTE and Sport Related Concussions or exposure to contact sports. As such, the notion that repeated concussion or subconcussive impacts cause CTE remains unknown" (McCrory et al., 2017). More research is needed to determine causation between concussive and subconcussive impacts and CTE (Hainline & Ellenbogen, 2017). Despite this, the media's representation of CTE research often is presented as having proven a direct relationship between CTE and contact sports, which has left many questioning the safety of sport participation at all age levels (Carson, 2017).

Underreporting of concussions among professional athletes

A common problem in diagnosing and treating concussions in athletes of all levels, including professional athletes, is the underreporting and nondisclosure of concussion symptoms to the appropriate medical personnel (Kerr et al., 2017). When an athlete does not report concussion symptoms, they are placing themselves at risk for exacerbating the present concussions or suffering another concussion, which has potentially devastating short- and long-term repercussions (De Beaumont et al., 2009; Guskiewicz et al., 2005; McCrory, 2001). The recent media attention and emerging research on the risks of concussions and continuing to play while symptomatic has led to an increase in interest on athlete education regarding the symptoms and risks of concussion, as well as the importance of disclosing symptoms. Despite the increased focus on education, underreporting still remains a prevalent issue, and it is critical to understand the reasons athletes choose (or choose not) to disclose their symptoms (Delaney et al., 2018).

Underreporting and the lack of education or understanding of concussions emerged as a growing issue in the early 2000s. One study reported that despite almost half of professional football players in the CFL experiencing concussion symptoms in the 1997 season, only 19% of these athletes recognized they had likely suffered a concussion (Delaney et al., 2000). Further, almost 70% of athletes who were believed to have suffered a concussion reported experiencing more than one episode of concussion-related symptoms during the same season (Delaney et al., 2000). This study was one of the first to acknowledge a potential gap in concussion education or understanding in professional sports, as well as the potential risks of suffering subsequent concussions. A similar lack of knowledge was found in a study conducted with university football and soccer athletes (Delaney et al., 2002). Despite participating in sports with a high risk for suffering a concussion, only 23% of football players and 20% of soccer players recognized they were experiencing concussion symptoms (Delaney et al., 2002). Attempting to identify the misconceptions that athletes held about concussions, one study found that four of the most common misconceptions identified were (1) there was no increased likelihood of repeat concussion after a player had sustained one, (2) brain imaging could detect concussions, (3) a concussion involves a direct hit to the head, and (4) there are no long-term health risks from multiple concussions (Williams et al., 2016). The study from Williams et al. (2016), in conjunction with research from Delaney et al. (2000, 2002), suggests that athletes across different sports and levels of participation lacked knowledge on concussion symptoms, the risks of playing while symptomatic, and the importance of reporting their symptoms to the proper medical personnel.

Another study on Canadian University athletes suggested that the main reason that athletes did not seek medical attention for possible symptoms of a concussion was that athletes did not feel their injury was serious enough and that they could continue playing without being a risk to themselves (Delaney et al., 2015). While this indicates that athletes may not fully understand the real dangers of continuing to play with a concussion, researchers have found that most high school and university athletes report adequate symptom and factual knowledge of concussions (Chrisman, Quitiquit, & Rivara, 2013; Conway et al., 2018). These findings suggest that even if athletes affirm that they understand the symptoms and risks, that does not necessarily mean they will disclose their symptoms to medical staff (Conway et al., 2018). While these important themes in underreporting of concussion emerged within university populations and provided crucial information on the need for better concussion education for athletes, research regarding underreporting in professional sport has been lacking.

Being a professional athlete comes with additional stressors that may impact an athlete's choice to not disclose their concussion symptoms. Professional athletes may feel pressure from coaches, teammates, or fans to uphold an athletic identify of being "tough" and may fear that reporting a concussion and being pulled from a practice or game may negatively impact their self-identity and the perceptions of those around them (Caron et al., 2013). Former professional hockey players who retired due to post-concussion symptoms revealed that they routinely hid their symptoms from teammates, coaches, and medical professionals to continue playing (Caron et al., 2013). Many were only removed from competition by their coaches and medical professionals when they were no longer able to hide their concussion symptoms (Caron et al., 2013). Among university athletes, identity and perceived norms about concussion reporting were suggested to influence an athletes' intention to disclose concussion symptoms (Kroshus, Kubanzansky, Goldman, & A et al.ustin, 2014). Previous research on university athletes has indicated that pressure from multiple external sources led athletes to report lower intentions to report concussion symptoms (Kroshus et al., 2015). Professional athletes may feel more pressure than athletes at other levels due to increased media attention, the financial ramifications of missing playing time, being labeled as a concussion-prone player, and potentially the fear of being forced into retirement due to a concussion (Caron et al., 2013). Many professional athletes sacrifice (or put on hold) their education to pursue a career in professional sport, which makes the implications of potentially losing their position on a team that much more complex.

A recent study by Delaney et al. (2018) found that although almost 30% of professional football players in Canada reported they felt they had suffered a concussion in the previous season, almost 80% of these athletes did not disclose their symptoms to the appropriate medical staff. Results also suggested that while the athletes were quite familiar with the league's protocol for concussion evaluation (removal from game, possibility of missing future games or practices) and showed improved knowledge on concussions as compared to previous research (Delaney et al., 2000), many of the players still chose to continue playing despite the known inherent risks. Similar to the research on university athletes, most CFL athletes who felt that they had suffered a concussion during the previous season indicated that they did not disclose their symptoms because they did not feel the concussion was serious enough and felt they could still continue to play with little danger to themselves. Another important reason for nondisclosure was the timing of when they suffered the injury. Approximately 20% athletes who hid their symptoms said they would normally have sought out medical attention, but they suffered the injury during an important time in the season (Delaney et al., 2018). It can be inferred that these professional athletes understood at least some of the risks of playing with a concussion, and it underscores the fact that increased knowledge does not necessarily translate to a change in reporting behavior. Interestingly, although the study examined professional athletes who receive a salary for playing professional football, the fear that being diagnosed with a concussion could affect their financial income now or in the future was listed as one of the more uncommon reasons for "hiding" a concussion. In fact, the percentage of professional football players and the reasons they did not report their self-diagnosed concussion is very similar to male and female university athletes studied across several different sports (Delaney et al., 2015). As such, lessons learned from professional athletes may be applicable to athletes across all levels of sports, as would research on how both concussion education and knowledge translation to professional athletes can be enhanced in order to improve overall player health and safety (Delaney et al., 2018).

Clinical issues of working in professional sports

For a healthcare provider, the majority of the clinical work and disposition decisions are similar when dealing with most recreational or high-level athletes. Sport medicine physicians and therapists who work for a professional team are often faced with a different dynamic. They have been hired by the team to care for the athletes and provide the team with a competitive advantage whenever possible. There is a flow of information about different medical conditions, including concussions, which occurs with the athletes, but also with the coaches and management as well. This can start during the preseason when past and ongoing injuries or medical conditions are discovered or discussed during the preseason pre-participation physicals performed by the medical staff. This information is released and discussed with the team and often the league with the athlete's consent, as most teams have athletes sign a release form at the end of the pre-participation physical. This release form allows the team medical staff to release this information to certain third parties, which usually includes team management, coaches, and the league. Such consent for release of information pertains only to the information included in the pre-participation sheets.

It is obvious that healthcare professionals must respect the confidentiality of all medical information and cannot divulge any information to media or others with a vested interest or curiosity in an athlete's state of health. During the year, however, the team medical staff may face moral dilemmas after a player has suffered an injury, such as a possible concussion, if that athlete does not want information released to the team. This is especially true for concussions that are diagnosed hours or days after an injury. The coaches and team management want to know the full extent of all injuries, so they may prepare for upcoming competitions or possibly use such information for contract and trade reasons. During these situations, the healthcare provider must realize that his or her ultimate responsibility is to the individual athlete. As with any patient, the team medical staff must realize that, ethically and medicolegally, if the player does not want this information released to outside parties, they must respect the patient's confidentiality. The only reason the medical staff can release or discuss preseason information with the team or other officials in the league is because the athlete has signed a release form allowing the physician to discuss the specific information contained in the pre-participation physical file.

When dealing with concussions (or any injury in general), most professional athletes want to return to competition as soon as possible. This may be problematic if an athlete does not want the medical staff to disclose such information to the team management or coaching staff. In reality, most athletes can be made to understand the need for proper healing, which involves stepping away from competition until full recovery has occurred. Explaining that many experts believe that the threshold for a subsequent concussion and brain injury is lower when they are still not fully recovered from a concussion is the first step (McCrory, 2001). The second step involves making the athlete understand that a lower concussion threshold means that they can suffer another concussion with much less force as compared to the force that caused the present concussion. Third, the athlete needs to understand that in general, the second concussion takes longer to recover than the first concussion, and the third concussion takes longer to recover than the second concussion, etc. (Delaney, Al-Kashmiri, & Correa, 2014). Finally, the athlete is made to understand that in fact, the way to play or compete as soon as possible and avoid more lost time to concussion is to ensure full healing from the present concussion and not risk a second injury that would likely result in a longer recovery period. Athletes who have these facts explained to them often understand the logic of making a formal diagnosis of concussion and ensuring full recovery from concussion by entering and following league-mandated concussion protocols.

Making the diagnosis of a concussion can be difficult under the best of circumstances. In a professional environment with teammates, coaches, fans, and media all observing and scrutinizing the medical team's behavior, it can create a stressful and sometimes intimidating situation. Many team sports such as American football and ice hockey allow for an easy in-game substitution during a concussion evaluation so the team is not penalized by playing with fewer players during the evaluation process. This allows for more time to relocate to the dressing room or another less distracting environment. In contrast, soccer rules allow the game to continue with one team a player short until the evaluation process is completed. Pressure to complete a rapid assessment can come from the athletes themselves, coaches, or other players. To help prepare for these stressful situations, the concussion evaluation process should be planned, practiced, timed, discussed, and approved in the preseason (or prior to competition) so that the staff, athletes, and coaches are aware of the protocols and the time required to complete the process. All of the sport medicine staff should adhere to the same procedures. Disposition decisions for concussed athletes should also be standardized and decided beforehand so that there is no confusion amongst the medical staff, athletes, or coaches when a diagnosis of a concussion is made. Some professional leagues now mandate the use of neutral physicians (often neurologists) and other healthcare professionals (i.e., neuropsychologists) when diagnosing and/or managing a concussion (Bradley, 2013; Christie, 2018; Ellenbogen et al., 2018). Concussions are unique in that this is the only injury which may require a "neutral" physician or other healthcare professional to be involved in the diagnosis and disposition decisions. The rationale is to provide the best care for athletes by having a qualified professional with no financial ties to the team assess and evaluate the athlete during the diagnosis and/or recovery process. As discussed previously, most professional leagues have protocols for concussion management—both for evaluation and disposition decisions. These protocols should be followed and documented to avoid any future conflicts or liability (Broglio et al., 2014).

Conclusions

Concussions in professional sports gather quite a bit of media attention and have served as a platform to help bring the science, management, and controversies of concussions to the public's attention. Despite this, robust research on the actual incidence of concussions in professional sports is wanting. While concussion education programs and formalized concussion protocols have increased in the past decade for most professional sports analyzed, research has shown that increased factual knowledge about concussions does not necessarily lead to safer behaviors and decisions by professional athletes. The media narrative of concussions in professional athletes has begun to change in recent years, with a focus more on the need to protect an athlete's health and well-being. With more media and fans calling on teams and leagues to better protect and manage concussed athletes, the hope is that this will help remove stigmas and barriers associated with athletes coming forward to be diagnosed and managed by team medical staff. Proper diagnosis and safe management of concussions in professional athletes will ideally set an example and standard of care that can serve as a model for all concussed athletes, regardless of their level of competition.

References

Anderson, E., & Kian, E. M. (2012). Examining media contestation of masculinity and head trauma in the National Football League. *Men and Masculinities, 15*, 152–173. doi: 10.1177/1097184X11430127.

Asken, B. M., Sullan, M. J., Snyder, A. R., Houck, Z. M., Bryant, V. E., Hizel, L. P., … Bauer, R. M. (2016). Factors influencing clinical correlates of chronic traumatic encephalopathy (CTE): A review. *Neuropsychology Review, 26*, 340–363. doi: 10.1007/s11065-016-9327-z.

Bloom, G. A., Horton, A. S., McCrory, P., & Johnston, K. M. (2004). Sport psychology and concussion: New impacts to explore. *British Journal of Sports Medicine, 38*, 519–521. doi: 10.1136/bjsm.2004.011999.

Bradley, B. (2013, September 3). *Independent concussion specialists ready to work NFL sidelines.* Retrieved from: www.nfl.com/news/story/0ap1000000237739/ article/independent-concussion-specialists-ready-to-work-nfl-sidelines.

Broglio, S. P., Cantu, R. C., Gioia, G. A., Guskiewicz, K. M., Kutcher, J., Palm, M., & Valovich McLeod, T. C. (2014). National Athletic Trainers' Association position statement: Management of sport concussion. *Journal of Athletic Training, 49*, 245–265. doi: 10.4085/1062-6050-49.1.07.

Brown, M. (2017, August 25). *Exclusive infographics show NFL, MLB, NBA, and NHL sponsorship growth over last decade.* Retrieved from: www.forbes.com/sites/ maurybrown/2017/08/25/exclusive-inforgraphics-show-nfl-mlb-nba-and-nhl-sponsorship-growth-over-last-decade/2/#6c4847437cf4.

Bruce, J. M., Echemendia, R. J., Meeuwisse, W., Hutchison, M. G., Aubry, M., & Comper, P. (2017). Development of a risk prediction model among professional hockey players with visible signs of concussion. *British Journal of Sport Medicine.* Advanced online publication. doi: 10.1136/bjsports-2016-097091.

Caron, J. G., Bloom, G. A., Johnston, K. M., & Sabiston, C. M. (2013). Effects of multiple concussions on retired national hockey league players. *Journal of Sport & Exercise Psychology, 35*, 168–179. doi: 10.1123/jsep.35.2.168.

Carson, A. (2017). Concussion, dementia and CTE: Are we getting it very wrong? *Journal of Neurology, Neurosurgery and Psychiatry, 88*, 462–464. doi: 10.1136/ jnnp-2016-315510.

Chrisman, S. P., Quitiquit, C., & Rivara, F. P. (2013). Qualitative study of barriers to concussive symptom reporting in high school athletics. *Journal of Adolescent Health, 52*, 330–335. doi: 10.1016/j.jadohealth.2012.10.271.

Christie, J. (2018, May 2). *NFL takes NHL's lead on concussions.* Retrieved from: www.theglobeandmail.com/sports/nfl-takes-nhls-lead-on-concussions/article4215606/.

Cochrane, G. D., Owen, M., Ackerson, J. D., Hale, M. H., & Gould, S. (2017). Exploration of US men's professional sport organization concussion policies. *The Physician and Sportsmedicine, 45*, 178–183. doi: 10.1080/00913847.2017.1305875.

Conway, F. N., Domingues, M., Monaco, R., Lesnewich, L. M., Ray, A. E., Alderman, B. L., ... Buckman, J. F. (2018). Concussion symptom underreporting among incoming National Collegiate Athletic Association Division I college athletes. *Clinical Journal of Sport Medicine.* Advance online publication. doi: 10.1097/JSM.0000000000000557.

De Beaumont, L., Theoret, H., Mongeon, D., Messier, J., Leclerc, S., Tremblay, S., ... Lassonde, M. (2009). Brain function decline in healthy retired athletes who sustained their last sports concussion in early adulthood. *Brain, 132*, 695–708. doi: 10.1093/brain/awn347.

Delaney, J. S., Al-Kashmiri, A., & Correa, J. A. (2014). Mechanisms of injury for concussions in university football, ice hockey, and soccer. *Clinical Journal of Sport Medicine, 24*, 233–237. doi: 10.1097/JSM.0000000000000017.

Delaney, J. S., Caron, J. G., Correa, J. A., & Bloom, G. A. (2018). Why professional football players chose not to reveal their concussion symptoms during a practice or game. *Clinical Journal of Sport Medicine 28*, 1–12. doi: 10.1097/jsm.0000000000000495.

Delaney, J. S., Lacroix, V. J., Leclerc, S., & Johnston, K. M. (2000). Concussions during the 1997 Canadian football league season. *Clinical Journal of Sport Medicine, 10*, 9–14.

Delaney, J. S., Lacroix, V. J., Leclerc, S., Johnston, K. M. (2002) Concussions among university football and soccer players. *Clinical Journal of Sport Medicine, 12*, 331–338.

Delaney, J. S., Lamfookon C., Bloom, G. A., Al-Kashmiri, A., & Correa, J. A. (2015). Why university athletes choose not to reveal their concussion symptoms during a practice or game. *Clinical Journal of Sport Medicine, 25*, 113–125. doi: 10.1097/JSM.0000000000000112.

Dixon, R. (2011, May 26). *Clarifying procedure in the NHL's concussion "quiet room."* Retrieved from: www.thehockeynews.com/news/article/clarifying-procedure-in-the-nhls-concussion-quiet-room.

Donnelly, P. (2004). Sport and risk culture. In K. Young (Ed.), *Sporting bodies, damaged selves: Sociological studies of sports-related injury,* (pp. 29–57). London: Elsevier.

Echemendia, R. J., Bruce, J. M., Meeuwisse, W., Hutchison, M. G., Comper, P., & Aubry, M. (2017a). Can visible signs predict concussion diagnosis in the National Hockey League? *British Journal of Sports Medicine.* Advanced online publication. doi: 10.1136/bjsports-2016-097090.

Echemendia, R. J., Meeuwisse, W., McCrory, P., Davis, G. A., Putukian, M., Leddy, J., ... Herring, S. (2017b). The Concussion Recognition Tool 5th Edition (CRT5): Background and rationale. *British Journal of Sport Medicine, 51*, 872–872. doi: 10.1136/bjsports-2017-097508.

Ellenbogen, R. G., Batjer, H., Cardenas, J., Berger, M., Bailes, J., Pieroth, E., ... Maroon, J. (2018). National Football League head, neck and spine committee's concussion diagnosis and management protocol: 2017–18 season.

British Journal of Sports Medicine. Advanced online publication. doi: 10.1136/ bjsports-2018-099203.

England Professional Rugby Injury Surveillance Project Steering Group. (2016). *England professional rugby injury surveillance project* (2015–2016 Season Report). Retrieved from: www.englandrugby.com/mm/Document/ General/General/01/32/25/17/1516_PRISP_Annual_Report_FINAL%28 withcontentspage%29_English.pdf.

Gibbs, N., & Watsford, M. (2017). Concussion incidence and recurrence in professional Australian football match-play: A 14-year analysis. *Journal of Sports Medicine*. Advance online publication. doi: 10.1155/2017/2831751.

Gouttebarge, V., Aoki, H., Lambert, M., Stewart, W., & Kerkhoffs, G. (2017). A history of concussions is associated with symptoms of common mental disorders in former male professional athletes across a range of sports. *The Physician and Sports Medicine, 45*, 443–449. doi: 10.1080/00913847.2017.1376572.

Green, G. A., Pollack, K. M., D'Angelo, J., Schickendantz, M. S., Caplinger, R., Weber, K., … Curriero, F. C. (2015). Mild traumatic brain injury in Major and Minor League Baseball players. *The American Journal of Sports Medicine, 43*, 1118–1126. doi: 10.1177/0363546514568089.

Guskiewicz, K. M., Marshall, S. W., Bailes, J., McCrea, M., Cantu, R. C., Randolph, C., & Jordan, B. D. (2005). Association between recurrent concussion and late-life cognitive impairment in retired professional football players. *Neurosurgery, 57*, 719–726. doi: 10.1093/neurosurgery/57.4.719.

Hainline, B., & Ellenbogen, R. G. (2017). A perfect storm. *Journal of Athletic Training, 52*, 157–159. doi: 10.4085/1062-6050-51.10.04.

Kerr, Z. Y., Register-Mihalik, J. K., Kay, M. C., Defreese, J., Marshall, S. W., & Guskiewicz, K. M. (2017). Concussion nondisclosure during professional career among a cohort of former National Football League athletes. *The American Journal of Sports Medicine, 46*, 22–29. doi: 10.1177/0363546517728264.

Kroshus, E., Garnett, B., Hawrilenko, M., Baugh, C. M., & Calzo, J. P. (2015). Concussion under-reporting and pressure from coaches, teammates, fans, and parents. *Social Science & Medicine, 134*, 66–75. doi: 10.1016/j. socscimed.2015.04.011.

Kroshus, E., Kubzansky, L. D., Goldman, R. E., & Austin, S. B. (2014). Norms, athletic identity, and concussion symptom under-reporting among male collegiate ice hockey players: a prospective cohort study. *Annals of Behavioral Medicine, 49*, 95–103. doi: 10.1007/s12160-014-9636-5.

Makhni, E. C., Buza, J. A., Byram, I., & Ahmad, C. S. (2014). Sports reporting: A comprehensive review of the medical literature regarding North American professional sports. *The Physician and Sports Medicine, 42*, 154–162. doi: 10.3810/ psm.2014.05.2067.

Manley, G. T., Gardner, A. J., Schneider, K. J., Guskiewicz, K. M., Bailes, J., Cantu, R. C., … Dvořák, J. (2017). A systematic review of potential long-term effects of sport-related concussion. *British Journal of Sports Medicine, 51*, 969–977. doi: 10.1136/bjsports-2017-097791.

Martland, H. S. (1928). Punch drunk. *Journal of the American Medical Association, 91*, 1103–1107.

McCrea, M., Hammeke, T., Olsen, G., Leo, P., & Guskiewicz, K. (2004). Unreported concussion in high school football players: Implications for prevention. *Clinical Journal of Sport Medicine, 14*, 13–17.

McCrory, P. (2001). Does second impact syndrome exist? *Clinical Journal of Sport Medicine*, *11*, 144–149.

McCrory, P., Meeuwisse, W. H., Aubry, M., Cantu, R. C., Dvořák, J., Echemendia, R. J., ... Turner, M. (2013). Consensus statement on concussion in sport: The 4th international conference on concussion in sport, Zurich, November 2012. *British Journal of Sports Medicine*, *47*, 250–258. doi: 10.1136/bjsports-2013-092313.

McCrory, P., Meeuwisse, W., Dvorak, J., Aubry, M., Bailes, J., Broglio, S., ... & Davis, G. A. (2017). Consensus statement on concussion in sport—The 5th international conference on concussion in sport held in Berlin, October 2016. *British Journal of Sports Medicine*, *51*, 838–847. doi: 10.1136/bjsports-2017-097699.

McCrory, P., Meeuwisse, W. H., Kutcher, J. S., Jordan, B. D., & Gardner, A. (2013). What is the evidence for chronic concussion-related changes in retired athletes: Behavioural, pathological and clinical outcomes? *British Journal of Sports Medicine*, *47*, 327–330. doi: 10.1136/bjsports-2013-092248.

McGannon, K. R., Cunningham, S. M., & Schinke, R. J. (2013). Understanding concussion in socio-cultural context: A media analysis of a National Hockey League star's concussion. *Psychology of Sport and Exercise*, *14*, 891–899. doi: 10.1016/j.psychsport.2013.08.003.

McKee, A. C., Cantu, R. C., Nowinski, C. J., Hedley-Whyte, E. T., Gavett, B. E., Budson, A. E., ... Stern, R. A. (2009). Chronic traumatic encephalopathy in athletes: Progressive tauopathy after repetitive head injury. *Journal of Neuropathology & Experimental Neurology*, *68*, 709–735. doi: 10.1097/nen.0b013e3181a9d503.

McKee, A. C., Stein, T. D., Nowinski, C. J., Stern, R. A., Daneshvar, D. H., Alvarez, V. E., ... Riley, D. O. (2013). The spectrum of disease in chronic traumatic encephalopathy. *Brain*, *136*, 43–64. doi: 10.1093/brain/aws307.

McLellan, T. L., & McKinlay, A. (2011). Does the way concussion is portrayed affect public awareness of appropriate concussion management: The case of rugby league? *British Journal of Sports Medicine*, *45*, 993–996. doi: 10.1136/bjsm.2011.083618.

Mez, J., Daneshvar, D. H., Kiernan, P. T., Abdolmohammadi, B., Alvarez, V. E., Huber, B. R., ... McKee, A. C. (2017). Clinicopathological evaluation of chronic traumatic encephalopathy in players of American football. *Journal of the American Medical Association*, *318*, 360–370. doi: 10.1001/jama.2017.8334.

Millspaugh, J. A. (1937) Dementia Pugilistica. *US Naval Medical Bulletin*, *35*, 303.

Nathanson, J. T., Connolly, J. G., Yuk, F., Gometz, A., Rasouli, J., Lovell, M., & Choudhri, T. (2016). Concussion incidence in professional football: Position-specific analysis with use of a novel metric. *Orthopedic Journal of Sports Medicine*, *4*, 1–6. doi: 10.1177/2325967115622621.

NFL.com. (2017, August 1). *Medical examination tents to debut on sidelines this season*. Retrieved from: www.nfl.com/news/story/0ap3000000823615/article/medical-examination-tents-to-debut-on-sidelines-this-season.

Omalu, B. I., Dekosky, S. T., Minster, R. L., Kamboh, M. I., Hamilton, R. L., & Wecht, C. H. (2005). Chronic traumatic encephalopathy in a National Football League player. *Neurosurgery*, *57*, 128–134. doi: 10.1227/01.NEU.0000163407.92769.ED.

Padaki, A. S., Cole, B. J., & Ahmad, C. S. (2016). Concussion incidence and return-to-play time in National Basketball Association players: Results from 2006 to 2014. *The American Journal of Sports Medicine*, *44*, 2263–2268. doi: 10.1177/0363546516634679.

Putukian, M., Aubry, M., & McCrory, P. (2009). Return to play after sports concussion in elite and non-elite athletes? *British Journal of Sports Medicine, 43,* 28–31. doi: 10.1136/bjsm.2009.058230.

Ragnarsson, K. T., Clarke, W. R., Daling, J. R., Garber, S. L., Gustafson, C. F., Holland, A. L., … Seltzer, M. M. (1999). Rehabilitation of persons with traumatic brain injury. *Journal of the American Medical Association, 282,* 974–983. doi: 10.1001/jama.282.10.974.

Seravalli, F. (2015, September 14). *NHL to use concussion spotters at all games.* Retrieved from: www.tsn.ca/nhl-to-use-concussion-spotters-at-all-games-this-season-1.360322.

Solomon, G. S., & Zuckerman, S. L. (2015). Chronic traumatic encephalopathy in professional sports: Retrospective and prospective views. *Brain Injury, 29,* 164–170. doi: 10.3109/02699052.2014.965205.

Wagner-McGough, S. (2015, Aug 9). *New NFL rule gives concussion spotters power to stop games.* Retrieved from www.cbssports.com/nfl/news/new-nfl-rule-gives-concussion-spotters-power-to-stop-games/.

Waldén, M., Hägglund, M., Orchard, J., Kristenson, K., & Ekstrand, J. (2013). Regional differences in injury incidence in European professional football. *Scandinavian Journal of Medicine & Science in Sports, 23,* 424–43. doi: 10.1111/j.1600-0838.2011.01409.x.

Wennberg, R. A., & Tator, C. H. (2008). Concussion incidence and time lost from play in the NHL during the past ten years. *Canadian Journal of Neurological Sciences, 35,* 647–651. doi: 10.1017/S031716710000946X.

Williams, J. M., Langdon, J. L., McMillan, J. L., & Buckley, T. A. (2016). English professional football players concussion knowledge and attitude. *Journal of Sport and Health Science, 5,* 197–204. doi: 10.1016/j.jshs.2015.01.009.

Yengo-Kahn, A. M., Johnson, D. J., Zuckerman, S. L., & Solomon, G. S. (2016). Concussions in the National Football League: A current concepts review. *The American Journal of Sports Medicine, 44,* 801–811. doi: 10.1177/0363546515580313.

13 Sociocultural aspects of concussion

Dominic Malcolm

Introduction

Fundamental to a social scientific approach is an emphasis on sociocultural factors. For sociologists of sport, concussion extends a well-established literature on subcultures of pain and injury in sport, including ideas about the relative tolerance of high levels of risk and violence that makes sport a unique sphere of social life (e.g., see Young, 2004). Concussion also resonates with the spectrum of issues that constitute the sociology of medicine, including the analysis of patient experience and illness behaviors; lay-professional relations (including the relative influence of competing bodies of knowledge); the professional dominance of medicine; analysis of the social construction of disease via medical research and practice; health inequalities (e.g., in relation to gender or socioeconomic status); cultural representations of health-related conditions; and the political context of public health interventions (e.g., see Nettleton, 2006). But the unique parameters of concussion—the relatively limited scientific understanding, the uncertainty over longer term neurocognitive decline, the "vague and heterogenous" symptoms (McNamee, Partridge, & Anderson, 2015, p. 193)—also make a sociocultural analysis particularly compelling.

However, it was only in the fifth and most recent Concussion in Sport Group (CISG) consensus statement (McCrory et al., 2017) that the significance of sociocultural factors in mediating experiences of mild traumatic brain injury was recognized. The statement explicitly stated that "psychological and sociocultural factors in sport play a significant role in the uptake of any injury-prevention strategy and require consideration in terms of the existing limitations of injury prevention strategies" (McCrory et al., 2017, p. 8). In particular, through references to learning styles and preferred learning strategies of target audiences there appears to be a growing awareness that "knowledge transfer" requires a broader and multidisciplinary skillset. The consensus statement from McCrory and colleagues (2017) also recognized the degree to which psychological research had enhanced understanding of the factors influencing the recovery from concussion. Indeed, in identifying the significance of factors such as sex, age, neurodevelopment, personal or family history of migraine, mental health problems, and past experiences of concussions, there was a more implicit recognition of how concussion, as it is currently understood, needs to be considered within its broad sociocultural context.

This chapter develops this belated recognition and charts the various ways in which sociocultural analyses have and can enhance our understanding of issues related to concussion. It focuses on five areas of brain injury-related research: athlete experience; medical practice; medical knowledge; public health; and cultural representations. Although each is addressed here discretely for heuristic reasons, it should be noted that ultimately the promise of a sociocultural approach is to provide the kind of holistic and comprehensive analysis of concussion that can only be achieved by seeing the interdependence of these different areas.

Athlete experience

Sociocultural analyses of athlete experiences of concussion first emerged in research focused on the cultures of risk in sport (Safai, 2003; Malcolm, 2009). This literature invokes ideas such as the "normalization" and "rationalization" of risk, pain, and injury as part of the "sport ethic" (Hughes & Coakley, 1991) or "culture of risk" (Nixon, 1992). While studies identify considerable similarities in the way that male and female athletes respond, gendered identities have been highlighted as significant in the social construction of injury (Messner, 1992; White & Young, 1999). In sum, athletes appear to talk about their bodies and understand injury in ways that are specific to sporting subcultures.

Sociologically, the key to understanding these forms of behavior is to investigate the distinct networks of relationships that characterize sport. While one of the first such studies from Safai (2003) identified a distinctly conservative orientation towards head injuries, this finding now appears to be the result of the approach espoused by a particular influential individual. More broadly, research suggests that brain injuries *do* evoke unique responses from athletes, but that these tend to be characterized by less—rather than more—caution. Specifically, in the precarious and insecure world of elite sports, where performance concerns are invariably prioritized over health, athletes tend to be particularly reluctant to present their symptoms of concussion to medical staff. Biomedical researchers (Broglio et al., 2010; Fraas et al., 2013; McCrea et al, 2004) have identified three reasons for this, namely athletes' (a) perceptions that their condition is not serious enough, (b) reluctance to leave the game and/or let down teammates, or (c) disbelief that a concussion has occurred. Because athlete reluctance to consult with medical staff is not unusual in sport (or even in the broader population), a sociocultural approach is required to explain why the rationales presented for such behavior are particularly pronounced in relation to concussion.

Malcolm's (2009) study of elite rugby explained how attitudes towards concussion were shaped by the individual's perception that their trajectory of recovery was undetermined and could have an unpredictable impact on their lives as athletes. Many reported that concussions did not necessarily impair playing performance, but uncertainty over what might happen if they revealed their concerns (would they, for instance, regain their place on the team?) meant that rugby players were reluctant to withdraw from sporting activities. Uncertainty also informed their decisions about whether to consult with medical staff. Players knew that clinicians could not offer relief from symptoms or enable their recovery or return-to-play except in the most severe cases. They also knew that alerting clinical staff to their concerns about having suffered a concussion would likely only disrupt their careers and identities through enforced withdrawal from sporting activities. In sum, while concussed players may experience unusual bodily sensations, "they seldom experience problems that they themselves cannot resolve and rarely, or only briefly, experience uncertainty in the form of concern about sporting performance" (Malcolm, 2009, p. 200).

Most recently, Liston, McDowell, Malcolm, Scott, and Waddington (2018) documented athletes' distinctly risky behaviors in relation to sport-related concussions. Their study of Irish amateur rugby players showed that individuals managed concussions by downplaying, ignoring, denying the significance, or concealing symptoms and "playing on." Post-injury consequences such as sleep disturbance, irritability, and mood swings were largely hidden from teammates, coaches, etc. There was, moreover, testimony to the effect of exhibiting a *preference* for receiving a concussion over musculoskeletal injuries. They argued that the former frequently entailed a more limited impact on a person's ability to play rugby and even rationalized the experiences of concussion-induced cognitive impairment as positive, "reverting" the individual to a "primal state" (deemed useful in the context of an aggressive sport such as rugby). Severity of injury, conversely, was assessed by these players as being directly related to the length of time one was unable to play sport and excluded considerations of longer-term neurocognitive decline. This "headstrong" attitude was derived "from within the subculture of rugby, that is, originating in the level of commitment made by players to each other and to the game" (Liston et al., 2018, p. 676).

Consequently, sociocultural studies of athlete experiences enable us to see the underlying logic to seemingly misguided or irrational behavior. The focus here is on the interrelations between actors (athletes, coaches, and clinicians) creating specific cultures of risk in which a marked tolerance towards head injuries is a notable feature.

Medical practice

A central premise of a sociocultural approach is that all healthcare treatment relies to a significant degree on social interaction. While the previous section briefly referred to the attitudes of athlete-patients towards clinicians, here the focus is on the impact of those interactions on the clinicians themselves. While essentially quantitative studies have identified how non-compliance with concussion protocols is not unusual in professional sport (Cusimano et al., 2017; Price, Malliaras, & Hudson, 2012), a qualitative approach provides (1) a detailed illustration of the frequently stated assertion that clinicians find cases of concussion particularly difficult to manage (McCrory et al., 2017); and perhaps more significantly, (2) a demonstration of how clinicians' actions are not simply a product of their training and professional instruction, but are fundamentally shaped through the interactions they encounter as part of their role in patient management (Malcolm, 2009, 2017).

Comparable to the uncertainty athletes feel when their careers and identities are threatened due to suspected concussion, healthcare professionals may experience uncertainty through being unable to master all aspects of medical knowledge and practice. Fueling their uncertainty in relation to concussion is the limited contemporary scientific knowledge base. Consensus statements are replete with provisos and reservations about what we currently do not know about concussion. For instance, it is notable how rarely, if at all, the position statements produced by either the National Athletic Trainers' Association (Broglio et al., 2014) or the American Medical Society for Sports Medicine (Harmon et al., 2013) provide recommendations based on "consistent and good quality experimental evidence" (Broglio et al., 2014, p. 246). Similarly, the 2017 CISG consensus statement notes that "critical questions remain … about the acute neurobiological effects of SRC on brain structure"; "insufficient evidence" for prescribing complete rest; and currently "limited evidence to support the use of pharmacotherapy" (McCrory et al., 2017, pp. 4–5). Guidelines on how to manage concussion have not only been repeatedly revised in recent years but continue to defer to the primacy of individual clinical judgment. Clinician interviewees reflect both their own uncertain knowledge and the difficulties of working in a context where the guidance and instruction they are given has frequently changed. For instance, they describe the difficulty of diagnosis, question the validity of existing protocols, and identify differences between sports as symptomatic of the lack of evidence (Malcolm, 2017).

The combination of uncertainty and skepticism linked to the changing regulatory environment generates three primary courses of action (Malcolm, 2009). First, clinicians may actively avoid the diagnosis of concussion. They may prefer to direct attention towards a different injury or treat the head injury but simply resist formally labeling it as a concussion. They may instead emphasize that a player should be withdrawn, as he would be unable to protect himself in contact. Secondly, clinicians tend to stress that their experiential knowledge of the sport has enabled them to develop their own guidelines for practice, which give primacy to particular signs and symptoms (Malcolm, 2009). Third, clinicians individualize treatment of their athletes, arguing that no two concussions are the same, and exerting their right to exercise clinical judgment over any textbook guidance or concussion identification tool. Prioritizing experiential knowledge and individualizing treatment essentially replaces a blanket "safety-first" approach with consideration of players' contributions to team performance. This effectively harmonizes the clinicians' approach with the concerns of players and coaches.

Ultimately, sociocultural studies show the distinct difficulties in implementing diagnostic and treatment guidelines in high-pressured elite sports environments. Clinicians' accounts reveal practices which are frequently removed from the conservative philosophies of existing protocols but which are compatible with the primacy given to individual clinical judgment (Malcolm, 2009; Malcolm, 2017;

see also Price, Malliaras, & Hudson, 2012). Clinical management problems essentially stem from the lack of strong evidential substance underpinning the relatively cautious recommendations.

Medical knowledge

A sociocultural approach further embraces the idea that concussion, like all such conditions, relies on biomedical research and practice to identify, define, and subsequently delineate its parameters. Simply put, people have expressed concerns about brain injuries incurred through playing sport for many years (Harrison, 2014), yet it is the specific actions of sporting and especially medical bodies that shape the contemporary understandings of the mild traumatic brain injuries that have relatively recently come to define as concussion. One can see this in the genesis of the CISG consensus statements, where one of the major initial concerns was to establish a definition of concussion around which researchers could focus their endeavors. As such, this section will try to understand concussion through its social construction in medical knowledge.

In "The Medicalization of Concussion," Malcolm (2017) argues that the sports medicine community has defined concussion as an issue which does and should fall under the provenance of medicine. The appointment of Paul McCrory as editor of the *British Journal of Sports Medicine* was a significant catalyst in this. McCrory capitalized on this influential position to rally, unify, and create a research agenda for a relatively disparate and divided set of scholars in the first years of the 21st century. From these actions stemmed the formation of the CISG, the production of consensus statements, the expansion of research, and, in particular, epidemiological studies. Epidemiology has certainly altered our understanding of the parameters of concussion as a social issue. Indicatively, epidemiology is a powerful tool for raising public awareness of concussion, and this in turn may (1) change people's perceptions of certain bodily sensations they experience; and (2) provide them with a socially-legitimate label through which to describe such sensations. The impact of this sociocultural critique goes beyond what was alleged to have been the deliberate and strategic attempts of the National Football League (NFL) through its Mild Traumatic Brain Injury Committee to have "fraudulently concealed" the risks of concussion and sub-concussive injuries to players (Hardes, 2017, p. 281). More simply, but no less systematically, through the identification of key risk variables, contemporary epidemiology tends to emphasize individual responsibility (e.g., poor tackling technique) and structural aspects of sports (e.g., the design of helmets, rules which allow certain forms of contact) rather than subcultural norms of being "headstrong" that ultimately "cause" concussions. Articles written by the NFL's aforementioned committee and controversially published in the journal *Neurosurgery* were allegedly written with a deliberate agenda to show that concussions were not a significant issue in the game (Fainaru-Wada & Fainaru, 2013).

A sociocultural analysis similarly questions the role consensus statements play in the social construction of knowledge. As Bercovitz (2000) argues, consensus statements "may be regarded as more a reflection of the desire of selected 'experts' and scientists to impose their world-view on research and practice" (p. 25). For example, Craton and Leslie (2014) have contested the evidence basis for some of the conservative recommendations in the CISG (2013) consensus statement, arguing that it: Contains inclusion criteria for diagnosis which are too broad and therefore could capture multiple other conditions; offers no supportive evidence for prescribing physical and cognitive rest (the latter now recognized as being a highly problematic concept, anyway); and is reliant on the notion of "asymptomatic" to guide graduated return to play, which is not operational, as most people are never fully asymptomatic of the inclusion criteria (p. 93). The content of consensus statements should thus be seen as a combination of medical "fact" and relatively subjective viewpoints informed by the concerns expressed in broader public debates.

However, to fully understand the medicalization of concussion, we must go beyond the actions of sports medicine personnel and explore the role of neuroscience (Hardes, 2017). Concern about concussion has developed in tandem with a "brain culture" (Thornton, 2011), where developments in knowledge, and particularly advances in imaging techniques, have offered the *potential* to provide a paradigmatic shift in our understanding of the human condition. However, neuroscience remains in its infancy, and public faith in its potential vastly outstrips its current efficacy. This was evident in the successful legal action brought forth by NFL players, although the case settled in the *absence* of compelling evidence of a sport-concussion-chronic traumatic encephalopathy (CTE) nexus.

In sum, a sociocultural approach is premised on a belief that scientific knowledge is not simply factual or neutral but subject to human or social processes. The current state of concussion science should therefore be seen as the product of the attempts of particular researchers to establish a common core of understanding in a relatively contested and pioneering medical field.

Public health

Sociocultural critiques of health promotion focus on three inter-related issues: *structure*, *surveillance*, and *consumption* (Nettleton & Bunton, 1995). *Structurally*, health promotion can be criticized for failing to recognize the importance of material (dis)advantage in mediating lifestyle and disregarding the significance of living conditions in contouring the choices that people can make. Typically, research in this area tends not to explore the heterogeneity in sporting populations' knowledge of concussion. *Surveillance* refers to the legitimacy of monitoring and regulating populations. This is especially complicated in relation to concussion as, by definition, the athlete-patient may not be able to make coherent decisions. But a sociocultural approach sensitizes us to the importance of recognizing that certain population cohorts actively seek out risk-taking behavior. Thus, while sociologists would agree that knowledge is often less important than the environment or relations in determining action (Kroshus et al., 2014), they would ask further and fundamental questions about whether such messages were unequivocally in "the interests" of the target group whose relatively voluntary behaviors are being restricted. Finally, health promotion has been criticized for blurring the boundaries between medicine and *consumer culture*. Specifically in relation to concussion, the representation of sport-related brain injury has created a significant market for both preventative equipment (e.g., helmets) and concussion assessment tools, which (1) creates opportunities for the commercial exploitation of sports participants; and (2) constructs distinct and socially desirable lifestyles which are only available to those who are already relatively economically empowered. Consequently, consumptive elements of public health often perpetuate social structural inequalities.

A sociocultural perspective provides a more rounded understanding and therefore a more reliable basis on which to orientate injury prevention strategies. For instance, rather than seeing coaches as either benign or indeed a force for more conservative concussion management (see e.g., Sarmiento, Mitchko, Klein, & Wong, 2010), these powerful individuals are viewed as a fundamental part of the problem. Similarly, a sociocultural perspective on public health highlights the dominance of psychological paradigms in health promotion. Not only do these lead to an advocacy of individual responsibility for health (Horrocks & Johnson, 2014), and consequently facilitate victim-blaming and stigmatization, they draw attention away from the underlying social causes of behavior. Moreover, because sociocultural evidence suggests that health promotion aimed at individual behavioral change is most effective in relation to populations in favorable social and economic conditions (Baum & Fisher, 2014), we can better understand the uneven uptake of concussion injury prevention programs. Currently, surveys of such interventions generally "suggest short-term improvements … while the long-term gains are mixed" (Mrazik et al., 2015, p. 1552). Rather, a sociocultural approach enables us to take a more holistic view of public health interventions, raising fundamental questions about equality, the legitimacy of population "control," and the potential for powerful commercial interests to exploit the opportunities that subsequently arise. By identifying how public health interventions replicate social structural inequalities, subject populations to high degrees of surveillance, and encourage them to engage in certain types of consumption, a sociocultural approach has the power to make injury prevention strategies more applicable and thus relevant to the lived experience of target populations.

Cultural representations

Finally, it is important to consider the cultural representations of concussion on the Internet, in the print media, and via film and television. Major themes documented on social media include personal experiences of concussion, the reported incidence amongst professional athletes, dissemination of research and education, and policy and safety implications (Sullivan et al., 2012; Workewych et al., 2017). Surveys of online content have found that CTE and Alzheimer's disease, dementia, or other cognitive problems are the most frequently cited consequences of concussion (Ahmed & Hall, 2017). Analyses of print media have highlighted the focus on athletes' personal experiences. Anderson and Kian (2012) argued that concerns over head injuries have led to a softening of American sporting masculinity, while McGannon, Cunningham, and Schinke (2013) highlighted how the psychological implications of head injury are largely ignored. Finally, Furness's (2016) analysis of *League of Denial* highlights how the film challenges dominant sport media narratives in which representations of concussion normalize violence, injury, and hegemonic masculinity. Instead the film documents the institutional failings of the NFL that led to the landmark establishment of a $1 billion compensation fund for former players.

More broadly, it can be argued that cultural representations of concussion have two primary consequences. First, the media tend to be relatively uncritical of the structural issues related to concussion. The consequence may be to underplay any broader political discussion of brain injury as a labor issue (Brayton et al., in press), or suggest that players are largely responsible for regulation failure. Some have argued that the media are therefore complicit in the sustained "antipolitics" of the NFL's messages, which hide a commodification of violence within "the dangerous moral contours of racial capitalism" (Benson, 2017, p. 307). Second, the media disseminates equivocal messages about the capacity of medicine to ameliorate public concerns about concussion. While on the one hand, media coverage has been accused of having "propagated an agenda of one-sided news and a sensationalised state of fear" (Kuhn et al., 2017, p. 1732), other accounts have been critical of the "overreliance on medico-scientific conceptions of CTE" (Ventresca, in press, p. 3), which both ignore the current limitations in scientific knowledge and in so doing exaggerate the potential of biomedicine to resolve both individual experiences and broader public concerns over sporting concussions (Malcolm, 2017).

A vital contribution of a sociocultural approach, therefore, is to locate athlete and clinician experiences, medical research, and health promotion within their cultural context. Analysis of the cultural representation of concussion enables us to consider concussion not just as a unique type of sports injury but as a condition which the population understands in ways that are structured according to broader social, political, and economic interests.

Conclusions

Building on what has only been a relatively recent recognition that sociocultural factors are significant in mediating the experience and management of concussion (McCrory et al., 2017), this chapter has sought to provide an overview of how concussion must be conceived of as impacting across a range of social domains—from cultural representations to public health, medical knowledge, medical practice, and athlete experience. Specifically, this chapter has identified how the peculiar social relations which form sports cultures shape the attitudes and behaviors of both the athletes and clinicians who negotiate the identification and management of concussion injuries. It has further examined how such social relations influence the construction and dissemination of medical knowledge (in relation to concussion) and how an awareness of sociocultural factors can enhance our design and delivery of public health messages designed to reduce the incidence and health costs of this particular sports injury. Noting how the populations' understanding of concussion is literally mediated through broader narratives of cultural representation reminds us of the interconnectedness of these apparently diverse social domains. Public perceptions, clinicians' actions, and even medical consensus statements do not develop in a vacuum. This point underscores the ultimate promise of a sociocultural approach; to provide a more comprehensive and systematic understanding of what is clearly a complex medical and social problem.

If the science of concussion can be said to still be in its infancy (McCrory et al., 2017), then sociocultural analyses of this medical and social phenomenon have barely been born. Consequently, there is a clear need to identify what research we need and how it might further our understanding of concussion. Complicating the establishment of this agenda is the existence of multiple disciplinary voices all speaking to the issue of concussion and making their pitch to be heard. As I have attempted to show here, sociocultural research should remain true to its disciplinary principles, and critical sociological researchers should not simply want to support or bolster the work of medicine (although clearly that is both worthwhile and will lead to important social benefits), but must also reflect upon and evaluate the concept and social functioning of health *per se*. This is what I attempt to illustrate in the concluding paragraphs.

In summarizing the breadth of potential sociocultural contributions to an understanding of concussion (see Table 13.1), it may be helpful to cite Stefan Timmermans' (2013) seven views (or warrants) about the unique contributions of qualitative health sociology and how this might be manifest in concussion research (Malcolm, 2018). Timmermans is a leading sociologist of health and illness and the senior medical sociology editor for the journal *Social Science and Medicine*. The first column of Table 13.1 reports each of Timmermans' seven warrants, and the second column describes how I imagine these might be applied to sociocultural research on sports concussion.

For many more familiar with the natural sciences, this array of aims and objectives may seem dauntingly broad, if not naively over-ambitious. But for those committed to a sociocultural analysis, they provide an antidote to the sometimes narrow and overly individualistic patient- or bodily-focused approach of biomedicine. Where sports medicine literature describes concussion as a particularly complex condition, a sociocultural approach *explains* how the network of interdependencies makes this so. Ultimately, it must be recognized that the social sciences have something different—advocates might say uniquely beneficial—to offer our understanding of concussion. It is both my contention that concussion, for various reasons (it seems to be a pressing social issue; it seems to be beyond simple or quick fixes; it seems that the social context in which it occurs places considerable strain on biomedical practices), is distinctively placed to become a

Table 13.1 A research agenda for sociocultural research on concussion

Warrant of health sociology (Timmermans, 2013)	Application to sports concussion research
Explore the social construction of beliefs	Illustrate the processes by which the diagnosis and management of concussion are shaped by the distinct characteristics of sport as a setting for medical practice
Reframe dominant perspectives	Question existing ideas that the "solution" to sport's "concussion crisis" lies solely or predominantly within the medical domain, and identify the potential contributions that might be made by alternative paradigms or ways of thinking
Chart the winners and losers of health interventions	Identify the existence and resultant impact of inequalities in medical provision between population cohorts, drawing attention to the way in which the medicalization of concussion may lead to aspects of social exclusion or social stratification of exercising populations
Identify the unfulfilled promises of medicine	Scrutinize the degree to which the claims made by medicine to be able to resolve concussion issues are evident in practice, and the degree to which existing practice is consistent with fundamental medical ethical promises such as "first do no harm"
Explore the experiences of medicine and health across multiple contexts	Illustrate cross-sport, cross-gender, and cross-cultural similarities and differences in concussion attitudes and behavior to reveal the spectrum of human experience and those practices which are distinct to, and therefore a product of, contemporary Euro-American contexts
Expose the impact of economic interests	Reveal which groups economically profit from the ever-increasing opportunities that arise from the threats posed by concussion injuries to both individuals and particular sports
Reveal how social relations mediate the impact of medical and health interventions	Provide a better understanding of how the social relations entailed in consultations about, and the diagnosis and management of, concussion can contribute fundamentally to the well-being of human populations

genuinely interdisciplinary field of study. It is my belief that this will benefit the many millions of people who sustain concussions each year and ensure that sport remains broadly popular and continues to confer distinct health benefits for the population. It is also my hope that that will occur. Now that the importance of the contribution of sociocultural approaches has been recognized by biomedical researchers (McCrory et al., 2017), it is vital that those who are fully conversant with such approaches actively begin to shape the concussion research agenda.

References

Ahmed, O., & Hall, E. (2017). "It was only a mild concussion": Exploring the description of sports concussion in online news articles. *Physical Therapy in Sport*, *23*, 7–13.

Anderson, E., & Kian, E. (2012). Examining media contestation of masculinity and head trauma in the National Football League. *Men & Masculinities*, *15*, 152–173.

Baum, F. & Fisher, M. (2014). Why behavioural health promotion endures despite its failure to reduce health inequalities. *Sociology of Health and Illness*, *36*, 213–225.

Benson, P. (2017). Big football: Corporate social responsibility and the culture and color of injury in America's most popular sport. *Journal of Sport & Social Issues*, *41*, 307–334.

Bercovitz, K. (2000). A critical analysis of Canada's "Active Living": Science or politics? *Critical Public Health*, *10*, 19–39.

Brayton, S., Helstein, M., Ramsey, M. & Rickards, N. (in press). Exploring the missing link between the concussion "crisis" and labor politics in professional sports. *Communication and Sport*.

Broglio, S., Cantu, R., Gioa, G., et al. (2014). National Athletic Trainers' Association position statement: Management of sport concussion. *Journal of Athletic Training*, *49*, 245–265.

Broglio, S., Vagnozzi, R., Sabin, M., Signoretti, S., Tavazzi, B., & Lazzarino, G. (2010). Concussion occurrence and knowledge in Italian football (soccer). *Journal of Sports Science and Medicine*, *9*, 418–430.

Craton, N., & Leslie, O. (2014). Time to re-think the Zurich guidelines? A critique on the consensus statement on concussion in sport, held in Zurich, November 2012. *Clinical Journal of Sports Medicine*, *24*, 93–95.

Cusimano, M., Casey, J., Jing, R., Mishra, A., Solarski, M., Techar, K., & Zhang, S. (2017). Assessment of head collision events during the 2014 FIFA World Cup tournament. *Journal of the American Medical Association*, *317*, 2548–2549.

Fainaru-Wada, M., & Fainaru, S. (2013). *League of denial*. New York: Crown Business.

Fraas, M., Coughlan, G., Hart, E., & McCarthy, C. (2013). Concussion history and reporting rates in elite Irish rugby union players. *Physical Therapy in Sport*, *15*, 136–142.

Furness, J. (2016). Reframing concussions, masculinity, and NFL mythology in League of Denial. *Popular Communication*, *14*, 49–57.

Hardes, J. (2017). Governing sporting brains: Concussion, neuroscience, and the biopolitical regulation of sport. *Sport, Ethics & Philosophy*, *11*, 281–293.

Harmon, K., Drezner, J., Gammons, M., Guskiewicz, K., Halstead, M., Herring, S. A., ... Roberts, W. O. (2013). American medical Society for Sports Medicine position statement: Concussion in sport. *British Journal of Sports Medicine*, *47*, 15–26.

Harrison, E. (2014). The first concussion crisis: Head injury and evidence in early American football. *American Journal of Public Health*, *104*, 822–833.

Horrocks, C., & Johnson, S. (2014). A socially situated approach to inform health and wellbeing. *Sociology of Health and Illness*, *36*, 175–186.

Hughes, R., & Coakley, J. (1991). Positive deviance among athletes: The implications of the sport ethic. *Sociology of Sport Journal*, *8*, 307–25.

Kroshus, E., Daneshvar, D., Baugh, C., Nowinski, C., & Cantu, R. (2014). NCAA concussion education in ice hockey: An effective mandate. *British Journal of Sports Medicine, 48*, 135–140.

Kuhn, A., Yengo-Kahn, A., Kerr, Z., & Zuckerman, S. (2017). Sports concussion research, chronic traumatic encephalopathy and the media: Repairing the disconnect. *British Journal of Sports Medicine, 51*, 1732–1733.

Liston, K., McDowell, M., Malcolm, D., Scott, A., & Waddington, I. (2018). On being "Head Strong": The pain zone and concussion in non-elite rugby union. *International Review for the Sociology of Sport, 53*, 668–684.

Malcolm, D. (2009). Medical uncertainty and clinician-athlete relations: The management of concussion injuries in rugby union. *Sociology of Sport Journal, 26*, 191–210.

Malcolm, D. (2017). *Sport, medicine and health: The medicalization of sport?* London: Routledge.

Malcolm, D. (2018). Concussion in sport: Public, professional and critical sociologies. *Sociology of Sport Journal, 35*, 141–148.

McCrea, M., Hammeke, T., Olsen, G. Leo, P., & Guskiewicz, K. (2004). Unreported concussion in high school football players: Implications for prevention. *Clinical Journal of Sports Medicine, 14*, 13–17.

McCrory, P., Meeuwisse, W., Dvorak, J., Aubry, M., Bailes, J., Broglio, S., … Davis, G. A. (2017). Consensus statement on concussion in sport—The 5th International Conference on Concussion in Sport held in Berlin, October 2016. *British Journal of Sports Medicine, 51*, 838–847.

McGannon, K., Cunningham, S., & Schinke, R. (2013). Understanding concussion in socio-cultural context: A media analysis of a National Hockey League star's concussion. *Psychology of Sport and Exercise, 14*, 891–899.

McNamee, M., Partridge, B., & Anderson, L. (2015). Concussion in sport: Conceptual and ethical issues. *Kinesiology Review, 4*, 190–202.

Messner, M. (1992). *Power at play: Sports and the problem of masculinity.* Boston, MA: Beacon Press.

Mrazik, M., Dennison, C., Brooks, B. Yeates, K. Babul, S., & Naidu, D. (2015). A qualitative review of sports concussion education: Prime time for evidence-based knowledge translation. *British Journal of Sports Medicine, 49*, 1548–1553.

Nettleton, S. (2006). *The sociology of health and illness* (2nd edition). Cambridge: Polity.

Nettleton, S., & Bunton, R. (1995). Sociological critiques of health promotion. In R. Bunton, S. Nettleton, & R. Burrows (Eds.), *The sociology of health promotion: Critical analyses of consumption, lifestyle and risk* (pp. 39–56). London: Routledge.

Nixon, H.L. II. (1992). A social network analysis of influences on athletes to play with pain and injuries. *Journal of Sport and Social Issues, 16*, 127–35.

Price, J., Malliaras, P., & Hudson, Z. (2012). Current practices in determining return to play following head injury in professional football in the UK. *British Journal of Sports Medicine, 46*, 1000–1003. doi: 10.1136/bjsports-2011-090687.

Safai, P. (2003). Healing the body in the "culture of risk": Examining the negotiations of treatment between sport medicine clinicians and injured athletes in Canadian intercollegiate sport. *Sociology of Sport Journal, 20*, 127–46.

Sarmiento, K., Mitchko, J., Klein, C., & Wong, S. (2010). Evaluation of the Centers for Disease Control and Prevention's concussion initiative for high school coaches:

"Heads up: Concussion in High School Sports." *Journal of School Health*, *80*, 112–118.

Sullivan, S., Schneiders, A., Cheang, C., Kitto, E., Lee, H., Redhead, J., ... McCrory, P. (2012). "What's happening?" A content analysis of concussion-related traffic on Twitter. *British Journal of Sports Medicine*, *46*, 258–263.

Thornton, D. J. (2011). *Brain culture: Neuroscience and popular media*. London: Rutgers University Press.

Timmermans, S. (2013). Seven warrants for qualitative health sociology. *Social Science and Medicine*, *77*, 1–8.

Ventresca, M. (in press). The curious case of CTE: mediating materialities of traumatic brain injury. *Communication and Sport*.

White, P., & Young, K. (1999). *Sport and gender in Canada*. Don Mills, ON: Oxford University Press.

Workewych, A., Muzzi, M., Jing, R., Zhang, S., Topolovec-Vranic, J., & Cusimano, M. (2017). Twitter and traumatic brain injury: A content and sentiment analysis of tweets pertaining to sport-related brain injury. *SAGE Open Medicine*, *5*, 1–11.

Young, K. (2004). *Sporting bodies, damaged selves: Sociological studies of sport-related injury*. Oxford: Elsevier.

14 Quantitative approaches in sport-related concussion research

Meredith Rocchi, Camille Guertin, and Scott Rathwell

Introduction

Sport-related concussions are generating increasingly more attention from the media, sport participants, and researchers, and are becoming an important part of the discussion surrounding player safety of all levels of sport. Currently, it is estimated that between 5–18% of all sport injuries are related to concussions (Gessel et al., 2007; O'Connor et al., 2017; Zuckerman et al., 2015). Due to the magnitude of concussion incidences, extensive research has been conducted to better understand the cognitive and physiological outcomes of a sport-related concussion such as headache, confusion, memory loss, and impaired mental processing (Echemendia et al., 2013; McCrea, Guskiewicz, & Marshall, 2003), as well as the length of time these symptoms persist (Broglio & Puetz, 2008). Currently, however, there is limited understanding of how sport-related concussions impact other outcomes for athletes, such as their depressive symptoms, their readiness to return to sport, or their concerns about re-injury (e.g., Mainwaring et al., 2010). To help address this gap, a call was made for research to move beyond assessing the cognitive and physiological outcomes of sport-related concussion and to expand to other concussion-related areas such as the psychological outcomes of concussions, concussion prevention strategies, and concussion education priorities (Bloom et al., 2004).

This emerging field of research presents a number of new questions for researchers to investigate. To help ensure this new field develops using strong evidence-based research, authors are encouraged to incorporate rigorous methodological designs and strong analytical approaches into their work in order to promote the replicability and transparency of their findings (Nature Supplement, 2014). The goal of the present chapter is to review popular quantitative research designs and discuss considerations for future sport-related concussion research. For each design, a brief explanation, the advantages and disadvantages, important considerations, and examples of past concussion research using that design will be presented. This chapter will focus on observational designs (i.e., researchers observe participants and variables of interest without intervening) and experimental designs (i.e., researchers intervene and observe the effects of their intervention on participants). Specifically, this chapter will cover cross-sectional, non-randomized groups, cohort (retrospective and prospective), experimental, and quasi-experimental designs (see Figure 14.1).

Observational designs

In observational research, the aim is to observe ongoing behavior and describe these observations. The type of data generated from observational research and the potential conclusions drawn are dependent on how observations are gathered. One key feature of observational research is that there is no attempt to manipulate variables or determine the actual causes of behavior. Instead, the goal is to understand how and when behavior occurs.

These observational designs are presented in order from the weakest level of evidence, where the goal is to observe and explore a phenomenon and generate hypotheses (i.e., cross-sectional, non-randomized group comparison studies), to the strongest, where the objective is to establish a temporal order of events (i.e., cohort studies, see Figure 14.1).

Cross-sectional studies

Cross-sectional studies consist of examining individuals at a single time point. These studies can be either *descriptive* in nature, where they aim to illustrate aspects of a specific condition or outcome, or *correlational*, in that they aim to identify relationships between variables. A researcher may use these types of

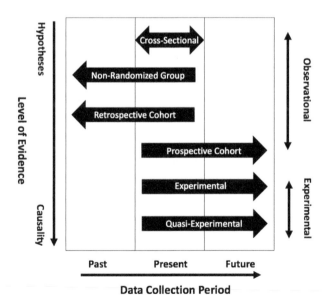

Figure 14.1 Overview of research designs by level of evidence and data collection period.

designs to describe a phenomena, determine the prevalence of cases in a population at a given point, explore the relationship between observed variables, or generate hypotheses for future research. For example, a researcher has a sample of athletes with concussions and an opportunity to collect data on their psychological symptoms at the end of the sport season. In a descriptive study, the researcher would ask the athletes to report on a variety of psychological symptoms and describe characteristics of the sample. Alternatively, in a correlational study, researchers would also ask athletes to report on a variety of symptoms, but in this case, they would aim to determine which factors were related to their concussion.

Advantages

The advantages of cross-sectional designs are that they can be conducted in a short period of time and they are relatively inexpensive to run (Mann, 2003). As there is no follow-up, participant dropout is not a concern, and less resources are required to run these studies. Cross-sectional studies are the best way to explore a new construct, determine prevalence of a given phenomenon, and they are useful at identifying associations that can then be more rigorously studied using a cohort, quasi-experimental, or experimental study. Since these studies do not aim to establish causation, an additional advantage is that they can be used to study multiple outcomes at the same time. Both descriptive (e.g., Davies & Bird, 2015; Register-Mihalik et al., 2013; Williamson & Goodman, 2006) and correlational (Kuehl et al., 2010; Bailey et al., 2010; Guskiewicz et al., 2007; Kroshus et al., 2017) designs have already been incorporated into a number of studies examining athletes who have suffered from a sport-related concussion (see Table 14.1). For instance, in a descriptive study examining athletes' concussion reporting behavior, researchers asked 1,532 high school football players about their concussion history, the number of concussions they had sustained that season, and whether they had reported the concussion (McCrea et al., 2004). The authors used the data to describe the percentage of athletes who had experienced a concussion and reported their concussion, and they found most athletes choose not to report it because they did not think it was serious enough. Cross-sectional research designs have also been implemented to identify associations between other variables and concussions. For example, in a correlational study, Beidler et al. (2017) asked a sample of 1,398 NCAA athletes to complete a survey about their personality characteristics (using the Big 5) and their concussion history. They grouped participants into those who had no history of concussion, those who reported one incident, and those who reported two or more. Overall, they found that personality characteristics were not related to having had a concussion or the number of concussions; however, they did find that agreeableness was associated with reporting concussions.

Disadvantages

In cross-sectional studies, researchers cannot provide an explanation for their findings; they simply look at frequencies of outcomes (descriptive) or associations

Table 14.1 Examples of additional research on concussion-related behaviors

Design	Purpose	Details	Analysis	Findings
Cross-sectional (correlational)				
Bramley, Patrick, Lehman, & Silvis (2012)	Evaluated the likelihood high school soccer players would identify themselves as having concussion-related symptoms during game situations.	183 high school soccer players completed a survey about their past concussion education and their likelihood of notifying their coach about a concussion.	Chi-square	Athletes who had previous concussion education training were more likely to report that they would notify their coach.
Kroshus, Garnett, Baugh, & Calzo (2016)	Whether there is an association between player beliefs about the consequences of continued play with a concussion and intentions to engage as a proactive bystander.	328 college athletes reported on their beliefs about continued play while symptomatic and their intentions as a bystander.	Multiple regression	Athletes who believed there were negative health consequences to continuing play were more likely to encourage teammates to seek help but not more likely to alert the coach or medical personnel.
Cross-sectional (descriptive)				
Guskiewicz, Weaver, Padua, & Garrett (2000)	Determine concussion incidence in high school and university football players.	242 athletic trainers recruited 17,549 collegiate and high school football players to report on their concussion symptoms.	Descriptive statistics	Overall, 5% of football players sustained at least one concussion, and 15% of those who sustained one sustained a second injury during the same season.
Torres et al. (2013)	Assess athletes' knowledge of signs and symptoms of concussion and also sought to estimate the potential frequency of underreporting in a collegiate athlete cohort.	262 athletes anonymously participated in this study about concussion symptoms and reporting	Frequencies	Of athletes who had a history of concussion, 43% knowingly hid symptoms to continue playing and 22% indicated that they would be unlikely to report a concussion.

(Continued)

Table 14.1 Continued

Design	Purpose	Details	Analysis	Findings
Non-equivalent groups (case-control designs)				
Kroshus, Baugh, Stein, Austin, & Calzo (2017)	Determine whether there are between-sex differences in concussion reporting intention and behavior.	328 college athletes reported on their intentions to report their concussions and likelihood of continuing to play with symptoms.	T-tests	Women had higher intentions to report than men, but there were no differences in their likelihood of continuing to play.
Non-equivalent groups (static group comparison)				
Covassin, Crutcher, Bleecker, Heiden, Dailey, & Yang (2014)	Compare the anxiety and social support of athletes with concussions and a matched group of athletes with orthopedic injuries.	Collegiate athletes (n = 63) with a diagnosed concussion were matched with athletes with orthopedic injuries (n = 63). Groups were matched for sex, sport, and time loss due to injury.	T-tests	Concussed athletes and those with orthopedic injuries reported similar anxiety and sources of social support post-injury.
Kontos, Elbin, Newcomer, Appaneal, Covassin, & Collins (2013)	Compared the coping responses of concussed athletes with those with an orthopedic injury and healthy controls and explored sex differences in coping behaviors following sport injury.	68 athletes with a concussion, 42 athletes with an orthopedic injury, and 33 healthy controls reported their coping behavior one week following their injury.	Independent ANOVA	Concussed athletes reported lower active, planning, acceptance, religion, self-distraction, venting, and self-blame coping than the orthopedic group, while the orthopedic group reported lower than the control group.

Design	Purpose	Details	Analysis	Findings
Cohort (prospective)				
Houston, Bay, & Valovich McLeod (2016)	Determine the relationship between post-concussion time lost and quality of life.	1,134 athletes completed a baseline assessment battery. During the study, 122 athletes sustained a concussion and underwent follow-up testing at three and ten days post-injury.	Multiple regression	Quality of life appears to play a role in time lost post-concussion and should be measured in combination with traditional concussion assessments.
Yang, Peek-Asa, Covassin, & Torner (2015)	Examine the impact of a concussion on psychological symptoms of collegiate athletes.	67 concussed collegiate athletes reported on their psychological symptoms.	Multiple Regression	Depression at baseline was the strongest predictor of depression and anxiety following concussion.
Cohort (retrospective)				
O'Rourke, Smith, Punt, Coppel, & Breiger (2017)	Explore psychosocial correlates of athletes' concussion symptoms during recovery.	51 youth athletes who participated in an outpatient concussion clinic completed assessments on average seven days post-concussion, as well as 14 and 21 days.	Hierarchical regression	Psychosocial variables accounted for 27% of variance in symptom change from Time 1 to Time 3.

(Continued)

Table 14.1 Continued

Design	Purpose	Details	Analysis	Findings
Cohort (matched retrospective)				
Turner, Langdon, Shaver, Graham, Naugle, & Buckley (2017)	To compare the psychological responses of student-athletes who have been diagnosed with a concussion to those of athletes diagnosed with musculoskeletal injuries with similar recovery duration.	15 collegiate athletes with a musculoskeletal injury, matched with 15 athletes who had sustained concussions, completed measures of mood profiles at three time points (acute, day one of exercise, and return to play).	MANOVA and ANOVA	Both groups reported improved mood profiles over time, but there were no significant differences between the two groups.
Experimental (randomized controlled trial)				
Echlin et al. (2010)	Evaluate the effectiveness of an educational intervention on concussion knowledge within a sample of junior fourth-tier ice hockey players.	67 male ice hockey players were randomized into three concussion education intervention groups (DVD, interactive computer, or control) and reported their knowledge at zero, 50, and 91 days.	Factorial ANOVA	No differences between groups at baseline, however, small differences emerged at 50 and 91 days later, supporting the effectiveness of the concussion education program.
Swartz, Broglio, Cook, Cantu, Ferrara, Guskiewicz, & Myers, (2015)	Evaluate the effectiveness of a helmetless tackling training program in reducing head impacts.	50 athletes were randomly assigned to the five-minute helmetless tackling drills group or the noncontact drills group.	Repeated-measures ANOVA	The results supported that a helmetless-tackling training intervention reduced head impacts in collegiate football players within one football season.

Design	Purpose	Details	Analysis	Findings
Quasi-experimental (non-equivalent groups)				
Hutchison, Mainwaring, Comper, Richards, & Bisschop (2009)	To determine if athletes with concussion and those with minor musculoskeletal injuries experienced differential emotional response to injury.	34 injured intercollegiate athletes (20 athletes with concussion, 14 athletes with musculoskeletal injuries) and 19 healthy active undergraduates assessed at baseline and on three non-consecutive days during a two-week period after.	Factorial ANOVA	Concussion produced an emotional profile characterized by elevated fatigue and decreased vigor. Athletes with musculoskeletal injuries displayed increased anger that resolved within two weeks.
Mainwaring, Hutchison, Bisschop, Comper, & Richards (2010)	To compare athletes' emotional response to concussion compared to anterior cruciate ligament (ACL) injury.	16 athletes with concussion, seven athletes with ACL injury, and 28 uninjured athletes completed pre-injury, post-injury and longitudinal measures of emotional functioning.	Factorial ANOVA	Athletes with ACL injuries reported higher levels of depression for a longer duration than athletes with concussion.

between constructs (correlational). Since they have no comparison group (i.e., no one to compare on the outcomes), these studies have limited validity outside the context of the study and cannot establish causation or the sequence of events. Additionally, studies that have low response rates (i.e., many participants were invited, but few participated) may be biased since the design may not capture important differences between the responders and non-responders. A final disadvantage of cross-sectional studies is that they are susceptible to common method variance where relationships are attributable to the measurement method used to assess the constructs (i.e., 1–7 Likert-type scales) and not necessarily relationships between the constructs (Lindell & Whitney, 2001). This type of systematic error can influence construct reliability and validity, as well as the strength of the correlational relationship between constructs (Podsakoff et al., 2003).

Considerations

Because the goal of this design is to describe or understand a phenomena, there are no minimum sample sizes required. Cross-sectional research designs can range from case studies of one participant to national surveys of thousands of participants. The analysis approach and potential conclusions that can be drawn depend entirely on the number of participants and the methods chosen for collecting the data. When using cross-sectional designs to assess relationships between variables, studies are often criticized for their susceptibility to common method variance. Fortunately, several methods can be used to reduce this form of bias. Statistically, researchers may wish to use a common latent factor when analyzing relational data in order to capture the variance explained by the common data collection method. There is debate, however, about the effectiveness of this statistical procedure (see Podsakoff et al., 2003, for a review). Alternatively, procedural remedies such as collecting data from different sources (athletes, coaches, parents) concurrently, or using secondary data, also exist for controlling common method bias. Finally, given that cross-sectional designs are not intended to determine cause and effect, researchers should ensure that they do not infer causation through the use of causal language in their results and conclusions. For example, researchers should avoid language like "influence" and "impact" in favor of words such as "related" and "associated."

Non-randomized group comparison studies

Non-randomized group comparison studies are typically retrospective in nature, meaning that participants who already have a certain condition are compared with others who do not (Mann, 2003). Similar to a cross-sectional design, participant data are collected at one time point only. However, the main objective is to compare the two groups and look for differences. Non-randomized group comparison studies typically use a *case-control design* or a *static-group comparison design*. The choice between these two designs depends on whether the comparison groups are the predictor (independent variable) or outcome (dependent variable) in the study. If researchers are interested in identifying the factors that lead to a given condition and determining the odds of developing the condition (i.e., the groups are the outcome), they will use a *case-control design* to compare groups on a given variable. For example, a researcher could identify potential risk factors such as sport type or gender and determine how these factors related to sustaining a concussion. If researchers plan to identify potential consequences of having a condition (i.e., the groups are the predictor), they will use a *static-group comparison design* to compare groups on different variables. For instance, researchers could compare athletes with a concussion to those without a concussion and examine whether they are more prone to depression or anxiety.

Advantages

Non-randomized group comparison studies are very useful for hypothesis generation and, when rigorously designed (i.e., the groups are matched on all key variables), for isolating important differences between groups. In a case-control study, Kroshus et al. (2017) examined college athletes to determine if there were differences between men and women in their intention to report concussions. The authors found that gender was a significant predictor of concussion reporting behavior where female athletes were more likely to indicate that they intended to report their concussion than male athletes. In a static-group comparison study examining collegiate athletes, Kuehl and colleagues (2010) compared athletes who reported 0, 1–2, or 3+ sport-related concussions on their reported body pain, vitality, and social functioning. Their results suggested that college athletes who had experienced previous concussions reported increased headaches and pain and decreased social functioning when compared to non-concussed athletes. The advantages of these studies are that they can be done quickly, are simple to administer, and are sometimes the only feasible option due to ethical reasons, sample availability, or the required resources (Mann, 2003). Furthermore, because individuals are sometimes deliberately chosen to participate in the research because they have the condition of interest, they can be more cost-effective since recruitment can be more targeted (Mann, 2003). Finally, non-randomized group comparison studies can help determine the relative importance of predictors and outcomes in relation to the presence or absence of the condition.

Disadvantages

One of the disadvantages of non-randomized group comparison studies is that they are inherently retrospective and participants join the study *after* they already have a condition. As a result, these study designs cannot directly determine the absolute risk of having a certain outcome; however, for case control studies, they can be used to calculate odds ratios (Mann, 2003). Furthermore, in some research designs, participants are assigned to their group based on self-reported history of sport-related concussions. As such, these types of designs are susceptible to recall bias, which can seriously impact the validity of the results. Finally, selecting the appropriate participants for the comparison group is a big challenge and can seriously bias the results if not done properly (Song & Chung, 2010). If participant matching cannot be guaranteed, it is essential to ensure that the comparison group is selected from the same population.

Considerations

Common to case-control and static-group designs is the aim of comparing groups. Thus, the quality of the data generated and the ability to generalize the results are largely dependent upon how closely matched the individuals are within the groups. The matching is ideally done at the individual level, where individuals in both groups are matched one-to-one on key variables such as age, gender, sport background, and sport experience (Hulley et al., 2001). However, for logistical and feasibility reasons, many researchers use an aggregate matching method where the two groups share similar composition overall on relevant characteristics (e.g., same mean age or proportion of females). Although an aggregate matching method is not as rigorous as a one-to-one approach, this approach substantially increases the reliability of the results over no matching. Finally, similar to cross-sectional study designs, researchers should ensure that their language does not imply causation when reporting on the results of their non-randomized group comparison studies.

Cohort studies

Cohort studies, also known as longitudinal studies, involve examining one or more samples (called cohorts) at multiple time points and can be either *prospective* or *retrospective* in design. In a *prospective* study, researchers measure a cohort on variables that might be relevant to the development of a certain outcome (i.e., a concussion), and then follow the cohort over time to see whether individuals develop the outcome and how it progresses. The key feature of this design is that participants have not already developed the outcome of interest at the beginning of the research process (i.e., baseline data). For example, in a prospective study design, a researcher could collect baseline psychological data (i.e., anxiety, depression, mood, etc.) at the start of a sport season with a group of athletes and then, for those that sustain a sport-related concussion, continue to monitor their psychological variables immediately following their concussion and into the future (i.e., three- and six-month follow-ups) to identify changes between pre- and post-concussion.

In a *retrospective* design, the cohort already has the condition at baseline and is followed moving forward. In this design, the researchers conceived the study and begin recruiting participants after the outcome has occurred. For instance, researchers can begin by collecting psychological data immediately after athletes sustain a concussion and then monitor changes across multiple time points (i.e., 3-, 6-, and 12-months post-concussion).

Advantages

Cohort studies have been used extensively to study concussion-related behaviors (e.g., Bagley et al., 2012; Booher et al., 2002; Caron et al., 2018; McCrea et al., 2004) and are currently considered the most popular design in sport-related concussion research (e.g., Echemendia et al., 2013). The advantage of any design that incorporates data from multiple time points is that it can provide information about the onset, continuity, and within-person changes of a given condition. For prospective studies specifically, they have the advantage of being designed with a research question in mind and, therefore, can be tailored to ensure that measurement is standardized and data collection is more complete. These designs are also easier and cheaper to run than experimental studies and, since the observations are conducted in temporal sequence, they can begin to identify potential causes from effects. For instance, Kontos et al. (2012) administered measures of depression and other related symptoms as part of a concussion surveillance program for high school and college athletes. During a 2-year period, if athletes experienced a sport-related concussion, they were asked to complete these measures again at 2 days, 7 days, and 14 days post-injury. Their results found that the 75 athletes who experienced a concussion reported increased depression scores up to 14 days following their concussion. Given that cohort studies are still observational in nature, they cannot be used to establish causation; however, prospective studies can be used to estimate risk factors when experimental studies are not possible. For Kontos and colleagues (2012), the use of a prospective longitudinal design allowed them to infer that concussions place athletes at risk for depressive symptoms.

For retrospective designs, the advantages lie in that the data is often available immediately and the studies are typically cheaper and shorter to run than prospective studies. In a retrospective longitudinal study, O'Rourke et al. (2017) looked at 51 young athletes who presented themselves to a concussion clinic within 14 days of sustaining their injury. They assessed athletes' symptoms, as well as psychosocial variables (motivation, achievement goals, athletic identity, coach behavior, and parent behavior) on that initial visit, as well as at two additional times points approximatively one and two weeks later. Overall, they found that athletes who demonstrated performance anxiety and low motivation at baseline exhibited more severe concussion symptoms at both follow-up assessments.

Disadvantages

Despite many advantages, cohort studies do have some important disadvantages. Regardless of whether using a prospective or retrospective design, collecting data over multiple time points increases the risk of participant attrition (i.e., dropout) and the presence of confounding variables (i.e., variables that the researchers failed to control for), which can seriously impact the validity and replicability of the results. An additional problem with prospective studies is that they require a large sample size since it is difficult (or impossible) to know which percentage of the initial sample will develop the condition. For retrospective designs, the primary disadvantage is that researchers may have limited control over what occurred before the condition started or how long the participant had the condition before they joined the study. This makes it difficult to control for confounding factors or other circumstances that affected the condition.

Considerations

For prospective designs in general, it is important to consider the latency period that may occur between baseline data collection and waiting for the condition of interest to occur. The longer the delay between baseline and onset of the condition (i.e., a concussion), the more vulnerable the study becomes to participant dropout. Thus, concussion researchers may consider using prevalence and incident rates when estimating sample sizes, although admittedly, these estimates may not be accurate. A related consideration that is specific to concussion research is the issue of collecting baseline data. Due to the logistical challenges related to the feasibility of screening all athletes (LeMonda et al., 2017) and the fact that many athletes do not take the screening seriously (Schatz et al., 2017), researchers may not be acquiring the most reliable and valid data. For retrospective designs, researchers can extend the rigor and validity of their findings by including a comparison group that is matched on key variables. For example, Turner and colleagues (2017) used a matched retrospective cohort design to compare the psychological mood profiles of 15 student-athletes who had been diagnosed with a concussion to those of 15 athletes diagnosed with musculoskeletal injuries with similar recovery duration. Athletes were assessed at the acute phase of their injury, on the first day they returned to exercise, and when they returned to play. Their results found that both groups' mood profiles improved at each measurement point; however, there were no significant differences between the two groups. For prospective designs, the inclusion of a comparison group would result in a quasi-experimental design (specifically, a pretest-posttest design), which is discussed in the next section. A final consideration for both designs is the number of assessments and the time interval between assessments once the data collection has begun. If participants are contacted too often, it could potentially promote dropout due to participant fatigue. If there is too much time between assessments, the study becomes susceptible to more extraneous and confounding variables. Researchers should aim to maximize efficiencies and reduce participant burden by conducting pilot or feasibility tests before officially beginning data collection.

Experimental designs

Experiments are the only reliable method available for determining cause-effect relationships between two or more variables (Reis & Judd, 2000). An experimental design involves measuring a variable of interest (dependent variable), some sort of manipulation to a different variable (independent variable), and then examining changes in the dependent variable following the manipulation of the independent variable, with the objective of determining cause and effect. Although experimental designs require multiple assessment points (like cohort designs), what makes them different is the presence of a manipulation. A manipulation can include a specific intervention like a training program or treatment technique but can also include the onset of a new condition, like a concussion. The key requirements for a true experimental research design, which are researchers' only method for inferring causal relationships, are the presence of a control group (i.e., a group of individuals who participate in the study but do not receive the manipulation) and randomization (i.e., where every participant has an equal opportunity to be in the experimental or control group).

Randomized controlled studies

Randomized controlled trials are the gold standard in determining whether a cause-effect relationship exists between the independent and dependent variables (Sibbald & Roland, 1998). These designs include a number of essential features. First, there must be at least one experimental group that receives the manipulation and a control group that participates in the research but does not receive the manipulation. Then, participants must be randomly assigned to either group. When possible, researchers should use a blind (i.e., participant is unaware of which group they are in) or double-blind (i.e., both participants and researchers are unaware of what group each participant is in) procedures to help reduce potential bias created by expectations of participating in the study. Randomization helps ensure that no systematic differences exist between the groups and thus reduces the potential bias caused by confounding variables.

For example, researchers may be interested in testing an intervention aimed at reducing depression symptoms in athletes who are recovering from a concussion using a single-blind design. Athletes who have sustained a sport-related concussion would provide baseline depression symptom information, then be randomly assigned to either the intervention group that would receive training and support in managing their depressive symptoms or to the control group that receives an unrelated training in concussion education. Then, the two groups will be compared on their reported depression symptoms at later time points.

Advantages

Randomized controlled trials are preferred because, through randomization, they minimize the risk that confounding variables impact the conclusions of the study. The use of a control condition ensures that variations due to extraneous factors are accounted for within the study design. The prospective design also minimizes recall error and selection bias for participants, thus improving the fidelity of the results. Finally, the best advantage is that the study design allows for causal inferences. For instance, Swartz and colleagues (2015) conducted a randomized controlled trial in a concussion prevention setting to test a helmetless-tackling behavior intervention for collegiate football players. A sample of 50 players were randomized to either the intervention (25 players) or control (25 players) group. The intervention group participated in a five-minute tackling drill without their helmets or shoulder pads twice a week during the preseason and once per week throughout the season. During the same period, the control group performed noncontact football skills. Their frequency of head impacts was recorded with an impact sensor in all games. Differences between the two groups were examined, and the results supported that a helmetless-tackling training intervention reduced head impacts in collegiate football players within one football season.

Disadvantages

Given the resources (e.g., multiple groups, controls, interventions, multiple data time points) required in running a randomized controlled trial, they can often be expensive and time-consuming. Similar to any study that requires multiple data time points, these trials are at risk of participant attrition. Additionally, randomized controlled trials can only examine one population at a time, as the examination of multiple populations could potentially introduce bias through confounding variables. Finally, in many cases, experiments cannot be conducted in real-life settings and are done in either clinical or experimental settings, which reduces their external (or ecological) validity. Furthermore, there are certain types of research questions that cannot be answered with a randomized controlled trial due to ethical constraints. For example, exposing a participant to an intervention that is believed to be inferior or intentionally giving an athlete a concussion is unethical. Presumably due to the aforementioned disadvantages, there are no published studies that have used a randomized controlled trial design to examine psychological aspects related to concussions (i.e., depression, anxiety, etc.).

Considerations

When designing randomized controlled trials, researchers should consider the type of control groups they use as a comparison (Kinser & Robins, 2013). For example, researchers can choose to have a *no-treatment control group*, where the control participants simply perform the assessments but receive no version of the intervention. This approach accounts for participant history during the intervention and any statistical bias related to completing repeated assessments; however, these participants are increasingly susceptible to dropout and may seek other treatment during the study. Researchers can also use a *wait-list control group*, where the intervention is delayed for the period of the study and control participants receive the intervention after the study is complete. This method is often used when it would be unethical for participants not to receive the intervention; however, the waiting period may make the study unfeasible if participants seek other treatment due to long wait times. Finally, researchers can use *attention control groups*, where the control participants receive some sort of related intervention, but not the one of interest in the study (i.e., a placebo treatment or alternative training). Researchers must choose this type of design if they want to use blind or double-blind procedures. These designs generally require more resources and must address ethical issues related to participants' expectations of receiving treatment but are most reliable for minimizing confounding variables.

Researchers should also consider the procedures for randomization they select (Doig & Simpson, 2005). As an example, blocked randomization, where participants are randomized within blocks of four to eight, ensures that there is an equal balance in the number of experimental and control participants throughout the study. Stratified block randomization refers to using important factors such as gender or sport to additionally categorize participants in order to ensure there is an equal balance between the experimental and control groups. These randomization procedures help reduce the likelihood of extraneous factors influencing the results of the study. An additional consideration is the sample size required to detect an effect (Lenth, 2001). Researchers should ensure that they conduct power analyses in order to determine the number of participants necessary to observe significant results. Finally, part of the gold standard protocol of conducting randomized controlled trials is to register the trial officially within a database before data collection begins (i.e., clinicaltrials.gov). This registration ensures that the design protocol and specific hypotheses are officially documented before data collection and gives confidence to end-users that the study was conducted as planned. As a general rule, researchers should consult and follow the consolidated standards of reporting trials (CONSORT) reporting guidelines (www.consort-statement.org) and checklists to ensure their results are to standard.

Quasi-experimental studies

As described above, due to logistical or ethical constraints related to concussion research, it is probable that when designing a study, the requirements of a true experimental design cannot be met, resulting in the need for a quasi-experimental design. Specifically, if a researcher does not have a control group, it is called a *pretest-posttest design*, where they recruit a sample of participants, conduct baseline tests, introduce a manipulation, then check for within-person changes from baseline measures. For example, in a pretest-posttest design, a researcher could be interested in testing the effectiveness of a concussion education program. They could test athletes' knowledge of concussion information, have athletes participate in the education program, then re-test their knowledge to determine whether there were any differences.

If a researcher has a control group but cannot ensure randomization, it becomes a *non-equivalent groups design*. In this type of design, participants become part of the experimental or control groups due to specific circumstances or as a result of their characteristics. Researchers still perform baseline assessments and introduce a manipulation; however, they are more interested in between-group differences. For example, researchers could be interested in determining the effectiveness of tackling training for football players who have a concussion history compared to those who do not. They could examine both groups' tackling behavior as a baseline measure, then conduct the tackling training, then re-assess their behavior after the training. This type of design would allow researchers to evaluate the effectiveness of their training program and determine whether it is more effective with one group or the other. Importantly, quasi-experimental designs can detect associations between the independent and dependent variables, but as with other designs, they cannot rule out the possibility that the results are caused by unknown confounding factors.

Advantages

The advantages of quasi-experimental designs are that they may be more feasible since they do not have the same logistical constraints (i.e., costs, recruitment, randomization, etc.) of true experimental designs. Additionally, since some phenomena are impossible to study from a fully experimental perspective without creating an artificial study environment such as a laboratory, a quasi-experimental design allows researchers to conduct experimental research in more naturally occurring settings, thus increasing the external validity of the results. These designs also limit ethical concerns surrounding pre-selection and random assignment, since it is unethical to manipulate certain things (i.e., to give athletes concussions). For instance, in an attempt to establish benchmarks of normal emotional recovery from concussion, Mainwaring and colleagues (2004) examined athletes' profiles of mood states before their injury and for a period following their concussion. Specifically, athletes reported their mood profiles (i.e., depression, confusion, and mood disturbances) as part of a preseason medical assessment (Time 1). For their study, it would be unethical to take a random sample of athletes and administer them a concussion. Thus, Mainwaring and colleagues waited for athletes to sustain a concussion and then recruited them to complete a measure of mood states in the first 72 hours following their concussion (Time 2), as well as approximately 14 (Time 3) and 21 days (Time 4) post-injury. The athletes' uninjured teammates who had also completed the Time 1 assessment served as the control group and completed the Time 2, 3, and 4 assessments on a similar interval schedule. Overall, the results found that at pre-injury, all athletes reported similar mood profiles, but that athletes who sustained a concussion reported elevated disturbances at Times 2 and 3, but that these disturbances subsided by Time 4.

Disadvantages

Given the presence of confounding variables (e.g., previous head injuries, other symptoms, etc.), quasi-experimental designs are not ideal when studying phenomena that is novel or multifaceted since it will be difficult to identify what changes have been caused by the manipulation in the study and what is due to other factors outside of the study (Axelrod & Hayward, 2006). Since there is no randomization or true control group, imbalances can occur between the two groups, and the generalizability of the results to the larger population will be limited by the sample that was collected, and statistical analyses can be rendered meaningless. In designs where the manipulation occurs naturally (i.e., a concussion), it can take a long time for the manipulation to occur, which increases the likelihood that confounding variables (e.g., time of season, group dynamics) are interfering with the results. Due to the complexity of the design, and the fact that researchers must wait for participants to suffer a concussion, it is not surprising that there have been limited quasi-experimental studies used in concussion research.

Considerations

Researchers can reduce the bias in a non-equivalent groups design and increase the generalizability of their results by using matching procedures. The more variables researchers use to match the groups, the more generalizable the results of the study will be. In a pretest-posttest design, researchers can ensure that their studies are large enough to perform the planned analyses and detect results by collecting big samples at baseline. For both types of designs, using clear inclusion and exclusion criteria can also help encourage homogeneity between the groups, thus improving the interpretability and reliability of the results. Finally, the analyses chosen must take into consideration the non-equivalent groups or lack of randomization and ensure that they include sufficient control for variability in the results that is caused by the design of the study. Failing to do this control could result in overestimating the size of the effect of the treatment.

Discussion

The strengths and weaknesses of each design were discussed and examples from current concussion studies were presented for each design. Concussion researchers have many opportunities to use these designs to ensure the rigor and validity of their research and improve the interpretability and replicability of their results. Although this chapter discussed research design, it did not dedicate significant attention to determining the study design that best fits a given research question or selecting the appropriate analytical approach once data is collected. Researchers can consult the PICOT (population, intervention, control, outcome, time) formulation for guidelines in determining which study design best fits the research question (Riva et al., 2012). These guidelines are especially relevant for randomized controlled trials. In terms of analytical approaches, the studies reviewed in this chapter used a number of approaches, including linear regression, nominal logistic regression, multiple regression, independent analysis of variance (ANOVA), factorial ANOVA, and MANOVA, among others. The type of analysis chosen depends not only on the design of the study (i.e., cross-sectional versus cohort) but also on the type of data that was collected and the number of variables of interest. These considerations are part of what is known as the statistical assumptions underlying each type of analyses.

When designing a study, it is essential for researchers to consider which analyses they will perform and to verify that their study design is in line with the assumptions of those tests before starting data collection. For some researchers who are less familiar with quantitative analyses, the use of a decision tree (see discoveringstatistics.com;

Field, 2009) can help identify the appropriate analysis plan. Statistical decision trees rely on the number of variables of interest (i.e., how many independent and dependent variables) as well as the level of measurement of each variable (i.e., categorical or continuous) to determine which test is most appropriate. In statistics, there are four levels of measurement that can be classified into *categorical variables*, where variables are made up of categories and a participant must clearly fall into one category (nominal, ordinal), or *continuous variables*, where participants' scores can take on any value (interval, ratio). When considering categorical variables, a researcher must determine whether the categories can be placed into a logical order. If there is no logical order, this is considered a nominal variable (i.e., gender, sport, favorite color). For nominal variables, if there are only two categories, it is also referred to as a dichotomous variable. If there is a logical order, it is an ordinal variable (i.e., letter grade, placement in a race). When considering continuous variables, a researcher must consider whether participants' scores have a true interpretable zero. If there is no interpretable zero, it is considered an interval variable (i.e., 1–7 Likert-type scales), whereas if the variable has a true zero (i.e., height, weight, race time), this is considered a ratio variable. Where possible, researchers should aim to collect data at the ratio level, since it is possible to convert ratio data into interval, interval into ordinal, and ordinal to nominal data, but it is impossible to go in the opposite direction.

Moving forward

In an ideal scenario, researchers would advance a new idea through all of the study designs discussed in this chapter, moving from the observational phase, where the objective is to understand prevalence and relationships between the variables, to the evidence phase in experimental designs. For example, a qualitative researcher may observe that an athlete who suffered from a concussion engaged in mindfulness exercises, and this helped them reduce their feelings of depression (see Chapter 15 in this book for more information about qualitative research). From there, a researcher could design a cross-sectional study to collect data from a number of athletes who have suffered from concussions and ask them to report on their mindfulness activities as well as their depressive symptoms. Through observational analyses, the researcher could learn that there is a link between mindfulness activities and reduced depressive symptoms. Next, a researcher could use a non-randomized group comparison design to compare athletes who have suffered from concussions who practice mindfulness with athletes who do not, to determine if there are lower instances of depressive symptoms in the mindfulness group. From there, a researcher could use a retrospective cohort design to assess athletes' mindfulness behavior and depressive symptoms in their recovery from a concussion. Through this design, the researcher could determine that mindfulness activities reduce depressive symptoms over time. Finally, the researcher could design an intervention based on building and practicing mindfulness skills and administer this training program to athletes as part of a randomized controlled study. As this example illustrates, all research designs play an important part in understanding and interpreting behavior. The most important consideration is that researchers follow up on their work with a more rigorous design in order to advance the evidence in their field. In doing this, researchers should critically examine their findings and evaluate how their results fit within the larger objectives of their field (see the ORBIT model for an example; Czajkowski et al., 2015).

Another important consideration is the use of theory in research. Theories are sets of concepts, definitions, and propositions that explain the relationships between variables (National Institutes of Health, 2017). Theories provide systematic approaches for understanding events, behavior, or situations. Without a strong theoretical framework, research becomes a guessing game to determine how factors relate to each other. Research in concussion related-behavior could be significantly advanced by the integration of theory into research. For this reason, we recommend consulting the chapter in this book dedicated to the use of theory in concussion research when designing future studies on concussion-related issues (see Chapter 6 in this book). From a study design and statistical analysis approach, using strong theoretical frameworks allows researchers to identify, integrate, and test for potential mediating and moderating variables. Specifically, mediating variables explain the process through which an intervention has an effect, while moderating variables account for why an intervention may have a different impact for certain individuals (Mackinnon, 2011).

Conclusion

In this chapter, an overview and examples were provided for observational (cross-sectional, non-randomized group comparisons, and cohort) and experimental (experimental and quasi-experimental) research designs. This chapter also listed key considerations for planning and designing studies, as well as guidelines for collecting, analyzing, and interpreting data in order to provide researchers with the necessary tools to incorporate these designs into their future work. With this in mind, it is hoped that researchers will take the opportunity to critically evaluate their own approaches and look for ways to improve and expand upon their existing methods with the goal of developing strong evidence-based research and of promoting the replicability and transparency of their findings.

Acknowledgment

We would like to extend our thanks to Dr. Shane Sweet for his extremely thoughtful and relevant comments on an earlier version of this chapter.

References

Axelrod, D. A., & Hayward, R. (2006). Nonrandomized interventional study designs (Quasi-experimental designs). In Penson D. F., Wei, J. T. (eds.), *Clinical Research Methods for Surgeons* (pp. 63–76). New York, NY: Humana Press.

Bagley, A. F., Daneshvar, D. H., Schanker, B. D., Zurakowski, D., d'Hemecourt, C. A., Nowinski, C. J., … Goulet, K. (2012). Effectiveness of the SLICE program for youth concussion education. *Clinical Journal of Sport Medicine*, 22, 385–389. doi: 10.1097/JSM.0b013e3182639bb4.

Bailey, C. M., Samples, H. L., Broshek, D. K., Freeman, J. R., & Barth, J. T. (2010). The relationship between psychological distress and baseline sports-related concussion testing. *Clinical Journal of Sport Medicine*, 20, 272–277. doi: 10.1097/JSM.0b013e3181e8f8d8.

Beidler, E., Donnellan, M. B., Covassin, T., Phelps, A. L., & Kontos, A. P. (2017). The association between personality traits and sport-related concussion history in collegiate student-athletes. *Sport, Exercise, and Performance Psychology*, 6, 252–261. doi: 10.1037/spy0000107.

Bloom, G. A., Horton, A. S., McCrory, P., & Johnston, K. M. (2004). Sport psychology and concussion: New impacts to explore. *British Journal of Sports Medicine*, 38, 519–521. doi: 10.1136/bjsm.2004.011999.

Booher, M. A., Wisniewski, J., Smith, B. W., & Sigurdsson, A. (2002). Comparison of reporting systems to determine concussions incidence in NCAA Division I collegiate football. *Clinical Journal of Sports Medicine*, 13, 93–95. doi: www.ncbi.nlm.nih.gov/pubmed/12629426.

Bramley, H., Patrick, K., Lehman, E., & Silvis, M. (2012). High school soccer players with concussion education are more likely to notify their coach of a suspected concussion. *Clinical Pediatrics*, 51, 332–336. doi: 10.1177/0009922811425233.

Broglio, S. P., & Puetz, T. W. (2008). The effect of sport concussion on neurocognitive function, self-report symptoms and postural control. *Sports Medicine*, 38, 53–67. doi: 10.2165/00007256-200838010-00005.

Caron, J. G., Rathwell, S., Delaney, J. S., Johnston, K. M., Ptito, A., & Bloom, G. A. (2018). Development, implementation and assessment of a concussion education programme for high school student-athletes. *Journal of Sports Sciences*, 36, 48–55. doi: 10.1080/02640414.2017.1280180.

Covassin, T., Crutcher, B., Bleecker, A., Heiden, E. O., Dailey, A., & Yang, J. (2014). Postinjury anxiety and social support among collegiate athletes: A comparison between orthopaedic injuries and concussions. *Journal of Athletic Training*, 49, 462–468. doi: 10.4085/1062-6059-49.2.03.

Czajkowski, S. M., Powell, L. H., Adler, N., Naar-King, S., Reynolds, K. D., Hunter, C. M., … Epel, E. (2015). From ideas to efficacy: The ORBIT model for developing behavioral treatments for chronic diseases. *Health Psychology*, 34, 971–982. doi: 10.1037/hea0000161.

Davies, S. C., & Bird, B. M. (2015). Motivations for underreporting suspected concussion in college athletics. *Journal of Clinical Sport Psychology*, 9, 101–115. doi: 10.1123/jcsp.2014-0037.

Doig, G. S., & Simpson, F. (2005). Randomization and allocation concealment: A practical guide for researchers. *Journal of Critical Care*, 20, 187–191. doi: 10.1016/j.jcrc.2005.04.005.

Echemendia, R. J., Iverson, G. L., McCrea, M., Macciocchi, S. N., Gioia, G. A., Putukian, M., & Comper, P. (2013). Advances in neuropsychological assessment of sport-related concussion. *British Journal of Sports Medicine*, 47, 294–298. doi: 10.1136/bjsports-2013-092186.

Echlin, P. S., Johnson, A. M., Riverin, S., Tator, C. H., Cantu, R. C., Cusimano, M. D., … Skopelja, E. N. (2010). A prospective study of concussion education in 2 junior ice hockey teams: Implications for sports concussion education. *Neurosurgical Focus, 29*, E6. doi: 10.3171/2010.9.FOCUS10187.

Field, A. (2009). *Discovering statistics using SPSS.* Sage publications.

Gessel, L. M., Fields, S. K., Collins, C. L., Dick, R. W., & Comstock, R. D. (2007). Concussions among United States high school and collegiate athletes. *Journal of Athletic Training, 42*, 495. doi: 10.1016/S0162-0908(08)79294-8.

Guskiewicz, K. M., Marshall, S. W., Bailes, J., McCrea, M., Harding, H. P., Matthews, A., … Cantu, R. C. (2007). Recurrent concussion and risk of depression in retired professional football players. *Medicine and Science in Sports and Exercise, 39*, 903–909. doi: 10.1249/mss.0b013e3180383da5.

Guskiewicz, K. M., Weaver, N. L., Padua, D. A., & Garrett, W. E. (2000). Epidemiology of concussion in collegiate and high school football players. *The American Journal of Sports Medicine, 28*, 643–650. doi: 10.1177/03635465000280050401.

Houston, M., Bay, C., & Valovich McLeod, T. (2016). The relationship between post-injury measures of cognition, balance, symptom reports and health related quality-of-life in adolescent athletes with concussion. *Brain Injury, 30*, 891–898. doi: 10.3109/02699052.2016.1146960.

Hutchison, M., Mainwaring, L. M., Comper, P., Richards, D. W., & Bisschop, S. M. (2009). Differential emotional responses of varsity athletes to concussion and musculoskeletal injuries. *Clinical Journal of Sport Medicine, 19*, 13–19. doi: 10.1097/JSM.0b013e318190ba06.

Hulley, S. B., Cummings, S. R., Browner, W. S., Grady, D. G., Hearst, N., & Newman, T. B. (2001). *Designing Clinical Research.* Philadelphia, PA: Lippincott Williams & Wilkins.

Kinser, P. A., & Robins, J. L. (2013). Control group design: Enhancing rigor in research of mind-body therapies for depression. *Evidence-Based Complementary and Alternative Medicine, e140467*, 1–10. doi: 10.1155/2013/140467.

Kontos, A. P., Covassin, T., Elbin, R. J., & Parker, T. (2012). Depression and neurocognitive performance after concussion among male and female high school and collegiate athletes. *Archives of Physical Medicine and Rehabilitation, 93*, 1751–1756. doi: 10.1016/j.apmr.2012.03.032.

Kontos, A. P., Elbin, R. J., Newcomer Appaneal, R., Covassin, T., & Collins, M. W. (2013). A comparison of coping responses among high school and college athletes with concussion, orthopedic injuries, and healthy controls. *Research in Sports Medicine, 21*, 367–379. doi: 10.1080/15438627.2013.825801.

Kroshus, E., Babkes Stellino, M., Chrisman, S. P., & Rivara, F. P. (2017). Threat, pressure, and communication about concussion safety: Implications for Parent Concussion Education. *Health Education & Behavior, 45*, 254–261. doi:1090198117715669.

Kroshus, E., Baugh, C. M., Stein, C. J., Austin, S. B., & Calzo, J. P. (2017). Concussion reporting, sex, and conformity to traditional gender norms in young adults. *Journal of Adolescence, 54*, 110–119. doi: 10.1016/j.adolescence.2016.11.002.

Kroshus, E., Garnett, B. R., Baugh, C. M., & Calzo, J. P. (2016). Engaging teammates in the promotion of concussion help seeking. *Health Education & Behavior, 43*, 442–451. doi: 10.1177/1090198115602676.

Kuehl, M. D., Snyder, A. R., Erickson, S. E., & McLeod, T. C. V. (2010). Impact of prior concussions on health-related quality of life in collegiate athletes. *Clinical Journal of Sport Medicine, 20*, 86–91. doi: 10.1097/JSM.0b013e3181cf4534.

LeMonda, B. C., Tam, D., Barr, W. B., & Rabin, L. A. (2017). Assessment trends among neuropsychologists conducting sport-related concussion evaluations. *Developmental Neuropsychology, 42,* 113–126. doi: 10.1080/87565641.2016.1274315.

Lenth, R. V. (2001). Some practical guidelines for effective sample size determination. *The American Statistician, 55,* 187–193. doi: 10.1198/000313001317098149.

Lindell, M. K., & Whitney, D. J. (2001). Accounting for common method variance in cross-sectional research designs. *Journal of Applied Psychology, 86,* 114–121. doi: 10.1037/0021-9010.86.1.114.

MacKinnon, D. P. (2011). Integrating mediators and moderators in research design. *Research on Social Work Practice, 21,* 675–681. doi: 10.1177/1049731511414148.

Mainwaring, L. M., Bisschop, S. M., Green, R. E., Antoniazzi, M., Comper, P., Kristman, V., … Richards, D. W. (2004). Emotional reaction of varsity athletes to sport-related concussion. *Journal of Sport and Exercise Psychology, 26,* 119–135. doi: 10.1123/jsep.26.1.119.

Mainwaring, L. M., Hutchison, M., Bisschop, S. M., Comper, P., & Richards, D. W. (2010). Emotional response to sport concussion compared to ACL injury. *Brain injury, 24,* 589–597. doi: 10.3109/02699051003610508.

Mann, C. J. (2003). Observational research methods. Research design II: Cohort, cross sectional, and case-control studies. *Emergency Medicine Journal, 20,* 54–60. doi: 10.1136/emj.20.1.54.

Marshall, S. W., & Guskiewicz, K. M. (2003). Sports and recreational injury: The hidden cost of a healthy lifestyle. *Injury Prevention, 9,* 100–102. doi: 10.1136/ip.9.2.100.

McCrea, M., Guskiewicz, K. M., & Marshall, S. W. (2003). Acute effects and recovery time following concussion in collegiate football players: The NCAA Concussion Study. *JAMA, 290,* 2556–2563. doi: 10.1001/jama.290.19.2556.

McCrea, M., Hammeke, T., Olsen, G., Leo, P., & Guskiewicz, K. (2004). Unreported concussion in high school football players: Implications for prevention. *Clinical Journal of Sport Medicine, 14,* 13–17. doi: 10.1097/00042752-200401000-00003.

Nature Supplement. (2014). Challenges in Irreproducible research. doi: www.nature.com/collections/prbfkwmwvz.

National Institutes of Health. (2017). What is theory. doi: https://www.nih.gov/

O'Connor, K. L., Baker, M. M., Dalton, S. L., Dompier, T. P., Broglio, S. P., & Kerr, Z. Y. (2017). Epidemiology of sport-related concussions in high school athletes: National Athletic Treatment, Injury and Outcomes Network (NATION), 2011–2012 through 2013–2014. *Journal of Athletic Training, 52,* 175–185. doi: 10.4085/1062-6050-52.1.15.

O'Rourke, D. J., Smith, R. E., Punt, S., Coppel, D. B., & Breiger, D. (2017). Psychosocial correlates of young athletes' self-reported concussion symptoms during the course of recovery. *Sport, Exercise, and Performance Psychology, 6,* 262–276. doi: 10.1037/spy0000097.

Podsakoff, P. M., MacKenzie, S. B., Lee, J. Y., & Podsakoff, N. P. (2003). Common method biases in behavioral research: A critical review of the literature and recommended remedies. *Journal of Applied Psychology, 88,* 879–903. doi: 10.1037/00219010.88.5.879.

Register-Mihalik, J. K., Guskiewicz, K. M., Valovich McLeod, T. C., Linnan, L. A., Mueller, F. O., & Marshall, S. W. (2013). Knowledge, attitude, and concussion-reporting behaviors among high school athletes: A preliminary study. *Journal of Athletic Training, 48,* 645–653. doi: 10.4085/1062-6050-48.3.20.

Reis, H. T., & Judd, C. M. (eds.). (2000). *Handbook of research methods in social and personality psychology.* Cambridge University Press.

Riva, J. J., Malik, K. M., Burnie, S. J., Endicott, A. R., & Busse, J. W. (2012). What is your research question? An introduction to the PICOT format for clinicians. *The Journal of the Canadian Chiropractic Association, 56,* 167–171. doi: www.ncbi.nlm.nih.gov/pmc/articles/PMC3430448/.

Schatz, P., Elbin, R. J., Anderson, M. N., Savage, J., & Covassin, T. (2017). Exploring sandbagging behaviors, effort, and perceived utility of the ImPACT Baseline Assessment in college athletes. *Sport, Exercise, and Performance Psychology, 6,* 243–251. doi: 10.1037/spy0000100.

Sibbald, B., & Roland, M. (1998). Understanding controlled trials. Why are randomised controlled trials important? *British Medical Journal, 316,* 201. doi: 10.1136/bmj.316.7126.201.

Song, J. W., & Chung, K. C. (2010). Observational studies: Cohort and case-control studies. *Plastic and Reconstructive Surgery, 126,* 2234–2242. doi: 10.1097/PRS.0b013e3181f44abc.

Swartz, E. E., Broglio, S. P., Cook, S. B., Cantu, R. C., Ferrara, M. S., Guskiewicz, K. M., & Myers, J. L. (2015). Early results of a helmetless-tackling intervention to decrease head impacts in football players. *Journal of Athletic Training, 50,* 1219–1222. doi:.10.4085/1062-6050-51.1.06.

Torres, D. M., Galetta, K. M., Phillips, H. W., Dziemianowicz, E. M. S., Wilson, J. A., Dorman, E. S., ... Balcer, L. J. (2013). Sports-related concussion: Anonymous survey of a collegiate cohort. *Neurology: Clinical Practice, 3,* 279–287. doi: 10.1212/CPJ.0b013e3182a1ba22.

Turner, S., Langdon, J., Shaver, G., Graham, V., Naugle, K., & Buckley, T. (2017). Comparison of psychological response between concussion and musculoskeletal injury in collegiate athletes. *Sport, Exercise, & Performance Psychology, 3,* 277–288. doi: . 10.1037/spy0000099.

Williamson, J. S., & Goodman, D. (2006). Converging evidence for the under-reporting of concussions in youth ice hockey. *British Journal of Sports Medicine, 40,* 128–132. doi: 10.1136/bjsm.2005.021832.

Yang, J., Peek-Asa, C., Covassin, T., & Torner, J. C. (2015). Post-concussion symptoms of depression and anxiety in Division I collegiate athletes. *Developmental Neuropsychology, 40,* 18–23. doi: 10.1080/87565641.2014.973499.

Zuckerman, S. L., Kerr, Z. Y., Yengo-Kahn, A., Wasserman, E., Covassin, T., & Solomon, G. S. (2015). Epidemiology of sports-related concussion in NCAA athletes from 2009–2010 to 2013–2014: Incidence, recurrence, and mechanisms. *The American Journal of Sports Medicine, 43,* 2654–2662. doi: 10.1177/0363546515599634.

15 Qualitative methods in concussion research

Kaleigh Ferdinand Pennock, Katherine A. Tamminen, and Lynda Mainwaring

Introduction

Concussions are complex injuries that have the potential to impact every facet of an athlete's life. Due to the complexity in the occurrence, etiology, and recovery from sport-related concussions, qualitative research approaches are particularly well-suited to explore the experience and meaning of sustaining a concussion in sport. In this chapter, we start by briefly reviewing the different methods and methodologies used within qualitative research. We then report the results of a review of qualitative research conducted on sport-related concussions and comment on the usefulness and benefits of various qualitative methods. We conclude by discussing some of the research trends and the uses of different qualitative approaches to advance sport-related concussion research.

Qualitative research approaches

Very broadly, qualitative research provides a method for understanding individuals' lived experiences and the meanings that people make about these experiences (Gubrium & Holstein, 1997; Sparkes & Smith, 2014). Qualitative researchers engage in naturalistic approaches and interpretive practices to make sense of how individuals develop meanings about their experiences—in this case, the experience of concussions in sport. As Denzin and Lincoln explain, "this means that qualitative researchers study things in their natural settings, attempting to make sense of, or interpret, phenomena in terms of the meanings people bring to them" (1994, p. 3). Qualitative research includes a range of approaches or methodologies, as well as diverse methods, strategies, and techniques for collecting and analyzing qualitative data. It is important to note that here we are distinguishing between the terms qualitative *methods* and *methodologies*—we use the term qualitative methods to refer to the tools, strategies, and techniques that researchers employ to collect, analyze, and present their data; whereas we use the term qualitative methodology to refer to the overarching tradition of inquiry of the qualitative research study. Each methodology provides a guiding framework for conducting qualitative inquiry: Methodologies provide a frame for the research question or focus of inquiry—they may entail different research methods to collect and analyze the data—and different methodologies produce different research findings and contributions to knowledge.

Qualitative researchers seek out the richest sources of information that will contribute to answering the research question; however, there is great variation in the methods used to collect qualitative data. Some of the most common approaches to collecting qualitative data include conducting semi-structured or focus group interviews, engaging in naturalistic observations of participants' behaviors and interactions, collecting textual documents (e.g., media/news reports), or collecting written or visual data from participants (e.g., photos, drawings, diary entries). Once these various forms of data have been generated, qualitative researchers may use a variety of approaches to analyze their data. However, the general process of analysis in qualitative studies often includes managing and organizing the data, reading or viewing the data and noting emergent ideas, describing and classifying notes into themes, developing interpretations about the data, and representing/writing the results of the analysis (Creswell & Poth, 2018). Through this process, the researcher is seeking to identify common as well as unique themes within the data, to identify patterns in the data, and to develop an understanding of the phenomenon, process, or experience of, in this case, sport-related concussions.

The most common methodologies for conducting qualitative inquiry include narrative approaches, ethnography, phenomenology, grounded theory, and case study (Kowalski et al., 2018; Sparkes & Smith, 2014). Methodologies are akin to a road map that provides direction and focus to the research questions, methods, and analytic approaches of a study, and they often have some characteristic approaches to data collection or analysis methods (e.g., the use of theoretical sampling and constant comparative method of analysis in grounded theory; the use of observation in ethnographic research). Qualitative methodologies often contain different variants, such as interpretative phenomenological analysis (Smith, Flowers, & Larkin, 2009) or existential phenomenology (Merleau-Ponty, 1969) as forms of phenomenology. However, researchers may also elect to use more generic qualitative descriptive approaches that are not tightly defined by specific data collection and analysis processes (also referred to as interpretive description or qualitative descriptive approaches; Sandelowski, 2010; Thorne, 2008). See Table 15.1 for an overview of several qualitative methodologies and typical variants, recommended readings, and example research questions that might be explored within these traditions of inquiry.

Whereas it is beyond the scope of this chapter, it is important to note that these various approaches to conducting qualitative research can be further situated within different paradigmatic or philosophical orientations, which encompass the researcher's worldview and assumptions that guide his or her research. Common paradigms or philosophical positions within sport and exercise psychology research include post-positivism or critical realism, constructivism/interpretivism, constructionism, feminist or critical theory, and postmodern approaches. We refer the reader to some key readings on the philosophical foundations of qualitative inquiry for more information regarding these paradigms and their

Table 15.1 Overview of qualitative research approaches

Methodology/Tradition of Inquiry (example variants in italics)	Purpose or Aim	Example of Approach	Example Concussion Studies	Suggested Readings
Narrative *Thematic narrative analysis* *Performative narrative analysis* *Structural narrative analysis* *Dialogical narrative analysis*	Understanding people's stories as representations of broader social experiences.	How do retired athletes make meaning of their history of concussions across the span of their sport careers?	Caron, Schaefer, André-Morin, & Wilkinson (2017)	Reissman (2008)
Ethnography *Cultural ethnography* *Institutional ethnography* *Visual ethnography* *Autoethnography*	Understanding cultures or cultural groups, behaviors, values, and beliefs.	How do athletes, coaches, and trainers understand, talk about, respond to, and manage sport-related concussions within a professional rugby team?	Smith & Sparkes (2009);Torres Colon, Smith, & Fucillo (2017)	Wolcott (1999); Atkinson (2016)
Phenomenology *Existential phenomenology* *Interpretative phenomenological analysis* *Empirical phenomenology*	Understanding a phenomenon or concept; understanding how people make sense of their personal and social world; understanding the essential structure of a phenomenon.	How do athletes experience the phenomenon of having an "invisible" injury such as a concussion?	André-Morin, Caron, & Bloom (2017)	Allen-Collinson (2016)

Approach	Purpose	Research Question	Example	References
Grounded Theory *Straussian grounded theory* *Constructivist grounded theory* *Glaserian grounded theory*	Constructing an explanatory theory of an event, process, action, or phenomenon.	What is the process by which athletes decide whether to disclose their concussion symptoms to coaches, trainers, or parents?	Hunt, Le Dorze, Trentham, Polatajko, & Dawson (2015)	Corbin & Strauss (2008); Charmaz (2014)
Case Study *Instrumental case study* *Intrinsic case study* *Collective case study*	Understanding the complexity or distinctiveness of a case as a bounded system (people, team, event, organization, community) that is of interest to researchers.	How are concussions managed at international high-performance sporting events such as the Olympics?	Anderson & Kian (2012)	Hodge & Sharp (2016); Stake (2005)
Generic Qualitative Approaches *Interpretive Description* *Qualitative Description* *Content analysis* *Thematic analysis*	Develop a comprehensive description of a phenomenon; identify and interpret patterns of meaning across a dataset.	What are the beliefs and attitudes about concussions among adolescent high-performance hockey players?	Kroshus, Gillard, Haarbauer-Krupa, Goldman, & Bickham (2017)	Sandelowski (2010); Thorne (2008)

underpinning assumptions (see Daly, 2007; Guba & Lincoln, 1994; Jones, Torres, & Arminio, 2014; Lincoln, Lynham, & Guba, 2017).

From the results of our review, it is evident that the use of qualitative research approaches contribute to our understanding of the experience and meaning of sport-related concussion, despite their relatively limited use thus far in the field of concussion research. The benefits of using qualitative approaches in this area can provide much-needed knowledge about the subjective experiences of those with concussion and those helping with the management of concussions, including parents, coaches, clinicians, and organizational leaders.

Review of qualitative research on sport-related concussions

We conducted a systematic search of the published, peer-reviewed qualitative literature on sport-related concussions. Five databases were searched (Embase, MedLine, PsycINFO, SportDISCUS, and CINAHL) using a combination of subject heading terms and key truncated text words. Search strings included terms for "concussion" (including "mTBI" and "head impacts"), and "qualitative research" (including "interviews," "focus groups," and "inquiry") as title, abstract, or key terms. In addition, we used Scopus to review the reference lists of included articles for additional texts. A total of 92 articles were retrieved and screened for inclusion; exclusion criteria included military populations, dissertations or conference proceedings, and mixed methods articles that lacked a substantive qualitative emphasis. A three-person team reviewed the articles for inclusion, reaching consensus through discussion. Seventeen articles were reviewed. Relevant data were extracted, including methods, population, the concussion sub-domain (e.g., post-concussion syndrome, concussions in the media), and primary findings.

Three main topics arose from reviewing the foci of the articles: (1) athletes' experiences of sport-related concussions ($n = 10$ articles); (2) caregivers' experiences related to sport concussions ($n = 3$); and (3) media analyses of sport-related concussions ($n = 4$).

Athletes' experiences of sport-related concussions

The "invisible" nature of sport-related concussion and the unique symptom presentation by each athlete makes it difficult to offer a one-size-fits-all approach of concussion management and support. Hearing directly about personal experiences with sport-related concussion offers rich insight about the impact of concussion on athletes' lives. Qualitative research offers opportunities to dig deeply into questions of *how* concussions influence athletes' lives: How do athletes experience concussion symptoms? How might social interactions or the culture of sport influence attitudes or beliefs about concussions in young athletes? How do athletes express their frustrations or fears when faced with career termination from multiple concussions?

Much of the qualitative research to date exploring athletes' sport-related concussion experiences has been framed in one of the following two spheres of interest: (1) the lived experiences following single, multiple, or protracted concussion experiences, or (2) the social, educational, and cultural factors associated with athletes' experiences beyond symptomology. The key findings of the research and the implications on our understanding of sport-related concussions are discussed.

Athletes living with sport-related concussions

A growing concern over the potential physical and cognitive consequences of sport-related concussions has dominated conversations in academia, sports media, and family dinner tables. Concerns stemming from repetitive hits to the head and multiple concussions have led to considerable research examining both short- and long-term implications of head injuries. The majority of the research has been from a quantitative perspective, with an emphasis on concussion rates, neurocognitive performance, and more recently, neurobiological markers of concussions. However, there is much to be gained with the use of qualitative methodologies. Beyond physical symptoms, the psychological consequences of sport-related concussions can have a profound effect on the lives of athletes.

Qualitative research provides opportunities to investigate the subjective experiences of athletes coping with concussion. It opens the door for investigators to ask how athletes experience concussion in consideration of their past experiences, their current state, and their future selves. For example, Caron et al. (2017) captured the experiences of a female university athlete with prolonged concussion symptoms through photography and nine audio logs. The narrative elucidated Daphnée's struggle with feelings of isolation and imprisonment from her concussion and her negotiation with a new sense of self. Caron et al. described how Daphnée grappled with developing a "*new* normal [life]" (2017, p. 511) and the distress of reframing her identity following sport career termination. A narrative approach offers the opportunity to see how self-identity changes over time and in the context of an injury. The use of narrative inquiry in Caron et al.'s study provides a pathway to examine how Daphnée reconsidered her sense of self and life in a new way after concussion. This richness and long-term perspective is difficult to achieve in quantitative work without conducting lengthy and resource-depleting longitudinal research, and even then, the subjective experience and meaning of injury is often missing.

Athletes' struggles with protracted recovery from concussions have implications that extend beyond sport. André-Morin, Caron, and Bloom (2017) examined the experiences of five female university athletes dealing with lengthy concussion recoveries using interpretative phenomenological analysis (IPA). Participants detailed the difficulties of managing a demanding course load and the importance of social support while managing persistent concussion symptoms. Work by Caron et al. (2013), also using IPA, explored the ripples from career-ending sport-related concussions in NHL players. Five retired professional male athletes shared their experiences with career termination and subsequent transition out of hockey after multiple concussions. These athletes chronicled their experiences, from the physical and emotional strain from concussions on their day-to-day lives, to the importance of the role of the spouse while struggling with symptoms. An inductive approach with IPA allows the researchers to use specific analysis techniques to make meaning of these life experiences. Specific data analysis techniques such as creating identity profiles of the athletes permits the researchers' interpretations and own experiences to guide the development of the themes and the stories of the athletes (Caron et al., 2013).

The recovery process from a sport-related concussion can impact the lives of young athletes as well as their support networks. Two studies used health-related quality of life (HRQOL) as a guiding framework to explore athletes' experiences post-concussion at two different stages: one-year post-concussion (Iadevaia, Roiger, & Zwart, 2015), and during the subacute phase (i.e., 15–30 days) post-concussion (Valovich McLeod et al., 2017). Both studies recruited adolescent athletes and their parents to participate in semi-structured interviews concerning their rehabilitation and post-concussion experiences. Using qualitative consensual review, Iadevaia et al. (2015) conducted a multiple-step analysis and reported four major themes concerning post-concussion quality of life: The significant effect of symptoms, feelings of frustration, school performance and enjoyment, and interpersonal relationships. Interestingly, the relationships between the adolescents and their close family members featured negative emotions like irritability, whereas the interactions between adolescents and their teammates were characterized largely as supportive and positive. These findings have implications for improving perceived quality of life for concussed athletes by addressing appropriate social support behaviors for families and teammates (Iadevaia et al., 2015). Similarly, Valovich McLeod et al. (2017) interviewed 12 adolescent athletes and their parents and used consensual qualitative research analysis methods. Findings focused on the psychosocial experiences of the participants. Athletes expressed difficulty adjusting after injury and felt isolated or excluded from daily events related to school and social activities. Valovich McLeod and colleagues noted that athletes reported a tendency to mask or minimize their symptoms in an attempt to "bring a sense of normalcy into their lives" (p. 8).

Although there are quantitative measures designed to assess HRQOL, these instruments may be unable to account for the inherent subjectivity of quality of life (Iadevaia et al., 2015). A qualitative approach creates opportunities for both the adolescents and parents to co-construct the implications and meanings of sport-related concussions in their daily lives. Using a collaborative analysis method allows for multiple researchers to analyze the data and reach a consensus on the findings; this technique is often used to help strengthen the validity of findings in post-positivist qualitative research.

The sociocultural context of concussions

The consequences of concussion on the lives of athletes are far-reaching. Parents, coaches, teammates, health-care providers, and educators all play various roles endorsing—and occasionally inhibiting—health-promoting behaviors.

Athletes may lack the prerequisite concussion knowledge to make informed decisions, or their choices may be at odds with the prevailing recommendations for return to sport or school. Children, in particular, may not receive age-appropriate concussion education, or may have difficulty expressing their symptoms. Addressing these issues, Pasek and colleagues (2015) worked directly with child athletes to understand post-concussion induced headaches—one of the most common symptoms—with the intentions to develop a tracking system for this population. The tool, the Headache Electronic Diary for Children with Concussion [HED-CC], was developed to improve communication between children, parents, and clinicians through the post-concussion rehabilitation phase, making it easier for children to track frequency, severity, and location of headaches, among other variables. By taking a qualitative approach in their study, the researchers were able to listen to young athletes describe their pain and learn which technology applications athletes felt would be most beneficial during recovery. Speaking directly to children about concussions can offer vital information to inform our development of educational programming. For example, Kroshus, Gillard, Haarbauer-Krupa, Goldman, and Bickham (2017) interviewed children six to eight years old about their concussion knowledge. Using a multi-step qualitative coding framework to identify themes, the authors found that the children had a general sense of the mechanisms of injury, such as a hit or impact to the head. The children were reported as logical and concrete in their thinking, providing specific examples with how someone could get hurt; however, the children had more difficulty identifying cognitive or emotional symptoms of a concussion. This exploratory study may be crucial for informing age-appropriate concussion education materials. Children this age may benefit more when given logical, clear examples and provided rules or specific instructions (e.g., ensure your helmet is always on when snowboarding) to minimize risk (Kroshus et al., 2017).

The development of comprehensive materials to educate athletes on the signs, symptoms, and protocols surrounding concussions are essential for their health and safety. Although there is evidence to suggest athletes are often uninformed about concussion symptoms, there is a growing body of research, supported by qualitative methods, that suggests athletes are aware of the common signs, symptoms, and risk associated with playing with a concussion but choose to stay in the game regardless (McCrea et al., 2004; Torres et al., 2013). When observing and speaking directly with athletes, the gaps between what athletes do and what athletes say become apparent. Chrisman, Quitiquit, and Rivara (2013) interviewed male and female high school athletes in focus groups about their beliefs and attitudes about sport-related concussions and found the majority would continue to play while symptomatic. Decisions to play in spite of symptoms are framed in context of the social process of the sport, including playing for a specific team, avoiding looking weak, and the relationship with the coach. Similar research into under-reporting in youth sports used semi-structured interviews and a grounded theory approach with male youth hockey players and parents, coaches, and trainers (Cusimano et al., 2017). Expectations of masculinity and strength, particularly in physically larger players, along with tacit pressure to perform from parents and coaches, emerged as powerful themes that influenced athletes' decisions not to report concussion symptoms. Referent others may also influence aggressive behaviors in young athletes and reinforce dangerous beliefs concerning revenge-seeking and winning at all costs (Cusimano et al., 2016). Although there are numerous survey-based studies that probe under-reporting attitudes and behaviors, they often lack the ability to provoke nuanced, contextualized answers from players and other social agents in sport.

The perceived beliefs and attitudes of referent others may also impact the decision-making of athletes on return to play (RTP) following sport-related concussion. Social influencers such as parents, teachers, coaches, and teammates have been shown to demonstrate compassion and support during RTP, which may help to improve athletes' experiences following a concussion and while they are recovering from their injury (McGuckin et al., 2016). McGuckin and colleagues interviewed five adolescent female hockey players on the social influencers during the RTP process after concussion. The authors used thematic content analysis and a phenomenological approach to help describe, rather than explain, the athletes' experiences (McGuckin et al., 2016). Although the athletes were mostly positive about their interactions with others during the RTP process, athletes did report some pressure from siblings and parents to rejoin play earlier than what felt comfortable. This study provides insight into the positive and negative influences on the RTP process for young female athletes and can serve as a framework for future research in this area.

By immersing themselves in the sport culture, speaking with, and observing athletes, qualitative researchers can begin to disrupt and challenge preconceptions about athletes in sport. Torres Colón, Smith, and Fucillo (2017) argued that those participating in sport at the recreational level share a passion for play and making connection in sport. Their research, which included participant observation and interviews, found that university-aged students who participated in sport recreationally are not ignorant or under-educated on concussion risks. Rather, students highly value the social benefits of sport participation and may be reluctant to report concussions or take time away to recover. Thus, reporting injuries or avoiding collision or contact sports due to the increased concussion risk are not viewed as favorable options. These nuanced views on participation in sport become clearer when qualitative research methods are selected, and participants can express how they thrive in a social sport environment.

Caregivers' experiences of sport-related concussions

In addition to exploring athletes' experiences of concussions, we also reviewed three papers examining the experiences and opinions of caregivers who provide support for individuals with concussions. These papers focused on two areas: sports medicine physicians' opinions of social media use for concussion support (Ahmed et al., 2013) and the experiences and practices of practitioners who treated brain-injured patients (Hunt et al., 2015; Walker Buck et al., 2013).

In these areas of research, grounded theory (Charmaz, 2006; Strauss & Corbin, 1998) and an interpretative description approach to the studies were employed.

Ahmed and colleagues (2013) interviewed eight general practitioners regarding the use of social networking sites (SNSs) to augment sport concussion management. Seven themes were distilled from an interpretative descriptive approach. The themes identified the use of (1) *social networking sites*, (2) *management of concussion*, (3) the *use of Facebook*, (4) the *use of technology for health (eHealth)*, (5) the need for *moderation* in SNS use, (6) awareness of *privacy issues*, and (7) the *risks and dangers* of using social media. Overall, SNSs were thought to be useful to communicate best practice information in a user-friendly manner, especially to youth, and an "ideal medium" (p. 41) through which sport concussion management at a community-based level can be facilitated. The qualitative approach to this study provided an opportunity to elicit practitioner wisdom about the value of using SNSs rather than imposing the researchers' ideas through a forced-choice questionnaire within a quantitative research framework. The answers given by the practitioners illuminated their perceived value of using SNSs in the management of concussions and shed light on their concerns as well.

Hunt et al. (2015) used grounded theory with reference to Charmaz's approach (2006) to examine how 13 occupational therapists facilitated goal-setting in acquired brain injury clients with cognitive impairments. The therapists were based in three different settings: Acute care hospitals, in-patient settings, and outpatient rehabilitation facilities. A continuum for goal-setting practices used by practitioners was conceptualized from the data: At one end of the continuum, client-centered goals were embraced by therapists, and at the other end of the continuum, organizationally-determined goals were prioritized (e.g., discharge from the program). Therapists who worked within a client-centered perspective encouraged clients to participate in rehabilitation goal-setting, thereby empowering both the client and the therapist. In contrast, therapists who worked toward organizational goals felt powerless and frustrated with the marginalization of client involvement. This study used grounded theory in a rigorous way to elucidate different goal sources, use of goal-setting practices, and a continuum to characterize the bipolar goal-setting sources. The qualitative method provided the opportunity to discover how the therapists approached goal-setting practices rather than imposing *a priori* established options on the therapists.

To examine the experience of 15 rehabilitation professionals who worked with outpatients with mild traumatic brain injury (mTBI), Walker Buck et al. (2013) used grounded theory techniques described by Straus and Corbin (1998). The constant comparison process of analysis (Glaser & Strauss, 1967) was employed by the authors, who concluded that rehabilitation workers are often required to help individuals with brain injury address psychosocial needs, and that professionals generally feel unprepared and undertrained to do so. Walker Buck et al. (2013) identified that there is "an acute need for mTBI-informed care, in which the psychosocial impact of this type of invisible injury is systematically addressed" (p. 749). The authors suggested that social workers are particularly well-suited to fill this gap, and that more research examining the impact of psychosocial issues on rehabilitation outcomes is needed. Although this research did not focus exclusively on sport concussion, the findings that knowledge of psychosocial aspects of recovery and rehabilitation are lacking and needed resonate with recommendations from those conducting research on psychological sequelae of sport concussion (Bloom et al., 2004; Broshek, De Marco, & Freeman, 2015; Kontos, Deitrick, & Reynolds, 2016; Mainwaring, Hutchison, Comper, & Richards, 2012; Moore, Lepine, & Ellemberg, 2017), and the latest consensus statement (McCrory et al., 2017). By using grounded theory, the researchers were able to identify the range of experiences, challenges, and insights related to psychosocial aspects of coping with mTBI. The personal observations of those working on the frontlines of rehabilitation came to light through the qualitative approach. Whereas the research identified an important issue, it did not develop the findings into a substantive grounded theory about rehabilitations professionals' experiences with mTBI patients. It is often the case that formal theories are not developed using grounded theory methods, but rather, a clearer picture of the issues and how they might be classified are identified.

Although only one of the three qualitative studies reviewed related directly to the clinical management of sport concussion, all studies provided valuable insights on the possibilities, directions, and need for qualitative research related to sport concussion management. Clinical management of sport concussion varies widely across medical and rehabilitation professionals; qualitative approaches to relevant questions would benefit the evolving science and practical management of sport-related concussions.

Media analyses of sport-related concussions

By turning their attention to media articles and documentaries about sport-related concussion, qualitative researchers have also examined the way that concussions are represented to broad audiences, which may reflect current concerns and understandings about concussions within society. Furthermore, in-depth analysis of media representations of sport-related concussion helps to draw connections between attitudes towards concussions and notions of aggression, risk, and masculinity in sport. In doing so, it is possible to understand how dominant notions of masculinity may influence athletes' attitudes towards concussions, and it is possible to identify instances where attitudes toward concussions may be shifting alongside changes to the dominant narrative of masculinity in sport.

In a study tracking the types of media reporting surrounding sport-related concussions, a thematic analysis of 541 news articles published between 1985 and 2011 in four newspapers in Canada and the United States was conducted by Cusimano and colleagues (2013). Their content analysis of these sport-related concussion news articles resulted in five main themes that were pervasive in the media articles: (1) *aggression* as a precursor to sport-related concussions, (2) *perceptions of brain injury*, (3) *equipment* that may help to prevent brain injuries, (4) *rules and regulations* to prevent concussions, and (5) the implications of brain injuries for *youth hockey players* and the need to keep young athletes healthy. The authors noted that early reports of concussions in hockey referred to equipment necessary to prevent brain injuries and the implications for teams when star players were injured; however, more recent news reports described the overall extent of concussions in hockey and their implications for young athletes. While news articles conveyed the seriousness of concussions, describing them as "needless," the newspapers also described them as "part of the game" and an unavoidable hazard in hockey. This thematic analysis helps to identify patterns in the way that media representations of sport-related concussions can shape the public's understanding of concussions, which may also reflect societal opinions about the nature and implications of concussions in hockey.

Taking a more in-depth look at media representations of concussion, Anderson and Kian (2012) examined media reports of concussions and injuries in American football surrounding the case of athlete Aaron Rodgers, who chose to remove himself from a game following a hit to the head. Their textual analysis of 10 published news articles covering Rodgers' concussion between 2010 and 2011 revealed that all but one article emphasized the significance of a teammate encouraging Rodgers not to continue playing and expressing support for his decision to withdraw from the game in the interest of his health. Through their analysis, the authors argued that concussions are not an inevitable part of sport and football in particular, but rather that they are produced through ongoing masculinization of the game that encourages the glorification of violence. However, they noted that the unquestioned acceptance of traumatic brain injuries may be waning due to increasing societal awareness of the impact of concussions for athletes; cultural changes wherein young men are less concerned about expressing emotional intimacy, fear, and pain; and increasing legal and financial concerns among sport governing bodies and associations regarding the health and safety of their athletes. Based on their analysis of the media reports surrounding the Rodgers case, Anderson and Kian (2012) suggested that attitudes toward concussions are changing, although athletes' attitudes may lag behind others because they wish to continue playing through pain and decide for themselves whether they wish to put themselves at risk of brain injury. This argument is echoed by Furness (2016), whose analysis of the documentary *League of Denial* also positions the phenomenon of sport-related concussions within the social and cultural context of sport and society. Furness' analysis demonstrates how the documentary challenges the dominant normalization of violence within football, contributing to "a progressive shift in the way that injury and vulnerability in professional football players is both discussed and remembered in popular culture" (p. 56).

McGannon, Cunningham, and Schinke (2013) also examined the social and cultural context within which sport-related concussions occur in their analysis of 68 news articles reporting on ice hockey athlete Sidney Crosby's concussion sustained during the 2010–2011 season. The authors found that in the media representations of Crosby's concussion, the content of the news articles reflected an overarching narrative of a culture of risk and its impact on athletes. This narrative encompassed three sub-narratives concerning Crosby's concussion as a cautionary tale, Crosby's concussion as a political platform, and concussion as an ambiguous injury. The authors also noted that in the media reports of Crosby's concussion, there was a large emphasis on the physical aspects of sport-related concussion and their treatment, in effect silencing any discussion about the emotional, social, and psychological repercussions of sustaining sport-related concussion. The authors' analysis of the reporting surrounding sport-related concussion sustained by high-profile players draws attention to the physical, cultural, and political implications of concussions in sport. Overall, there is a relatively limited body of research examining media accounts of sport-related concussions; however, those studies are important in drawing attention to the social and cultural context of brain injuries in sport. Crucially, such studies explore the often taken-for-granted assumptions about injuries and sport-related concussions, and they raise important questions about the acceptability of risk at the expense of athlete health and well-being. That work is valuable in identifying changes in discourses about sport-related concussion and opportunities for the media to contribute to changing the narrative around athletes' acceptance of risk and injury in sport and prioritizing athlete health and safety.

Commentary and discussion

Overall, the most common qualitative approaches used to study sport-related concussion include methods frequently used in the field of sport psychology (Culver, Gilbert, & Sparkes, 2012), such as semi-structured interviews and content analyses or thematic analyses of interview data. However, the research demonstrates a wide array of methodological approaches, including thematic analysis, ethnographic analysis, grounded theory, and phenomenological and narrative approaches. The studies included the voices of athletes themselves, as well as supportive others and caregivers, which sheds light on the social context of sport-related concussions. The inclusion of three studies which considered the media reports of concussions adds to our understanding of how concussions are shaped by, and contribute to, broader societal discussions of risk, aggression, and masculinity in sport. In the studies we reviewed, there was an emphasis on examining concussions in hockey at both the youth and professional levels across a range of sports, and there was surprisingly little research with football players, a well-studied population in quantitative research. There is a dearth of studies on high-performance athletes or older adults, and no studies that addressed the experiences of concussions among LGBTQ athletes, athletes with physical impairments, or athletes of color.

In order to advance qualitative research on sport-related concussions, we urge researchers to consider the breadth of qualitative methodologies available to them and the possible research questions that may be pursued using these different approaches. For example, adopting life history or narrative approaches would enable researchers to explore how older, retired athletes make meaning of their history of concussions and how the experience of multiple concussions and impaired cognition (or the possibility of impaired cognition) may influence one's identity and sense of self. Similarly, adopting a narrative approach, researchers may question how discourses such as achievement at all costs (e.g., performance narrative; Douglas & Carless, 2015; and career termination, Caron et al., 2013) are used to understand and make sense of concussion experiences.

Other methodological approaches that may be useful to explore sport-related concussions include ethnography and grounded theory. Ethnographic research could be used to gain insight into the subcultures of various sports that influence athletes' attitudes and opinions about concussions, as well as the ways that athletes, coaches, and trainers talk about, respond to, and manage sport-related concussions. Such approaches could shed light on the ways that individuals make sense of concussions and normalize the risk of concussions in some sports (e.g., football, hockey, etc.), and it may also help provide information about how to best tailor concussion intervention or harm-reduction approaches to various sport contexts. Grounded theory research is well-suited to developing theoretical explanations of a phenomenon or social process (Corbin & Strauss, 2008); therefore, it would be particularly useful to use grounded theory to examine the process by which athletes gain information and knowledge about sport-related concussions or to examine the process of athletes' decisions to report or not report concussion symptoms. Similarly, grounded theory could be used to understand how effective concussion management and prevention programs are executed and delivered within sport organizations.

In conclusion, the qualitative research examining sport-related concussions is relatively new (e.g., the earliest article reviewed was published in 2012), but from our review we find that these studies have made important contributions to understanding the ways in which athletes and support providers (e.g., coaches, clinicians, parents) experience and make sense of sport-related concussions. This body of research also situates sport-related concussions within the broader social, cultural, and political context of sport and draws attention to the implications of dominant discourses of masculinity, aggression, and risk acceptance in sport. Findings from the reviewed studies demonstrate the impact of sport-related concussions on participants' identities, athletic careers, and long-term health and well-being. Qualitative approaches provide important information about athletes' experiences with sport-related concussions, while also highlighting the complexity of the injury. Ongoing research with qualitative approaches will continue to provide a rich, comprehensive, and thorough understanding of athletes' sport-related concussion experiences.

References

Ahmed, O., Sullivan, S. J., Schneiders, A., Moon, S., & McCrory, P. (2013). Exploring the opinions and perspectives of general practitioners towards the use of social networking sites for concussion management. *Journal of Primary Health Care, 5*, 36–42. doi: 10.1071/HC13036.

Allen-Collinson, J. (2016). Breathing in life: Phenomenological perspectives on sport and exercise. In B. Smith & A. C. Sparkes (Eds.), *Routledge handbook of qualitative research in sport and exercise* (pp. 11–23). New York, NY: Routledge.

Anderson, E., & Kian, E. M. (2012). Examining media contestation of masculinity and head trauma in the National Football League. *Men and Masculinities, 15*, 152–173. doi: 10.1177/1097184X11430127.

André-Morin, D., Caron, J. G., & Bloom, G. A. (2017). Exploring the unique challenges faced by female university athletes experiencing prolonged concussion symptoms. *Sport, Exercise, and Performance Psychology, 6*, 289–303. doi: 10.1037/ spy0000106.

Atkinson, M. (2016). Ethnography. In B. Smith & A. C. Sparkes (Eds.), *Routledge handbook of qualitative research in sport and exercise* (pp. 49–61). New York, NY: Routledge.

Bloom, G. A., Horton, A. S., McCrory, P., & Johnston, K. M. (2004). Sport psychology and concussion: New impacts to explore. *British Journal of Sports Medicine, 38*, 519–521. doi: 10.1136/bjsm.2004.011999.

Broshek, D. K., De Marco, A. P., & Freeman, J. R. (2015). A review of post-concussion syndrome and psychological factors associated with concussion. *Brain Injury, 29*, 228–237. doi: 10.3109/02699052.2014.974674.

Caron, J. G., Bloom, G. A., Johnston, K. M., & Sabiston, C. M. (2013). Effects of multiple concussions on retired National Hockey League players. *Journal of Sport & Exercise Psychology, 35*, 168–179. doi: 10.1123/jsep.35.2.168.

Caron, J. G., Schaefer, L., André-Morin, D., & Wilkinson, S. (2017). A narrative inquiry into a female athlete's experiences with protracted concussion symptoms. *Journal of Loss and Trauma, 22*, 501–513. doi: 10.1080/15325024.2017.1335150.

Charmaz, K. (2006). *Constructing grounded theory: A practical guide through qualitative analysis.* London, UK: Sage.

Charmaz, K. (2014). *Constructing grounded theory* (2nd ed.). London, UK: Sage.

Chrisman, S. P., Quitiquit, C., & Rivara, F. P. (2013). Qualitative study of barriers to concussive symptom reporting in high school athletics. *Journal of Adolescent Health, 52*, 330–335. doi: 10.1016/j.jadohealth.2012.10.271.

Corbin, J., & Strauss, A. (2008). *Basics of qualitative research: Techniques and procedures for developing grounded theory* (3rd ed.). Thousand Oaks, CA: Sage.

Creswell, J. W., & Poth, C. N. (2018). *Qualitative inquiry and research design: Choosing among five approaches* (4th ed.). Los Angeles, CA: Sage.

Culver, D. M., Gilbert, W., & Sparkes, A. C. (2012). Qualitative research in sport psychology journals: The next decade 2000–2009 and beyond. *The Sport Psychologist, 26*, 261–281. doi: 10.1123/tsp.26.2.261.

Cusimano, M. D., Ilie, G., Mullen, S. J., Pauley, C. R., Stulberg, J. R., Topolovec-Vranic, J., & Zhang, S. (2016). Aggression, violence and injury in minor league ice hockey: Avenues for prevention of injury. *PLoS ONE, 11*, 1–15. doi: 10.1371/ journal.pone.0156683.

Cusimano, M. D., Sharma, B., Lawrence, D. W., Ilie, G., Silverberg, S., & Jones, R. (2013). Trends in North American newspaper reporting of brain injury in ice hockey. *PLoS ONE, 8*, e61865. doi: 10.1371/journal.pone.0061865.

Cusimano, M. D., Topolovec-Vranic, J., Zhang, S., Mullen, S. J., Wong, M., & Ilie, G. (2017). Factors influencing the underreporting of concussion in sports: A qualitative study of minor hockey participants. *Clinical Journal of Sport Medicine, 27*, 375–380. doi: 10.1097/JSM.0000000000000372.

Daley, K. J. (2007). *Qualitative methods for family studies and human development.* Thousand Oaks, CA: Sage.

Denzin, N., & Lincoln, Y. (1994). Introduction: Entering the field of qualitative research. In N. Denzin & Y. Lincoln (Eds.), *The Sage handbook of qualitative research* (1st ed., pp. 1–17). Thousand Oaks, CA: Sage.

Douglas, K. & Carless, D. (2015). *Life story research in sport: Understanding the experiences of elite and professional athletes through narrative.* Abingdon, NY: Routledge.

Furness, Z. (2016). Reframing concussions, masculinity, and NFL mythology in League of Denial. *Popular Communication, 14,* 49–57. doi: 10.1080/154057 02.2015.1084628.

Glaser, B., & Strauss, A. (1967). *The discovery of grounded theory.* London, UK: Weidenfeld and Nicolson.

Guba, E. G., & Lincoln, Y. S. (1994). Competing paradigms in qualitative research. In N. Denzin & Y. Lincoln (Eds.), *The Sage handbook of qualitative research* (1st ed., pp. 105–117). Thousand Oaks, CA: Sage.

Gubrium, J. F., & Holstein, J. A. (1997). *The new language of qualitative method.* New York, NY: Oxford University Press.

Hodge, K., & Sharp, L. A. (2016). Case studies. In B. Smith & A. C. Sparkes (Eds.), *Routledge handbook of qualitative research in sport and exercise* (pp. 62–74). New York, NY: Routledge.

Hunt, A. W., Le Dorze, G., Trentham, B., Polatajko, H. J., & Dawson, D. R. (2015). Elucidating a goal-setting continuum in brain injury rehabilitation. *Qualitative Health Research, 25,* 1044–1055. doi: 10.1177/1049732315588759.

Iadevaia, C., Roiger, T., & Zwart, M. B. (2015). Qualitative examination of adolescent health-related quality of life at 1 year postconcussion. *Journal of Athletic Training, 50,* 1182–1189. doi:10.4085/1062-6050-50.11.02

Jones, S. R., Torres, V., & Arminio, J. (2014). *Negotiating the complexities of qualitative research in higher education: Fundamental elements and issues* (2nd ed.). New York, NY: Routledge.

Kontos, A. P., Deitrick, J. M., & Reynolds, E. (2016). Mental health implications and consequences following sport-related concussion. *British Journal of Sports Medicine, 50,* 139–140. doi: 10.1136/bjsports-2015-095564.

Kowalski, K. C., McHugh, T.-L. F., Sabiston, C. M., & Ferguson, L. J. (2018). *Research methods in kinesiology.* Don Mills, Canada: Oxford University Press.

Kroshus, E., Gillard, D., Haarbauer-Krupa, J., Goldman, R. E., & Bickham, D. S. (2017). Talking with young children about concussions: An exploratory study. *Child: Care, Health and Development, 43,* 758–767. doi:10.1111/cch.12433

Lincoln, Y. S., Lynham, S. A., Guba, E. G. (2017). Paradigmatic controversies, contradictions, and emerging confluences, revisited. In Denzin, N. K., Lincoln, Y. S. (Eds.), *The Sage handbook of qualitative research* (5th ed., pp. 108–150). Los Angeles, CA: Sage.

Mainwaring, L., Hutchison, M., Comper, P., & Richards, D. (2012). Examining emotional sequelae of sport concussion. *Journal of Clinical Sport Psychology, 6,* 247–274. doi: 10.1123/jcsp.6.3.247.

McCrea, M., Hammeke, T., Olsen, G., Leo, P., & Guskiewicz, K. (2004). Unreported concussion in high school football players: Implications for prevention. *Clinical Journal of Sport Medicine, 14,* 13–17. doi:10.1097/00042752-200401000-00003

McCrory, P., Meeuwisse, W., Dvořák, J., Aubry, M., Bailes, J., Broglio, S., ... Vos, P. E. (2017). Consensus statement on concussion in sport—The 5th international conference on concussion in sport held in Berlin, October 2016. *British Journal of Sports Medicine, 51,* 838–847. doi: 10.1136/bjsports-2017-097699.

McGannon, K. R., Cunningham, S. M., & Schinke, R. J. (2013). Understanding concussion in socio-cultural context: A media analysis of a National Hockey League star's concussion. *Psychology of Sport and Exercise*, *14*, 891–899. doi: 10.1016/j. psychsport.2013.08.003.

McGuckin, M. E., Law, B., McAuliffe, J., Rickwood, G., & Bruner, M. W. (2016). Social influences on return to play following concussion in female competitive youth ice hockey players. *Journal of Sport Behavior*, *39*, 426–445.

Merleau-Ponty, M. (1969). *The visible and the invisible* (A. Lingis, Trans.). Evanston, IL: Northwestern University Press.

Moore, R. D., Lepine, J., & Ellemberg, D. (2017). The independent influence of concussive and sub-concussive impacts on soccer players' neurophysiological and neuropsychological function. *International Journal of Psychophysiology*, *112*, 22–30. doi: 10.1016/j.ijpsycho.2016.11.011.

Pasek, T. A., Locasto, L. W., Reichard, J., Fazio Sumrok, V. C., Johnson, E. W., & Kontos, A. P. (2015). The headache electronic diary for children with concussion. *Clinical Nurse Specialist*, *29*, 80–88. doi: 10.1097/NUR.0000000000000108.

Reissman, C. K. (2008). *Narrative methods for the human sciences*. Los Angeles, CA: Sage.

Sandelowski, M. (2010). What's in a name? Qualitative description revisited. *Research in Nursing and Health*, *33*, 77–84. doi: 10.1002/nur.20362

Smith, J. A., Flowers, P., & Larkin, M. (2009). *Interpretative phenomenological analysis: Theory, method, and research*. Los Angeles, CA: Sage.

Smith, B., & Sparkes, A. C. (2009). Narrative inquiry in sport and exercise psychology: What can it mean, and why might we do it? *Psychology of Sport and Exercise*, *10*, 1–11. doi: 10.1016/j.psychsport.2008.01.004.

Sparkes, A. C., & Smith, B. (2014). *Qualitative research methods in sport, exercise and health: From process to product*. New York, NY: Routledge.

Stake, R. E. (2005). Qualitative case studies. In N. K. Denzin & Y. S. Lincoln (Eds.), *The Sage handbook of qualitative research* (3rd ed., pp. 443–466). Thousand Oaks, CA: Sage.

Strauss, A., & Corbin, J. (1998). *Basics of qualitative research: Techniques and procedures for developing grounded theory* (2nd ed.). Thousand Oaks, CA: Sage.

Thorne, S. (2008). *Interpretative description*. Walnut Creek, CA: Left Coast Press.

Torres, D. M., Galetta, K. M., Phillips, H. W., Dziemianowicz, E. M. S., Wilson, J. A., Dorman, E. S., ... Balcer, L. J. (2013). Sports-related concussion: Anonymous survey of a collegiate cohort. *Neurology Clinical Practice*, *3*, 279–287. doi: 10.1212%2FCPJ.0b013e3182a1ba22

Torres Colón, G. A., Smith, S., & Fucillo, J. (2017). Concussions and risk within cultural contexts of play. *Qualitative Health Research*, *27*, 1077–1089. doi: 10.1177/1049732316669339.

Valovich McLeod, T. C., Wagner, A. J., & Welch Bacon, C. E. (2017). Lived experiences of adolescent athletes following sport-related concussion. *Orthopaedic Journal of Sports Medicine*, *5*, 1–10. doi: 10.1177/2325967117745033.

Walker Buck, P., Spencer Sagrati, J., & Shapiro Kirzner, R. (2013). Mild traumatic brain injury: A place for social work. *Social Work in Health Care*, *52*, 741–751. doi: 10.1080/00981389.2013.799111.

Wolcott, H. (1999). *Ethnography: A way of seeing*. New York, NY: Altamira.

Index

Page numbers in *italics* refer to figures. Page numbers in **bold** refer to tables.